Praise for *Re-Engineering the Kitchen*®

"*Re-Engineering the Kitchen* is a standout among food & nutrition books, offering a logical solution to the problems that create our bad eating habits."

"What I liked most about this book is that Steele doesn't just stop at suggestions in her book but works to provide readers with ways to take action. She's not shying away from the monumental task she's asking readers to do: address their hopes and fears about how they run their own kitchen. But she also provides readers with the information they need to do better, and that comes in the form of nutritional facts as well as worksheets and new information in a simple and digestible way."

"High nutritional content, low waste, and cost efficiency are at the top of Steele's priorities, and she nails them with over 100 Agile Recipes in this book. It's a nice break-up to the informational portions of *Re-Engineering the Kitchen*."

"*Re-Engineering the Kitchen* is a book that will help you feel more in control of your kitchen and, perhaps, the rest of your life."

– Independent Book Review

Full editorial review is available at independentbookreview.com

Re-Engineering the Kitchen®

A simple method to put Real Food on your table faster, easier, and cheaper

Alin E. Steele, BSE, MBA, PE

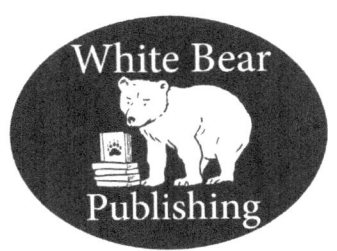

White Bear Publishing

Agile Figure Illustrations: Guy Harvey

Cover Design: Simon Thompson

Editors: Becky Alexander
         Emily Kearns

Interior Design: White Bear Publishing

ISBN-13: 979-8-9893475-3-7

Library of Congress Control Number: 2024918495

First Edition – October 2024
Printed in the United States of America

Published by White Bear Publishing
Ramsey, MN

Table of Contents

INTRODUCTION

This book will show you a step-by-step method to achieve better nutrition for less cost and effort. By applying process improvement techniques to the process of how we feed ourselves, we can put more Real Food on the table faster, easier and cheaper.

Why should you care what I have to say about food? I am not a medical professional, and I am not giving you medical advice (please read the Medical Disclaimer on the copyright page, again). I am not a fitness influencer, professional chef, nor actress/model/celebrity-turned-cookbook-author. I am not a dietician or nutritionist who can advise you personally on what to eat. I can't tell you how to lose weight (as lucrative as that might have been). I don't seem to be an expert in anything you traditionally associate with a book about food. What in the world could I possibly have to offer? I am here to offer you something new. A new approach to eating. I'm an engineer obsessed with process improvement. What I will share with you is a systematic method to help you make better food a reality: more nutritious, quicker to prepare, and less expensive. We are going to Re-Engineer the Kitchen to make the entire food process work for you and your life. Let me tell you how I got here.

The food landscape of my childhood in middle-class Detroit in the 60s and 70s was bleak. Casseroles were the hot ticket: tuna-noodle casserole with, if you were lucky, crushed potato chips on top, or scalloped potato and ham with the new-fangled dehydrated potatoes out of the box. I was fortunate that my parents had lived in a variety of places, so we had a broader range of foods on rotation than most of our neighbors. We were considered odd for eating very few things out of a box (even cold cereal, which my father thought was the ultimate food industry scam), and instead, enjoyed things like seafood, lamb, exotic veggies such as broccoli, and "foreign" foods like Chinese or Mexican. My mom worked (again, unusual for my neighborhood) so whatever I prepared – no matter how inexpertly – was one thing she didn't have to. But I didn't want to waste my time on boring, tasteless food – I wanted flavor! I wanted pizazz! I wanted something edible for dinner before 9 pm.

They say necessity is the mother of invention and my parents were, in today's terminology, highly functioning alcoholics. They loved me dearly, held responsible jobs and were never intoxicated at work. (Rest in peace, Mom and Dad.) However, when they got home at 6 pm, the evening meal was a very low priority. The Old Crow flowed like iced tea. I was in college before I learned that most people thought that one drink meant one shot of hard liquor, not half of a tumbler. After 10-12 ounces of bourbon, dinner was a long time in the making and generally unimpressive by the time it was done.

So, I learned to cook. I also learned to improvise because we never seemed to have key ingredients to make anything. Julia Child, ever fearless in the kitchen, was my inspiration. She made cooking Real Food seem like a quest within my reach. The 1964 edition of *Joy of Cooking* by Irma Rombauer and Marion Rombauer Becker was my textbook. With over 800 pages of recipes and, probably even more valuable, detailed sections explaining ingredients and techniques, I eventually developed some understanding of food and a basic competence in cooking.

Perhaps inevitably, I had issues with my weight. As insignificant as it seems now, I vividly remember the agony in high school when I went from a size 5 to size 7. The absolute numbers were secondary to the feeling of losing control. I've had years of relative thinness and years of, shall we say, not-thinness. However, no matter what the scale is saying, it always feels like I'm losing the battle. I suspect that I am not alone in this regard. This has, at least in part, fueled my continuing and intense interest in health and nutrition.

I earned a degree in chemical engineering and then an MBA with a concentration in finance and business economics. I'm a licensed professional engineer. I enjoyed a demanding 30-year career in the energy industry. My husband and I raised two amazing sons. For the first time in history, women were (sort of) encouraged to "have it all" which, in fact, meant doing it all. I was determined to live that dream, and my husband was with me every step of the way. We had some crazy-busy years in there. It makes me tired now just thinking about it!

Through everything I was trying to provide the best food possible for my family and keep my sanity intact. Figuring out one's own diet is hard enough, but trying to feed a family is a whole new can of worms. While I had accepted that adults could make their own decisions about food, I wasn't ready for how processed foods were pushed and marketed to kids. Suddenly, nutrition, and food culture in general, took on new relevance for me. I read about health and diet and nutrition and cooking. And then I read some more. After more than 100 books, as well as countless articles, studies, and reference papers, I'm still reading. I earned a Certificate in Nutrition and Healthy Living from Cornell University.

One thing became clear: the proliferation of food and nutrition-related information does not necessarily make it easier to decide how to feed one's family, or yourself. Nutritional information in the popular press tends to be complex, biased, out of context, or so simplistic that it feels patronizing. One study confirms a hypothesis and the next seems to conclude differently. Every week a new nutrient appears that supports the health of a particular body system. And diets! All sorts of people and organizations advocate certain types of diets to achieve a certain result, from losing weight to managing specific health issues to adhering to certain theories or ethics. How can we possibly wade through all the noise?

I've always been good at analyzing volumes of data and turning it into actionable information. After so much research, I've concluded that there is a core of basic nutritional information that can be applied to any "diet". When you slice and dice the data, it becomes apparent that we can prioritize, and quantitatively manage, the most important nutrient-dense foods. The consolidated basic nutrition information included here in this book is in an easy-to-use format that you can apply to your life, regardless of the latest headline. I've tried to include just enough of the underlying science to understand why something is important, with further references if you'd like to delve deeper into that area.

While I learned to be a competent home cook, I always resented the amount of time, money, and energy it took to manage the whole process of getting decent food on the table. Being an engineer with a process mindset, I am always looking for ways to improve any, and every, process. For me, process improvement includes:

- Establishing clear objectives
- Eliminating extra steps
- Improving quality
- Reducing waste
- Reducing costs.

I have developed a method: the Re-Engineered Food Cycle, to make better food more attainable for anyone: easier, healthier, and less expensive. This method, complete with the necessary tools, techniques, strategies, and the new and innovative Agile Recipes™, is what I want to share with you.

Even those of you who have successfully fed a family for decades might learn something new. I know there are plenty of people out there, like you, like me, who want a fresh, fact-based approach to food. Together, we can sift through the overwhelm, and make a clear plan that works. As we Re-Engineer the Kitchen®, I hope you will look at your process for planning, procuring, and preparing food from a new perspective.

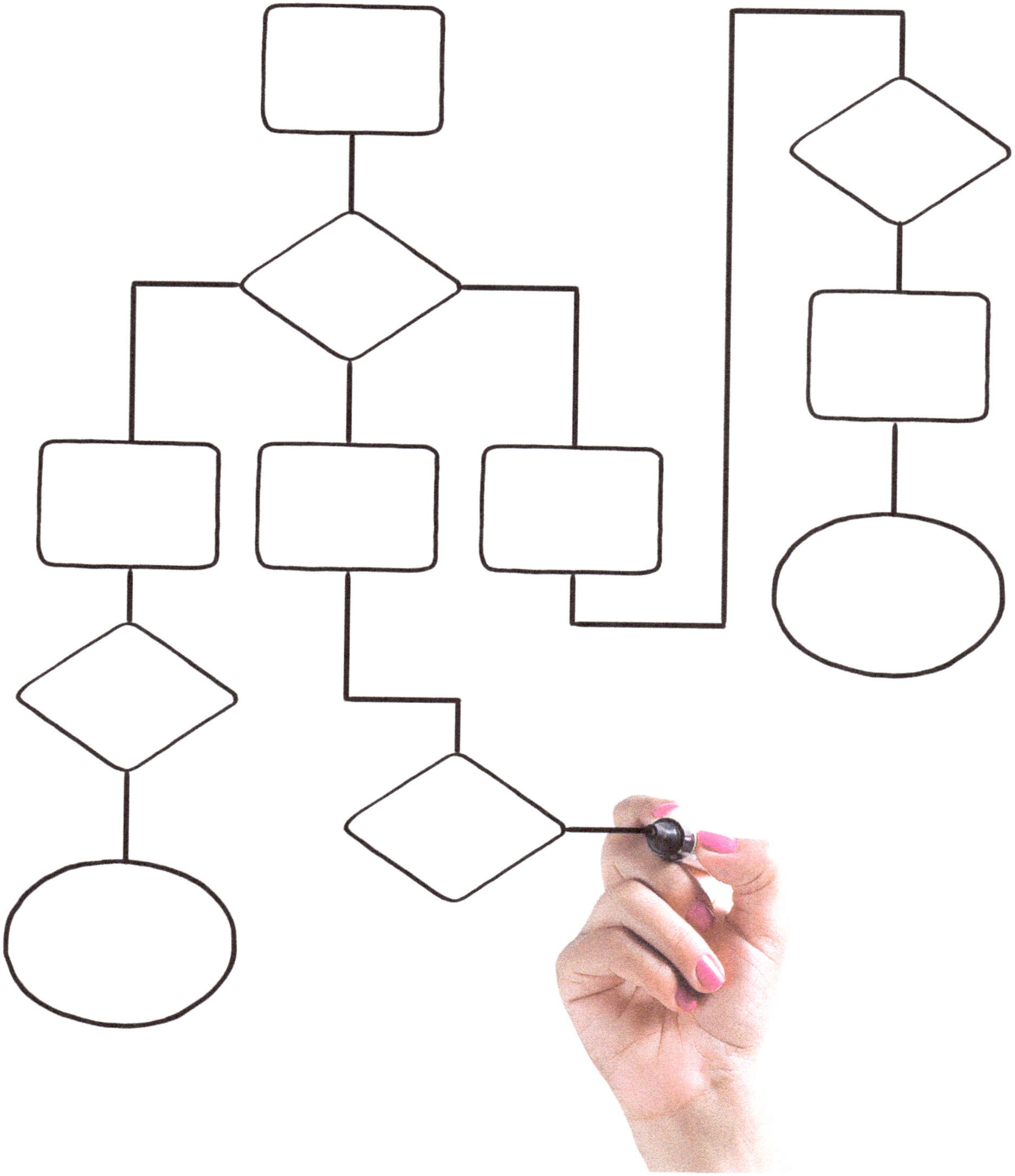

CHAPTER 1

WHAT IS RE-ENGINEERING THE KITCHEN®?

Think about your overall food process. Take a moment to answer the following questions:

- Where does your food come from?
- How much time and money do you spend on it?
- Does it taste good?
- Are you happy with the nutrition?
- Are you throwing too much food away?

If you are like many people, your food process leaves significant room for improvement. It simply takes too much time, money, and effort to get great food on the table, and often with suboptimal results. Last-minute takeout, throwing food away because it wasn't eaten and over-reliance on convenience foods are just a few indicators that your food process could be better. This book is for anyone who would like to improve their personal process of planning, procuring, and preparing food.

In general, we want our food to be delicious, nutritious, inexpensive, and easy. Every day our food choices are influenced by our environment and our culture. We have professionals who advise us on food preparation. (There are over 70,000 cookbooks listed on Amazon and several television channels devoted strictly to food!) We have health experts telling us what we should eat. We have various agenda-driven advisors telling us what food is "morally" acceptable. We have restaurants constantly tempting us with a wide array of delicious dishes. And lastly, we have the prepared-food industry touting the advantages of every convenient (and profitable) food product they can think of. While all these voices are eager to tell you what to eat and how to cook, none of them are focused on optimizing your overall food planning, procurement, and preparation process to meet your time, cost, nutritional and taste goals.

Our food landscape has become so complicated that it is easy to feel overwhelmed. The proliferation of food-related media content, along with the ever-growing diet industry, proves that many people are struggling to achieve some level of mastery over their food. While most nutrition advice is well-intentioned, it can seem confusing, complex, and contradictory. The food we end up eating is influenced by many external factors beyond our control, not the least of which is the proliferation of highly processed foods coupled with relentless time and resource constraints. If we could visualize the typical chaotic process of procuring food in modern society, it might look like Figure 1.

Figure 1 – Typical Food Planning, Procurement, and Preparation Process

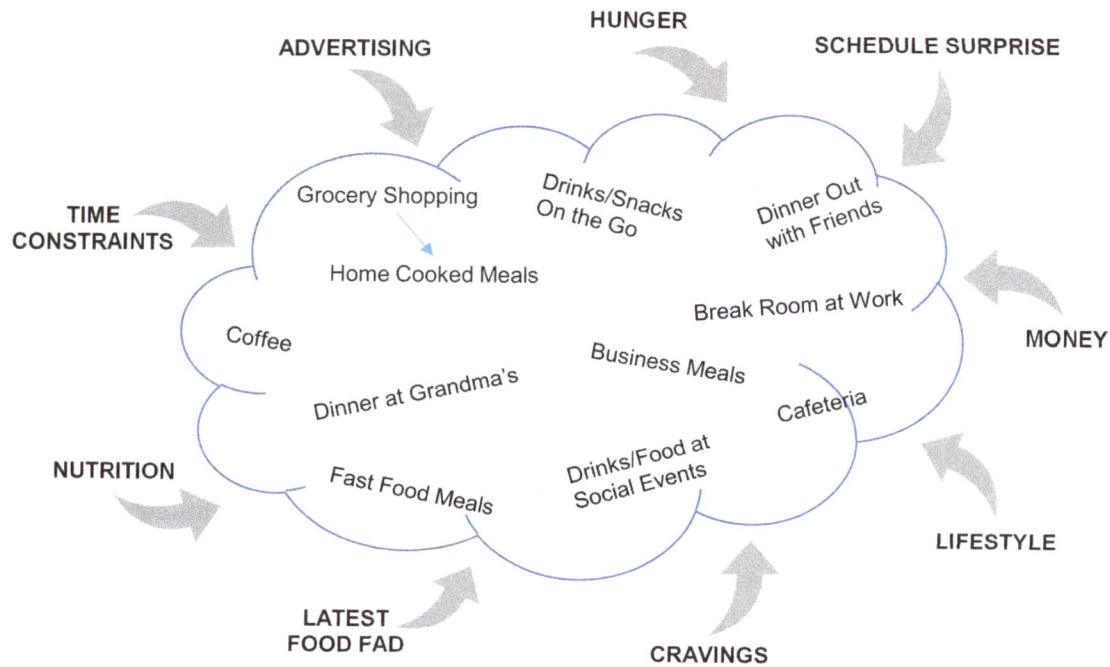

In each situation, we may try to "make good choices" but the options can be limited; often there are no good choices to be made. We may have planned for several nutritious meals, but their benefit is undermined by impulsive snacks or eating out. Trying to avoid certain foods is challenging if you have not proactively planned for the foods you do want to eat. Simply knowing what to eat is meaningless without strategies to make buying and preparation manageable. We need to pull all the pieces of food planning, procurement, and preparation into one integrated process with clear, prioritized objectives.

It is interesting to note that no convenient word or phrase describes the entire process of providing nutrition for ourselves. There are a lot of verbs that describe parts of the process: plan, procure, shop, provision, cook, store, prepare, serve, dispose (of waste), diet, feed, nourish, and maybe manage. It is hard to optimize a process that we have trouble even naming, much less defining. What we are talking about here is the whole process of feeding ourselves from start to finish. This includes everything from nutrition-based planning, to procurement, cost management storage, preparation, waste management, kitchen equipment management, eating, to cleaning up. For simplicity, we will call this whole process the Food Cycle.

Process Improvement

Businesses the world over have benefited greatly from the rigorous application of process-improvement principles. Feeding ourselves and our families – the Food Cycle – is certainly one of the most important processes we will ever manage. We will Re-Engineer the Kitchen® by optimizing the Food Cycle to meet your time, cost, nutritional goals. We will provide the actionable information and tools you need to make better food a reality!

The techniques of process optimization are well-established and are applied to business and manufacturing processes everywhere. You have probably heard of many of the business process improvement frameworks such as Kaizen, Six Sigma, 5S, Value Stream Mapping, DMAIC (define, measure, analyze, improve, and control), and so on. Details of the process improvement frameworks may differ, but they all have certain elements in common. That first common element is to define the process. Defining the process means identifying the inputs, the outputs, and the required steps. It may sound simple, but it can be challenging to put the lines around a process in the right place. We must decide what is part of the process and what is an outside factor. For example, we will assume that going to work to earn money to buy food is outside of the Food Cycle, but the associated budget and time constraints are inputs that affect the process.

To be effective, the Food Cycle we've defined needs to show us the big picture, the bird's-eye view. We need to see the forest, not just the trees. It needs to be comprehensive and integrated with our life. We cannot effectively improve a process by focusing on small bits and pieces here and there. We need to see the whole and it needs to make sense to us.

By looking at the big picture, we can develop an integrated plan to manage food from all our sources. The Re-Engineered Food Cycle will allow us to focus on our most important goals and develop a flexible plan to achieve them.

Figure 2 – The Re-Engineered Food Cycle

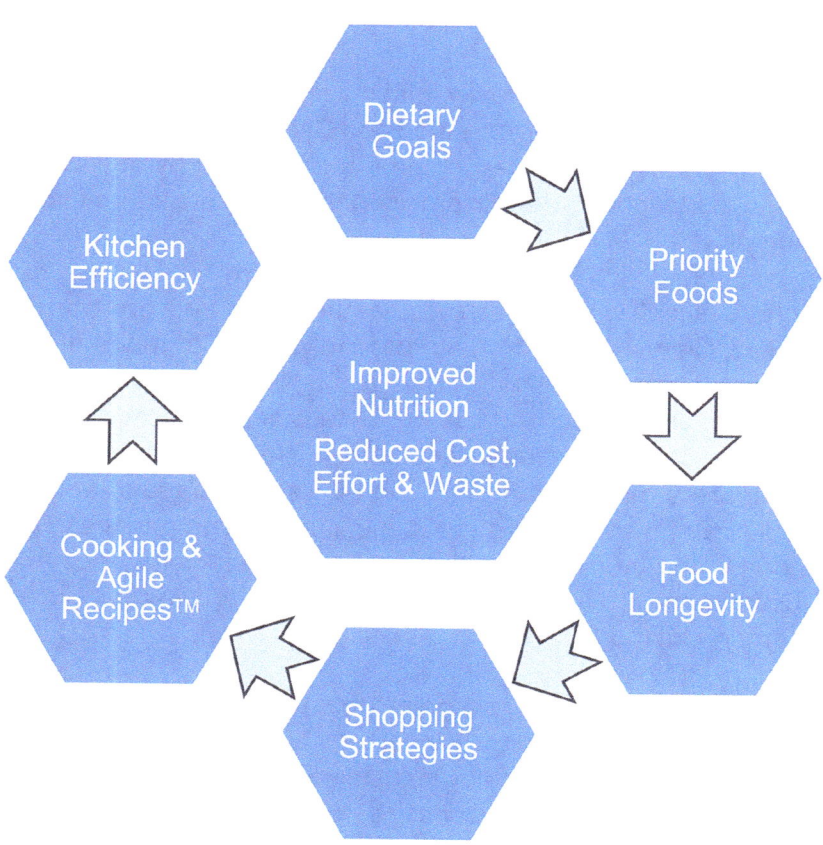

Our process improvement efforts will start with a needs assessment; determining exactly what factors are important and why. These broad objectives include:

- Improved nutrition
- Reduced cost
- Minimized food waste
- Reduced time and effort

Process Improvement Implementation

Phase I – Managing Priority Foods: We will develop the Re-Engineered Food Cycle planning process to meet your nutritional objectives. We will start with nutrition fundamentals and distill this down to actionable information. The planning stage includes determining required quantities for the most important foods: the Priority Foods (defined in Chapter 5). Priority Foods are the foods that you do want in your diet and are often the most difficult to manage. Then we will show you how to plan where your Priority Foods are going to come from and how to shop most effectively. We will also show you how to optimize your food value and reduce the amount of food wasted.

Phase II – Improving Carbohydrates and Dietary Fats: We will show you how to shift your carbs from highly processed grains and sugars to whole foods/whole grains. Next, we will give you the tools to work healthier fats and oils into your diet while reducing the level of the unhealthy, highly processed ones.

Phase III – Shopping and Cooking: We will cover shopping strategies to meet both your nutritional goals and lifestyle objectives. We will show you how to buy the right amount of the right foods while managing food longevity and budget considerations. Next, we will give you techniques to prepare whatever you've bought with streamlined, flexible recipes. All the recipes in this book have been re-engineered to be uncomplicated, quick, reliable, and flexible. The number of steps and ingredients have been whittled down to the bare minimum. Even the recipe format has been redesigned for quick, visual comprehension, in print or on a screen. These recipes are flexible so that you can easily substitute ingredients for what you have on hand, add optional flavors, and adjust to meet dietary requirements. Many include a theme and several variations allowing you to use the same basic recipe to achieve various results. These are so much more functional than your typical recipe that we will call them Agile Recipes™!

Phase IV – Efficient Kitchen Management: Lastly, we will give you techniques for a more productive kitchen and to make cooking Real Food easier. We will include strategies to save time and effort while reducing food waste.

This book will give you a new perspective on how you provide food for yourself and your family. Let's start Re-Engineering your Kitchen®!

My friend Agile will help show the way.

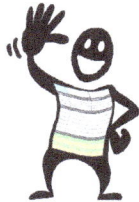

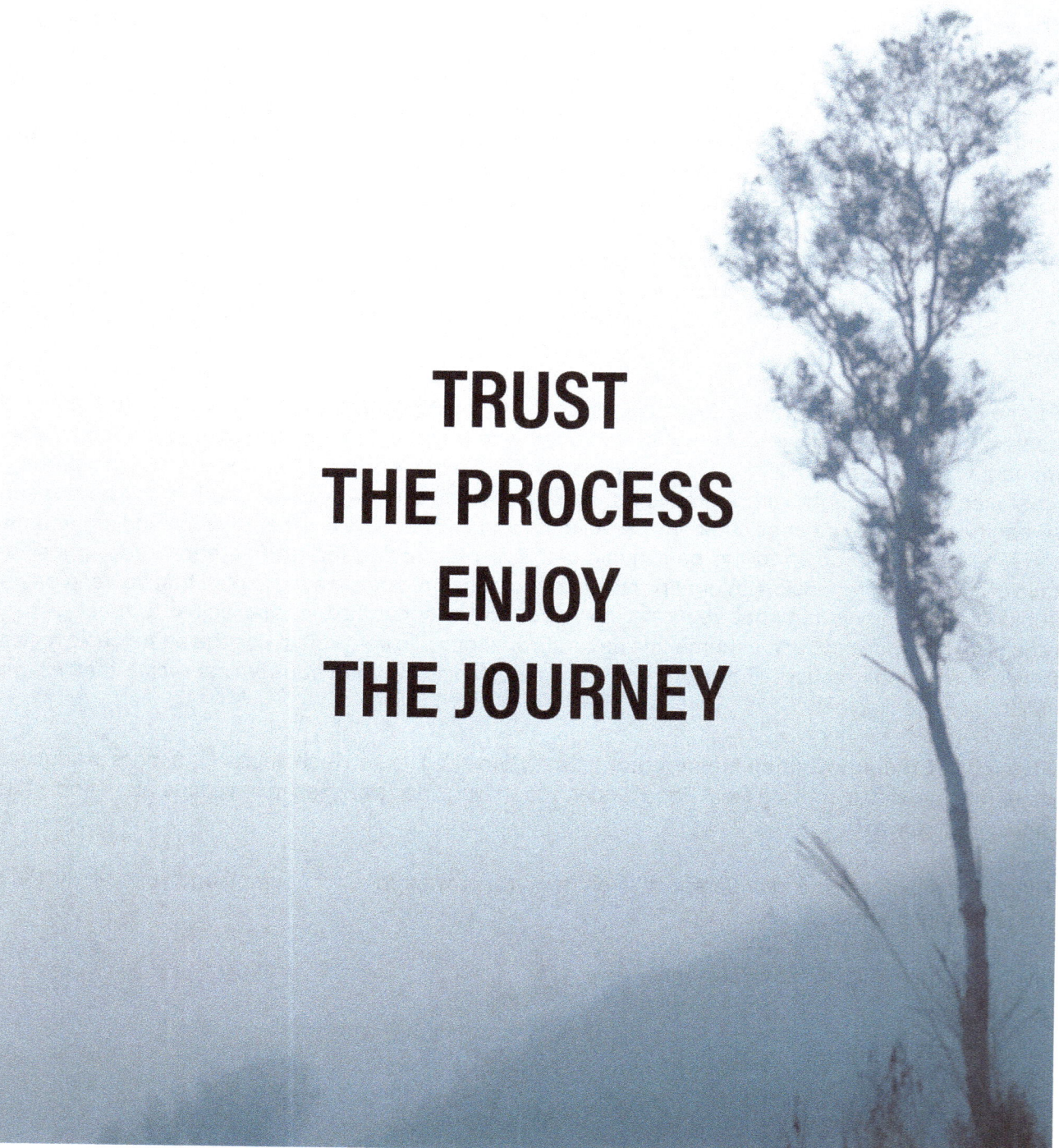

**TRUST
THE PROCESS
ENJOY
THE JOURNEY**

Re-Engineering the Kitchen® – Key Points

Typical food process is chaotic with suboptimal results

Process improvement
- » **Optimized process for all food sources**
- » **The Re-Engineered Food Cycle**

Primary objectives
- » **Improve nutrition**
- » **Reduce cost and eliminate waste**
- » **Reduce time and effort**

Process improvement implementation
- » **Phase I – Managing Priority Foods**
- » **Phase II – Improving Carbohydrates and Dietary Fats**
- » **Phase III – Shopping and Cooking**
- » **Phase IV – Efficient Kitchen Management**

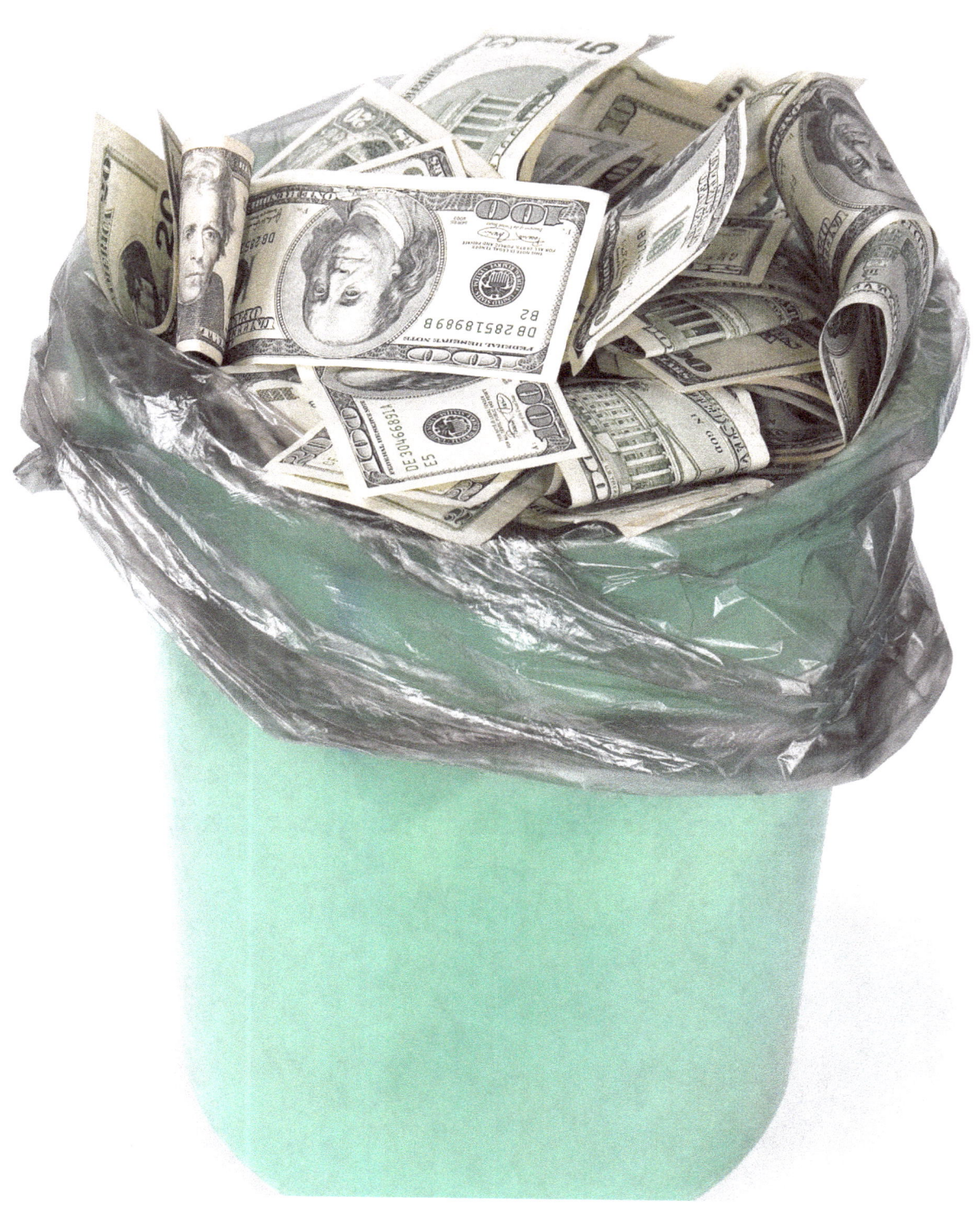

CHAPTER 2

THE IMPACTS OF FOOD WASTE

You may be wondering why we are discussing the reduction of food waste already. Aren't we supposed to be focused on improving nutrition and saving time and money doing so? True enough, but food waste is a clear indicator of a broken Food Cycle. When you are throwing away food for any number of reasons, it is a symptom of a process that is not working well. The expense and effort associated with the wasted food was squandered, and the nutrition was never realized. You may even feel guilty about it and vow to "try harder" next week, as though it is a personal failure. It's not you; it's your process.

Figure 3

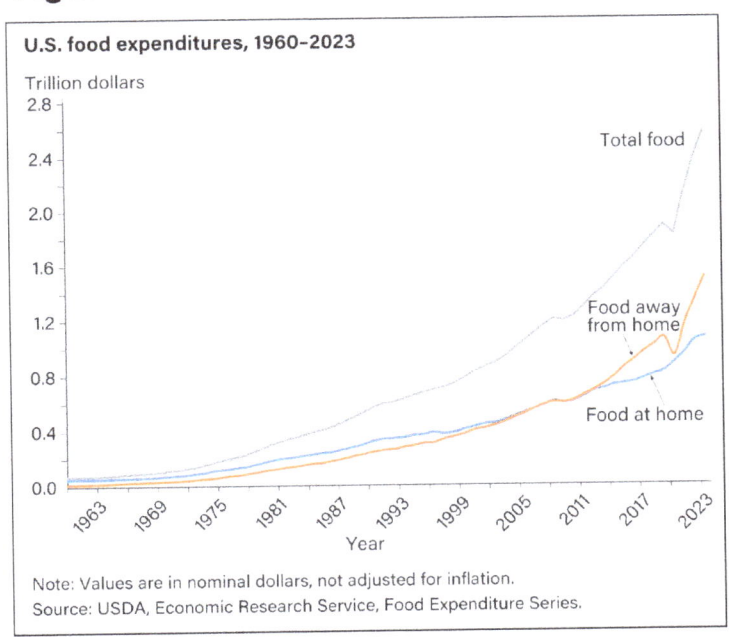

U.S. food expenditures, 1960–2023

Note: Values are in nominal dollars, not adjusted for inflation.
Source: USDA, Economic Research Service, Food Expenditure Series.

Globally, about 30% of food production is wasted and, in America, that number is about 40%. This includes losses through the entire process from harvest to the final commercial and residential end users. Besides the huge social and economic costs, the environmental impact is huge. The Intergovernmental Panel on Climate Change[1] estimates that food loss and waste was responsible for about 10% of the greenhouse gases for the period 2010–2016.

A 2020 study by Yang Yu and Edward C. Jaenicke of Pennsylvania State University[2] showed that the average amount of food wasted at the household level is about 30%, which translates to an annual value of $330 billion in 2023.

Using the U.S. population of 336.7 million from census.gov, and the data on U.S. food-at-home expenditures, this equals $3,920 worth of food wasted per year for an average family of four. That is equivalent to $326 every month; enough to finance a vacation or maybe even a car payment! Or, in these times of high inflation, it just may fill the gap where your ends don't meet.

From a household perspective, wasted food can have a significant domino effect. When one food item has spoiled, there is often a corresponding impromptu meal eaten out. The planned home-cooked meal is replaced by a more expensive restaurant or takeout meal. In addition, the other fresh ingredients for the planned meal are now at risk.

The cost of wasted food goes well beyond your own bank account. Almost all wasted food in the U.S. ends up in landfills, increasing the cost of municipal garbage processing and taking up ever-decreasing landfill space. The EPA[3] estimates that decomposing organic matter in landfill sites generates 16% of the U.S. carbon emissions. These secondary costs of food waste are hidden in higher food costs, higher garbage service costs, and greater environmental impacts.

We will reduce food waste by implementing methods to purchase, store, and use foods so that there is less to throw out. Some of these waste-reduction strategies include:

- Buying the right amount of the right food (Priority Foods)
- Tailoring food purchases to match food longevity with your lifestyle
- Agile Recipes™:
  - tailored to package sizes
  - featuring fewer essential ingredients
  - showing substitutions so you can use what you have
- Using storage techniques to keep ingredients fresh longer

As we become increasingly aware of our collective environmental footprint, we are embracing ways to reduce waste in packaging, plastics, and energy. Food waste is a high-impact waste stream that we, as individuals, have the power to minimize. Do it for yourself; do it for the planet.

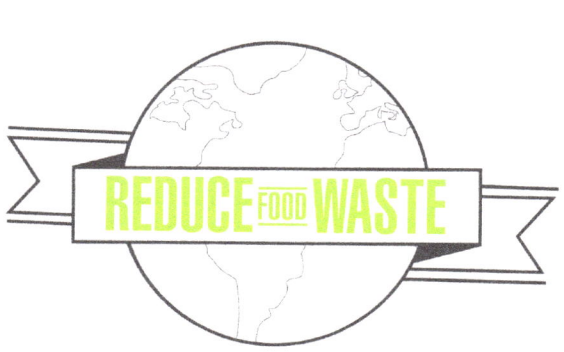

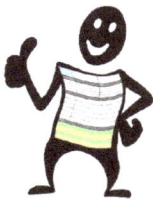

The Impacts of Food Waste – Key Points

Wasted food indicates a poor process

In the U.S. 30-40% of food is wasted
>> **Creates significant greenhouse gas emissions**
>> **Family of four could be wasting $3,920 of food per year**

Strategies to reduce waste
>> **Buy the right amount of the right foods**
>> **Match food longevity to your lifestyle**
>> **Agile Recipes™**
>> **Kitchen techniques to reduce spoilage**

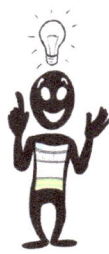

Some thoughts on nutrition . . .

"Let food be your medicine and medicine be your food."
– Hippocrates

"I don't think I'll ever grow old and say, 'What was I thinking eating all those fruits and vegetables?" – Nancy S. Mure

"I believe in eating real food." – Martha Stewart

"Those who think they have no time for healthy eating will sooner or later have to find time for illness." – Edward Stanley

"Don't eat anything your great-grandmother wouldn't recognize as food."
– Michael Pollan

"To eat is a necessity, but to eat intelligently is an art."
– La Rochefoucauld

CHAPTER 3

HOW DO WE IMPROVE NUTRITION?

It is widely accepted that the American diet, frequently called the Western diet, is poor at best, and is a contributing factor to, if not the cause of, the many chronic, degenerative diseases we face. We are also bombarded with diet advice that offers solutions: Mediterranean, DASH, vegan, keto, paleo, gluten-free, pro-biotic, raw, low-glycemic, and so forth. Managing your own nutrition is challenging. Managing nutrition for your whole family is even harder. This book is intended to support your specific dietary goals – whatever they are.

While this book does not advocate one diet regime over another, improved nutrition is an important goal. All the strategies presented here support the following nutritional principles:

A. Less ultra-processed foods

B. More nutrient-rich foods

C. More control over your food composition

D. Personal change in an imperfect world

A. Less Ultra-Processed Foods

We are all familiar with the term "junk food": highly processed food products with too many calories and too little nutrition. However, to study the effect of junk food on human health, a more detailed and consistent method to classify processed foods was required. The NOVA classification was developed by researchers at the University of Sao Paolo[4] to define the extent of processing for foods. This classification assigns foodstuffs to four groups according to the extent and purpose of industrial food processing. It is now used by scientists worldwide to study the impact of food processing on health. The four NOVA classifications categorizing the degree of food processing are shown in Figure 4 on page 18.

Figure 4 – The NOVA Food Classification System		
Group	Classification	Food Groups
1	Unprocessed or minimally processed foods	Fruit, vegetables, legumes, milk, eggs, yogurt, meat, nuts, poultry, seafood, grains and flours, spices, tea, juice, coffee, and water.
2	Processed culinary ingredients	Salt, white and brown sugar, honey, vegetable oils, butter, lard, and coconut fat.
3	Processed foods	Condensed milk, cream, cheese, traditionally cured ham and bacon, canned fruit, canned vegetables, canned fish, freshly made unpackaged bread, beer, cider, and wine.
4	Ultra-Processed Foods	Processed meats, ice cream, breakfast cereals, pizza, margarine, commercially baked breads and pastries, cookies, chips, chocolate, candies, carbonated drinks, instant soups, milkshakes, mayonnaise, fruit drinks, artificially sweetened drinks, and pudding/custard.

An important distinction between ultra-processed (UPF) and processed foods is that UPFs are not whole foods that have been modified by cooking and combining (for example, a jar of spaghetti sauce). Rather, UPFs are formulations of inexpensive industrial ingredients derived from food that are then recombined to create a hyper-palatable, convenient, and long-lasting food product. Note that on average, Americans get 60% of their calories from UPFs.

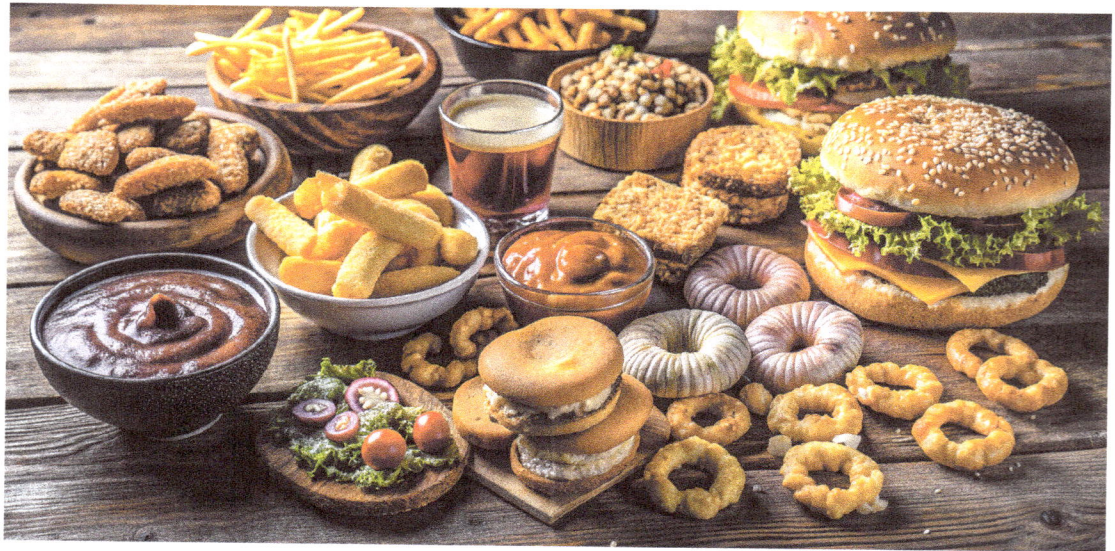

A recent study published in the *British Medical Journal*[5] studied almost 20,000 individuals for five years to determine the relationship between mortality and consuming UPFs. The study showed some startling results. People who consumed over four servings per day of UPFs experienced a 62% increased probability of early mortality from all causes during the study period.

Evidence against UPFs continues to mount. An umbrella review of epidemiological meta-analysis linking UPFs to adverse health outcome was published in early 2024. The researchers analyzed 45 studies from 2009 to June 2023 and concluded that, "Greater exposure to ultra-processed food was associated with a higher risk of adverse health outcomes, especially cardiometabolic, common mental disorder, and mortality outcomes."[6]

So, just why are UPFs linked with negative health effects? Is it:

- Due to their tendency to be high calorie/low nutritional value (e.g., empty calories)?
- Because they are so nutritionally imbalanced, with an over-representation of a few low-quality ingredients?
- The increased processed oils, sugar, MSG, and salt added for flavor?
- That we have processed essential nutrients and fiber out of food products?
- That industrial processing causes chemical changes to the food and/or changes how it is metabolized?
- That artificial additives and trace contaminants make a difference?
- All of the above?

We don't need to know the precise answers to each of these questions; the takeaway message is that less processed food is better for us. I believe that anything made at home is a better option than the ultra-processed version (even cake).

THE BOTTOM LINE

Always opt for natural or minimally processed foods and homemade meals over ultra-processed foods.

Which brings us to this question: "How do we find unprocessed – or at least less processed – food?" Walk into a large grocery store and it can be hard to navigate the choices presented to us. Very few items in the grocery store fall into the unprocessed or minimally processed category, but at least they are identifiable: produce, meat, dairy, whole legumes, and grains. Processed ingredients and foods often sit right next to – and look very similar to – the UPFs we should be avoiding. Consider butter versus the various butter-like spreads. Or how about all the products labeled as peanut butter? Some contain only ground peanuts and maybe a bit of salt, which are a pretty good choice, while others include up to 20% "other stuff". In both cases, the nutrition label would imply that they are darn-near equivalent in terms of fat and calories. However, looking at the list of ingredients, we can see that they are not similar at all. If an ingredient sounds more like a chemical than a food, that's a clue. If the ingredient list sounds like the inventory of an organic chemist's lab, you are probably holding an UPF product. A key objective of this book is to help you make that choice, to buy and prepare less-processed foods.

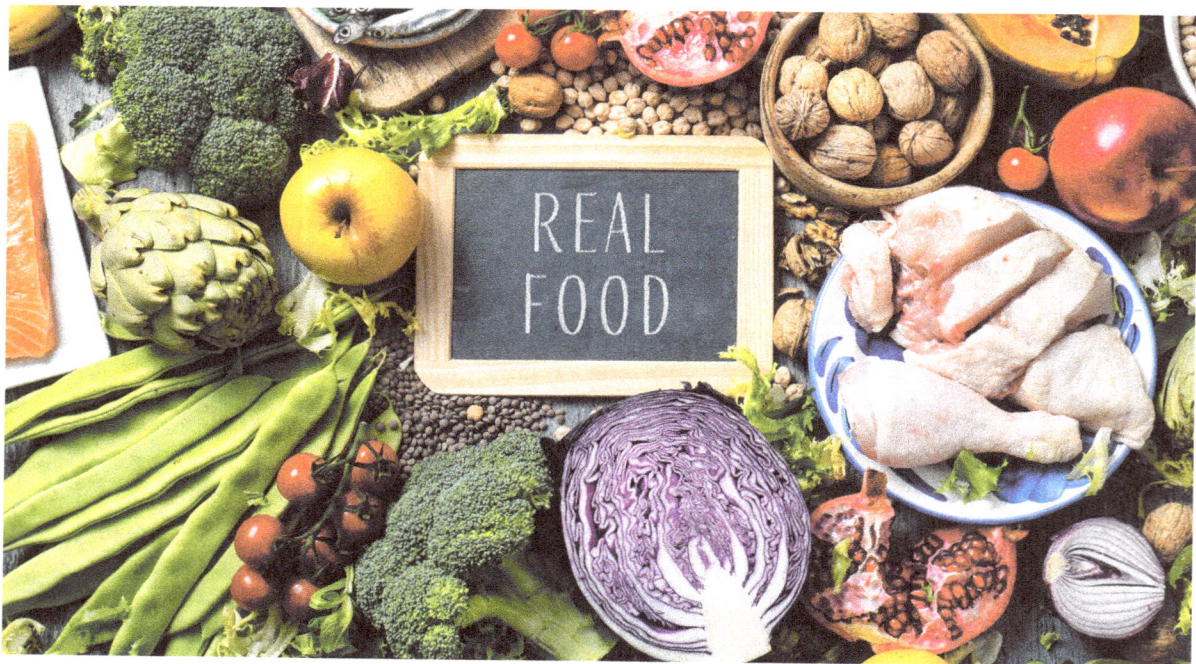

B.   Prioritizing Nutrient-Rich Foods

At the highest level, nutritional guidance can be summarized as follows: minimize the junk food (UPFs) and eat a balanced diet of whole, unprocessed foods with high-quality protein, and significant veggies and fruits. However, this is not specific enough to be very useful. The concept makes sense, but how can we make this happen? Won't it be more time-consuming and expensive? Where do we start?

Here, we will review generally accepted nutritional guidelines and show you how to translate these into an action plan that fits your life. To accomplish this, we will prioritize the nutrient-rich foods that are most important to work into your life: vegetables, fruit, and high-quality protein.

You often hear that you should get five to nine servings of vegetables and fruit each day. In today's busy world, this can be a tall order. Fast-food outlets seldom offer more than a couple of iceberg lettuce salads. Even with a nice restaurant meal, you might get eight green beans (is that even a "serving"?). This is often because fruit and vegetables are unforgiving to manage and somewhat expensive in significant quantities. A whole package (two stalks) of broccoli only provides about four cups of florets; less than two adults' daily vegetable requirement. If you always eat at home, you'd have to buy enough fresh, frozen and canned produce to serve at least 17.5 cups of veggies and 14 cups of fruit (about two gallons, combined!) for each adult every week. After you acquire all this, you still must store, prepare, and serve it. I am fond of saying that my favorite veggie or fruit is the one that someone else prepared!

Giving you strategies to work the right amount of vegetables and fruit into your diet, managing their longevity, and providing streamlined, appetizing recipes is a key focus of this book.

You probably hear a lot of advice related to protein these days: you should eat more protein or less, this type or that. Protein can be costly and must be handled carefully to avoid waste. We will first focus on determining the right quantity of protein to meet your needs. The good news is that there are many healthy protein sources available, and we will give you methods to buy the right amount of high-quality protein, while reducing cost and waste.

Lastly, we will give you tools to increase the amount of healthy fats and whole-food carbohydrates in your diet.

C.   Planning for More Control

How do you decide what to eat? For many people getting food is just one of many priorities, competing with your job, school, and family obligations. There are so many fast-food options available to us that we have got into the habit of not needing to plan in advance. How often do you find yourself hungry and end up choosing the most expedient option? Once you grab the burger or energy bar, your hunger is gone, only to be replaced by food regret. You promise yourself that you will do better next time.

Letting meals become a last-minute compromise is a prescription for poor decisions. The decision criteria become time or money or expedience: anything except nutrition. If you have planned ahead and have some easy options, you increase the odds of making a better decision.

It is easy to assume that the food you get in a restaurant has the same nutritional value as that prepared at home. Maybe it does and maybe it doesn't. Some restaurants provide extremely high-quality, fresh ingredients. However, they all must make a living in a tough and competitive environment, and their food must taste good. Really good. With ever-increasing palatability expectations, even the most conscientious restaurants are probably using more salt, sugar, processed ingredients, MSG, and highly processed vegetable oils than you would at home. In most cases, you just don't know. (Honestly, sometimes I don't want to know!) It is very easy to look at mashed potatoes or French fries on a restaurant plate and assume that they are nutritionally equivalent to the potatoes you would prepare at home. This is highly unlikely as shown in Figure 5 below.

Figure 5 – French Fry Comparison

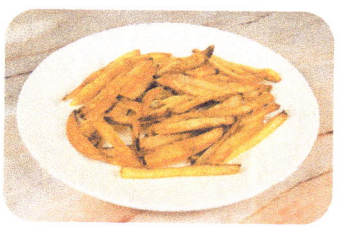 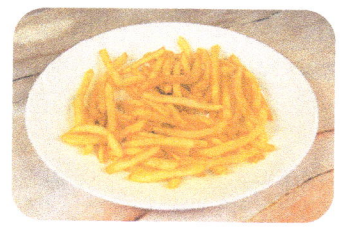 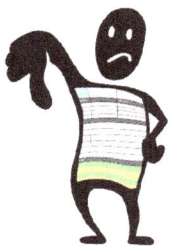

Ingredients:

Potatoes
Olive oil
Salt

Ingredients:

Potatoes
Canola oil
Salt
Soybean oil
Hydrogenated soybean oil
Natural beef flavor
Hydrolyzed wheat
Hydrolyzed milk
Citric acid
Dimelthylopolysiloxane
Dextrose
Sodium acid pyrophosphate
Corn oil
TBHQ

It wasn't that long ago that finances played a larger role in deciding whether to eat out. The decision was easy when going out simply did not fit in the budget. The price of eating out, particularly at fast-food/take-away restaurants, can now be almost competitive with eating at home. This is an amazing feat of food industry efficiency! It is quick, easy, cheap, filling, and tastes good: what's not to like?

Besides the nutritional issues, each and every fast-food visit reinforces your expectation (or your child's) that this is what food is supposed to taste like. It is hard to resist the artificial palatability of ultra-processed food, whether in the form of snacks, fast food, or even commercially prepared "normal" foods. Activating the same reward processes in our brains as an addictive drug, these foods are designed to be irresistible: I think of it as "crack-food". (For additional information on this topic read **Hooked: Food, Free Will, and How the Food Giants Exploit Our Addictions** by Michael Moss) We need to reset our expectations about what food should taste like. It is OK for food to taste like, well, food. Faced with the sheer volume of highly processed food, understanding the makeup of our food is essential to making good choices.

It is an understatement to say that there are profound issues with food supply, modern culture, public policy, and related health implications in the US and, indeed, the whole world. If you'd like to explore some of the complicated issues of the global food supply system, I recommend the following two books:

The Way We Eat Now by Bee Wilson is an excellent book, weaving the various elements together into a clear picture of our modern food ecosystem and how we got here.

Metabolical: The Lure and the Lies of Processed Food, Nutrition and Modern Medicine by Robert H. Lustig, MD, MSL. This book presents the reader with a meticulously researched analysis of the relationships between modern food and disease. Dr. Lustig does an excellent job of explaining how the body metabolizes different foods and the resultant impact on health, particularly chronic non-communicable diseases. He further demonstrates how the food industry, government, and the medical establishment are deeply invested in maintaining the status quo.

D.   Personal Change in an Imperfect World

Change is hard, even with lots of support. Don't expect much initial enthusiasm from your family; change is hard for them too. But do ask them to go on this journey with you. The more they understand about the what and the why, the more likely they are to get on board. Do expect to become frustrated as you try to source less processed food. It is not your imagination: the deck is stacked against you. Highly processed foods are everywhere: vending machines, fast-food outlets, cafeterias, restaurants, grocery stores, gas stations, sports venues... Sugar-laden junk food is marketed relentlessly, even to our children. In the face of systemic obstacles, it would be easy to give up. But you can't wait for the system to change. You have the power to improve your food process and your nutrition now. Let the system catch up with you!

Understanding these big-picture forces will make you a more informed consumer and citizen. It will also give you a healthy appreciation of the challenges ahead of us, collectively and individually.

However, the objective of this book is to help you manage your personal Food Cycle in the best way possible. Today. Part of that equation is making informed choices and trade-offs despite a deeply flawed food-supply landscape and finite resources. Wherever you are starting from, you can take a step in a positive direction today.

Putting ideas into practice:

Much has been written about what's wrong with our modern diets and recommendations about what we should and should not eat. However, there is little written about the integrated process to achieve a better nutritional result; the how. This book is for the individual who wants some tools and strategies to eat better, and to save time and money doing it. This book gives you the how; it is the bridge between intentions and results.

Nutritional advice often admonishes us to eat more or less of certain foods and is often based on what the average person eats. However, none of us are exactly average. The advice that applies to the whole of society may apply to you, or it may not. Advice in the form of "more and less" is not actionable. How much more? How much less? If we want to make changes in our own diet, we first must understand our current status compared to our goals. This means we need to look at amounts of food quantitatively and do some math. We will start this process in the next chapter.

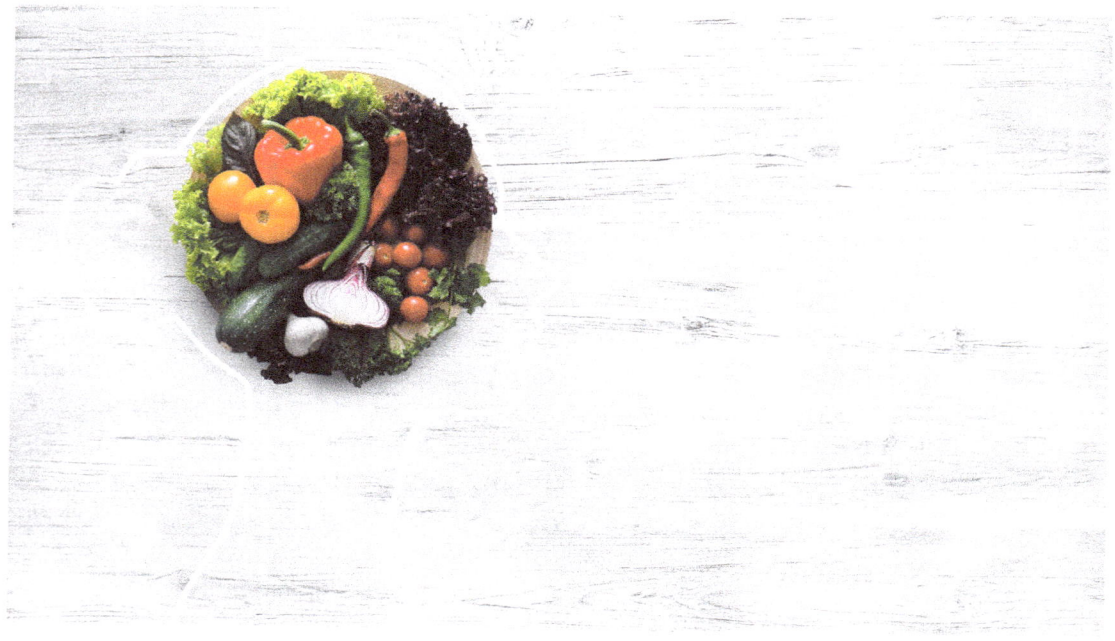

How Do We Improve Nutrition? – Key Points

Reduce ultra-processed foods
- » Formulations of inexpensive industrial ingredients derived from food, engineered to be hyper-palatable, convenient, and long lasting.
- » Make up about 60% of calories in US diet
- » Increase risk of mortality from all causes

Prioritize nutrient rich foods
- » Vegetables and fruits
- » High-quality proteins
- » Whole-food carbohydrates/healthy fats

Improved planning for better control of your foods

Personal change in an imperfect world
- » Our food supply system and food culture are not ideal
- » You can improve your personal food process now

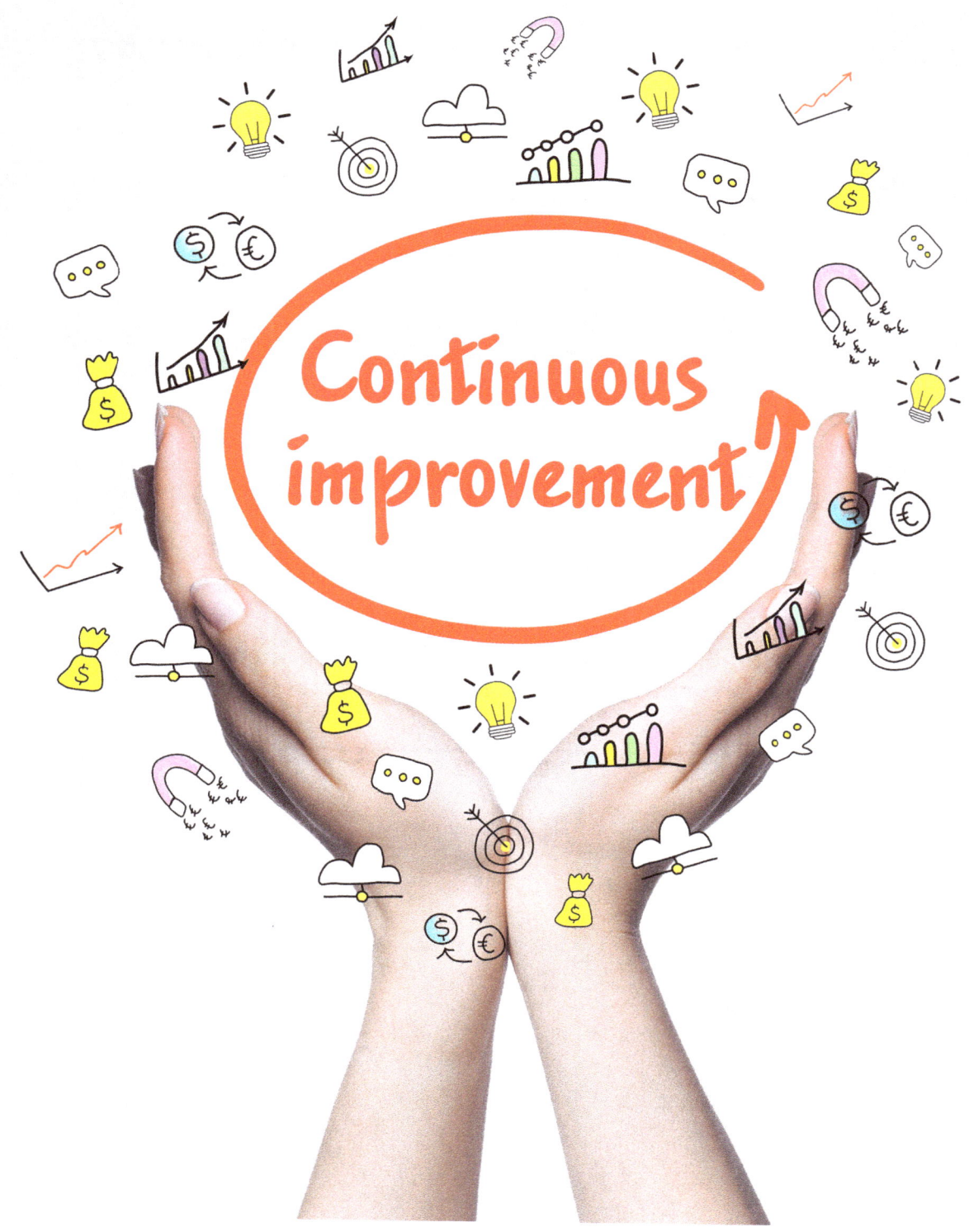

CHAPTER 4

PROCESS IMPROVEMENT: THE FOOD CYCLE

Most of us start our Food Cycle (the food planning, procurement, and preparation process) with vague objectives: we would like our food to be tasty, nutritious, cheap, and easy. Oh, and it would really nice if we could lose a little weight too. Then we just start buying and cooking and eating — and hope it all turns out OK. We never defined specific objectives, so how could we judge success anyway? Is it any wonder that we are often disappointed with the result?

A Quantitative Approach to Process Improvement

If we want to improve our Food Cycle, we need to get serious and employ the same techniques used to improve any process:

1. Define/design the process.
2. Set measurable goals.
3. Measure performance.
4. Adjust based on feedback.

1. Define/Design the Process

When it comes to food planning, most people use a meal-based approach. They make sure that some meals are covered, and then try to manage the meals to be nutritious or at least acceptable. This approach has some key shortcomings:

- it is not driven by high-level nutrition objectives.
- it does not plan well for non-meal food and beverages.
- there will be situations where the choices are poor.

By focusing on the end point (meals), we are going about the process backward. To improve our process, we need to start at the beginning: food procurement. I think it is helpful to remember:

You eat what you buy

Well, duh! As obvious as this seems, it is not how many of us operate. In general, we start food planning with ideas to make certain dishes, and then work backwards to a shopping list. The food and beverages associated with snacks, break rooms, coffee shops, cafeterias, convenience stores, etc. are never really included in any planning process. We need to turn this process around completely. Instead, we need to let our dietary goals drive our food planning and purchases.

Buy what you want to eat – not what you want to make

For example, if we have a goal of eating five servings per day of vegetables, we must have a plan to buy veggies for 35 servings each week. If we need to have all the recipes first, we'll never buy enough vegetables. Once we plan to acquire the right amount of the right foods from all sources, everything else falls in line.

The old chaotic food cycle was focused on purchases and preparation. The Re-Engineered Food Cycle adds nutrition-based planning at the beginning of the process and a results evaluation and feedback loop at the end.

Figure 6 – Re-Engineered Food Cycle Steps

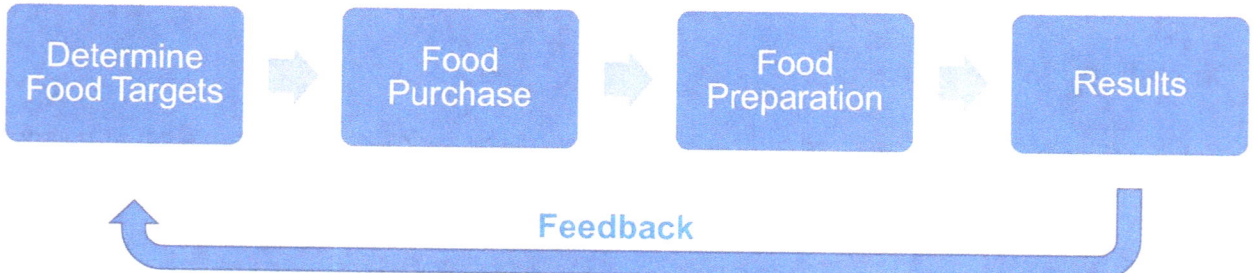

2. Set Measurable Goals

When it comes to food, there are a multitude of variables for which we could set goals: calories, food groups, carbs, fiber, sugar, fats, proteins, even food colors. Often our food goals are guided by numerous and conflicting sources: everything from advertisements, the latest story on the Internet, our friends and, so very powerfully, our personal culture and family history.

The secret to any successful process-improvement effort is to find the key important variables that truly drive the process objectives. We will focus on managing only the most impactful parts of the process. First, we will focus on and measure our nutrient-dense Priority Foods (defined later in Chapter 5). We will set measurable goals, plan our food purchases and preparation, and then evaluate results for these Priority Foods. Once we are doing well managing our Priority Foods, we will focus on the next phases to continue improving nutrition.

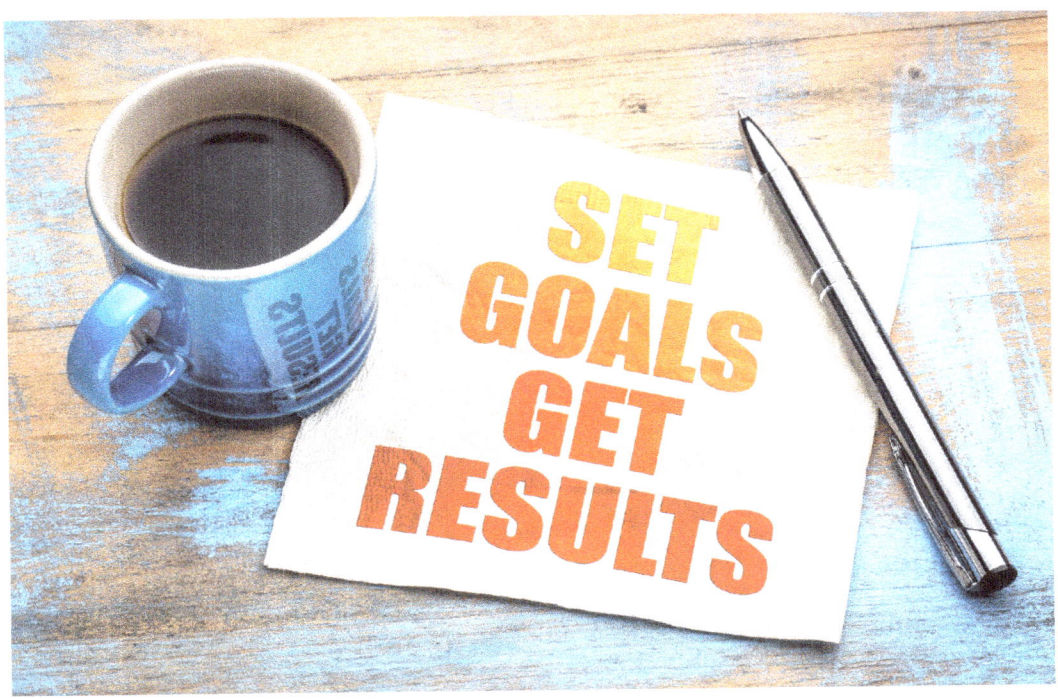

3. Measure Performance

This is the easy part. We will measure our performance each week by simply looking at whether we have eaten the Priority Foods we have purchased. This will tell us if we need to buy more or less of certain types of food or change the implementation part of the process.

4. Adjust Based on Feedback

When we talk about "process improvement", most of us think about a business environment with fancy "dashboards" charting progress and perhaps performance goals providing guidance. Our personal "processes" are just habits; how we do something. Habits are deeply ingrained and difficult to change. A simple and accessible feedback loop is essential if we have any hope of improving our personal processes (habits). Our feedback loop will tie directly into planning for the next week. Our results from one week (Priority Foods consumed) will inform us quite directly what needs to change for the following week.

Do not expect everything to work out perfectly the first week, or even the tenth. However, do expect continuous improvement over time. The steps outlined here will allow you to work toward your goals, continuously refining your Food Cycle as you learn what works best for you.

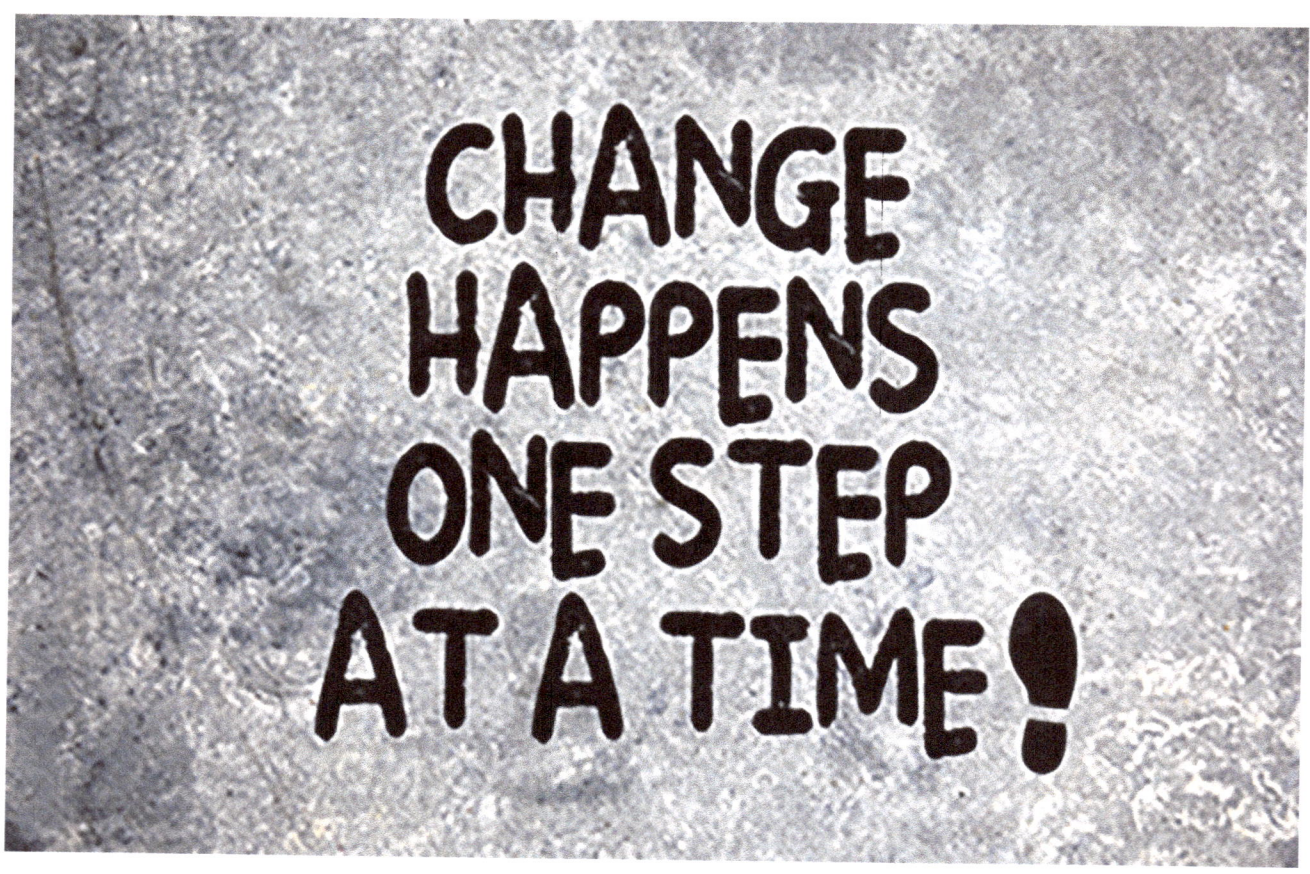

Process Improvement: The Food Cycle – Key Points

You need a quantitative approach to process improvement

Define the process
> » **Re-Engineered Food Cycle – includes all food sources**
> » **Start planning with nutritional goals, not meals**
> » **Buy what you want to eat, not what you want to make**

Define goals
> » **Focus on nutrient-dense Priority Foods**

Measure performance
> » **Was the right amount of Priority Foods consumed?**

Adjust process based on feedback
> » **Adjust Priority Food purchases or food preparation**
> » **Continuous improvement over time**

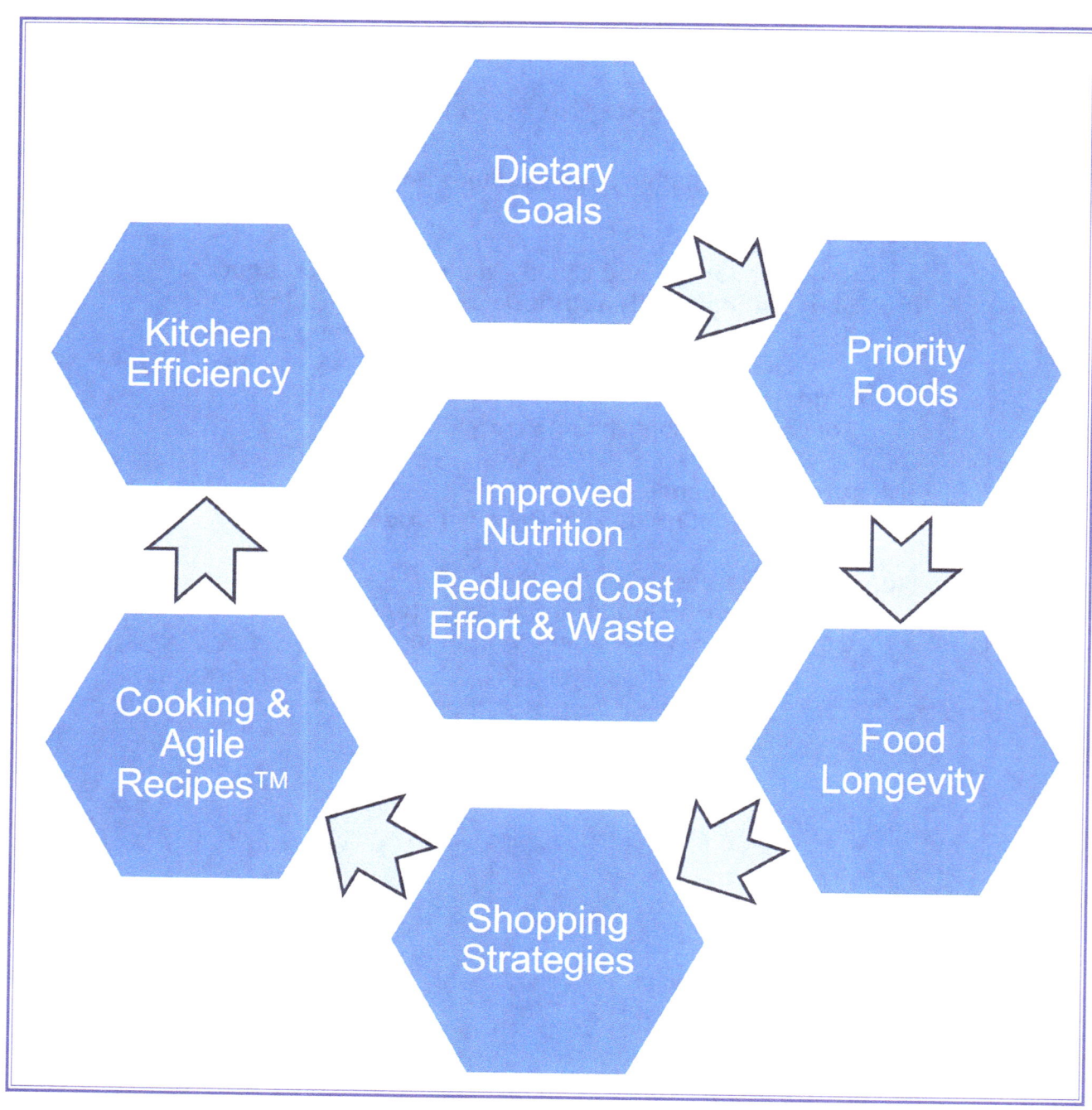

CHAPTER 5

THE RE-ENGINEERED FOOD CYCLE

The Re-Engineered Food Cycle brings together all your food and beverages from all sources into one, coherent process. The process is driven by your overarching food-related objectives, including nutrition, cost, and time. Food planning starts with the foods that are most important to work into your diet: high-quality vegetables, fruit, and protein. Chances are good that most people are not eating the optimum amount of these high-quality, nutritious foods. By ensuring enough of these Priority Foods are consumed, there is less room for junk food. These Priority Foods are the foundation of the Re-Engineered Food Cycle. There are four phases:

- In Phase I we will develop the plan to manage Priority Foods each week.
- In Phase II we will systematically replace low-quality carbohydrates and fats with high quality.
- Phase III will give you shopping strategies and preparation alternatives including Agile Recipes™ to achieve your food objectives.
- Phase IV will focus on efficient kitchen management techniques.

So, how is this different from the typical meal-driven planning process? Essentially, this is a top-down approach. It is an integrated, food-first process where we determine what food we intend to eat and then proceed to make that happen.

Figure 7 – Food Cycle Phases

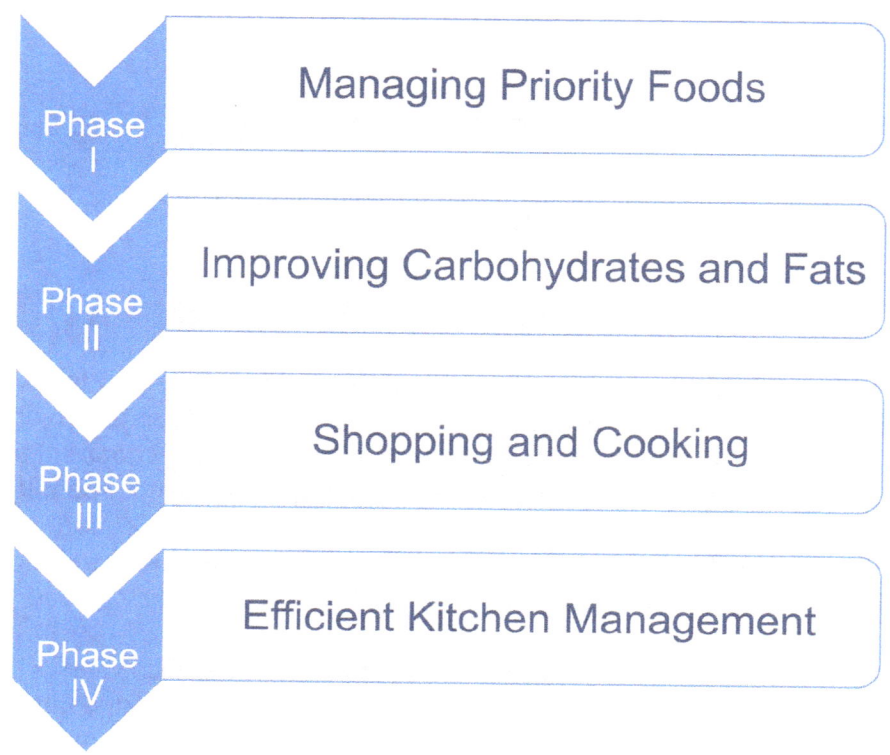

Phase I – Managing Priority Foods

We are going to approach changing our Food Cycle in phases. Getting the right amount of Priority Foods in our diet is the foundation of the Re-Engineered Food Cycle so we will do this first.

To get a handle on our integrated food process, we need to set clear objectives and then be able to evaluate how we are doing. We will manage the Food Cycle by keeping it very simple to start and optimizing only the most important variable, PFs. Our primary control variable is the quantity of these PFs consumed. With one key variable-set to manage, the process becomes straightforward:

- Step 1 – Determine your target quantity of PFs for your lifestyle
- Step 2 – Shop, cook, eat
- Step 3 – Compare the actual amount of PFs consumed to the target
- Step 4 – Evaluate and adjust the process accordingly

Figure 8 – Priority Foods Control Loop

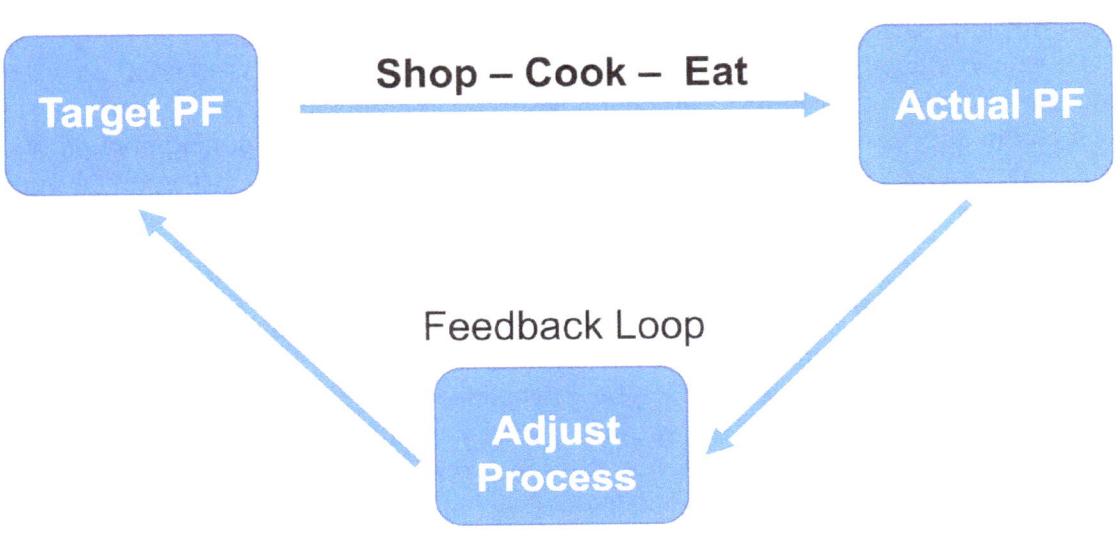

This looks easy but does it work? Yes, it does work because we have chosen to manage the hardest part of the whole process: PFs. Why are they "difficult"? These are the foods that are most challenging to work into your life; they are not cheap or universally available, have a short shelf-life, and need preparation and cooking. Fresh broccoli takes a bit more effort than, say, peanut butter crackers. We will make getting these PFs easier and more manageable.

In the following chapters, you will go through a step-by-step process to determine the best combination of PFs for you. By buying the right quantity of PFs, there is simply less room for lower quality, less nutritious food. After you have established a baseline PFs target, your weekly planning step will be adjusting your PFs for your immediate schedule. Your grocery list will focus on food types and volumes as opposed to a multitude of specific items. Focusing on food types as opposed to specific items facilitates buying the lower cost/higher quality option.

Every good process needs a feedback mechanism: a review of what is working well and what is not. At the end of the week, you can evaluate how you did by reviewing whether the target amount of PFs was, in fact, cooked and eaten. Is a detailed food diary necessary? Nope! Success can be quickly judged by simply looking at how much PFs is left or discarded by the end of the week. If you are running out of food early or discarding too much at the end of the week, you will need to adjust next week. The right adjustment will be fairly obvious as there are only so many levers to pull: shift what you buy or shift what you prepare and eat.

Phase II – Improve Carbohydrates and Fats

What about those "whole grains and healthy fats" you hear so much about? Yes, it is vitally important to choose the right carbohydrates and fats for your diet. These are particularly important since carbohydrates and fats often come in the form of ultra-processed foods. In Phase II, we will focus on improving carbs and fats. Low-quality carbohydrates (refined grains and sugar, in particular) and fats tend to be cheap and readily available. The challenge is often not about getting enough but, rather, improving quality and achieving balance. We will give you information and strategies to work toward a healthier combination of carbs and fats.

Phase III – Shopping and Cooking

Knowing what to eat is of no value if you don't have a feasible plan to procure and prepare it. Most people want great food (Every. Single. Day.) but have limited time and resources to make it happen. Phase III will focus on implementation: providing shopping strategies and streamlined recipes to efficiently prepare the foods you've chosen in the first two phases. The Agile Recipes™ in this book will give you simple preparation options for almost anything you purchase.

Phase IV – Efficient Kitchen Management

Let's make it easier to cook Real Food more often.

Reduced Time, Cost and Food Waste

Let's briefly consider the objectives that are not directly measured in our process, such as time, cost, and food waste. These variables do not need to be managed directly because they will, for the most part, naturally fall in line. If we buy the right amount of the right foods with the appropriate longevity, we will use everything and waste little. Food waste and food costs will automatically decrease as a result. Shopping for food types, rather than specific items, allows buying what is available, in season, or on sale. By optimizing quantity, you avoid over-buying expensive items. If your process is working well, you will see better value, time efficiency, and less food waste.

The Re-Engineered Food Cycle – Key Points

Integrated, *food first* process

Driven by overall food objectives

Considers food from all sources

Phase I – Managing Priority Foods
  » Set Priority Food targets, measure results, adjustments

Phase II – Improving Carbohydrates and Dietary Fats

Phase III – Shopping and Cooking
  » Shopping strategies
  » Agile Recipes™

Phase IV – Efficient Kitchen Management
  » Kitchen management strategies

Results: Less time, money, and food waste
  » Achieved by buying the right amounts of the right foods and managing them efficiently

But Does the Re-Engineered Food Cycle Work?

Well, it's working for us! My husband and I have faithfully implemented the Re-Engineered Food Cycle for two years now. At first it seemed unusual, even awkward, to calculate target amounts of food and shop this way. However, after about 3 weeks the process became routine.

The first result we noticed was that we had not been eating the volume of produce that we thought we were. We really believed that we were eating *at least* the recommended amount of veggies. Ha! Try about half to two-thirds on a good day. The target volume of produce turned into a driving force which influenced where and how we shopped. We needed a lot more veggies, so we ended up each week at the stores that reliably had the best selection, price, and quality of fresh and frozen produce. On the other hand, we ended up buying protein less frequently but in larger quantities and then storing/freezing it. We feel that we are getting better value for our grocery dollars as well as saving shopping time.

The next thing we noticed is that now we only go out to eat on purpose. In the past, eating out was frequently a result of not being up to cooking for some reason: we'd look at each other, shrug and someone would say "I guess we could go out...?". Missing ingredients, spoiled food, no good plan for what to cook, not enough time to prepare the planned recipe, or not being interested in cleaning the kitchen were all reasons to go out. Frequently those impromptu restaurant meals were not even enjoyed, they were simply expedient. Too often, the meal out was followed by regret that a bunch of money was wasted on food I never intended to eat. Don't get me wrong; we still go out to eat and pretty much whenever we want to. The key is that we go out when we want to enjoy a certain restaurant, preferably in a social context. It turns out that going out to eat like this happens much less frequently than before.

Lastly, our food waste has dramatically declined. It's not zero, but we are getting close. Sure, we still end up discarding a few slimy green onions in the bottom of a bag or the last crumbly, dried-out tortilla. However, we have not discarded new, packaged fresh food in well over a year. Food longevity, how long a food will last, is now considered before buying every grocery item. Cooked food is almost always 100% eaten, largely because there are options for every leftover to become part of an upcoming meal.

So, the bottom line is that we are eating better, spending less time and money, and wasting less food. Perhaps even more valuable, since I know I always have food and easy preparation options available, I am finding the whole Food Cycle infinitely less stressful!

"Change is not an event, it's a process."

— Cheryl James

PHASE I

RE-ENGINEERING THE KITCHEN®

MANAGING PRIORITY FOODS

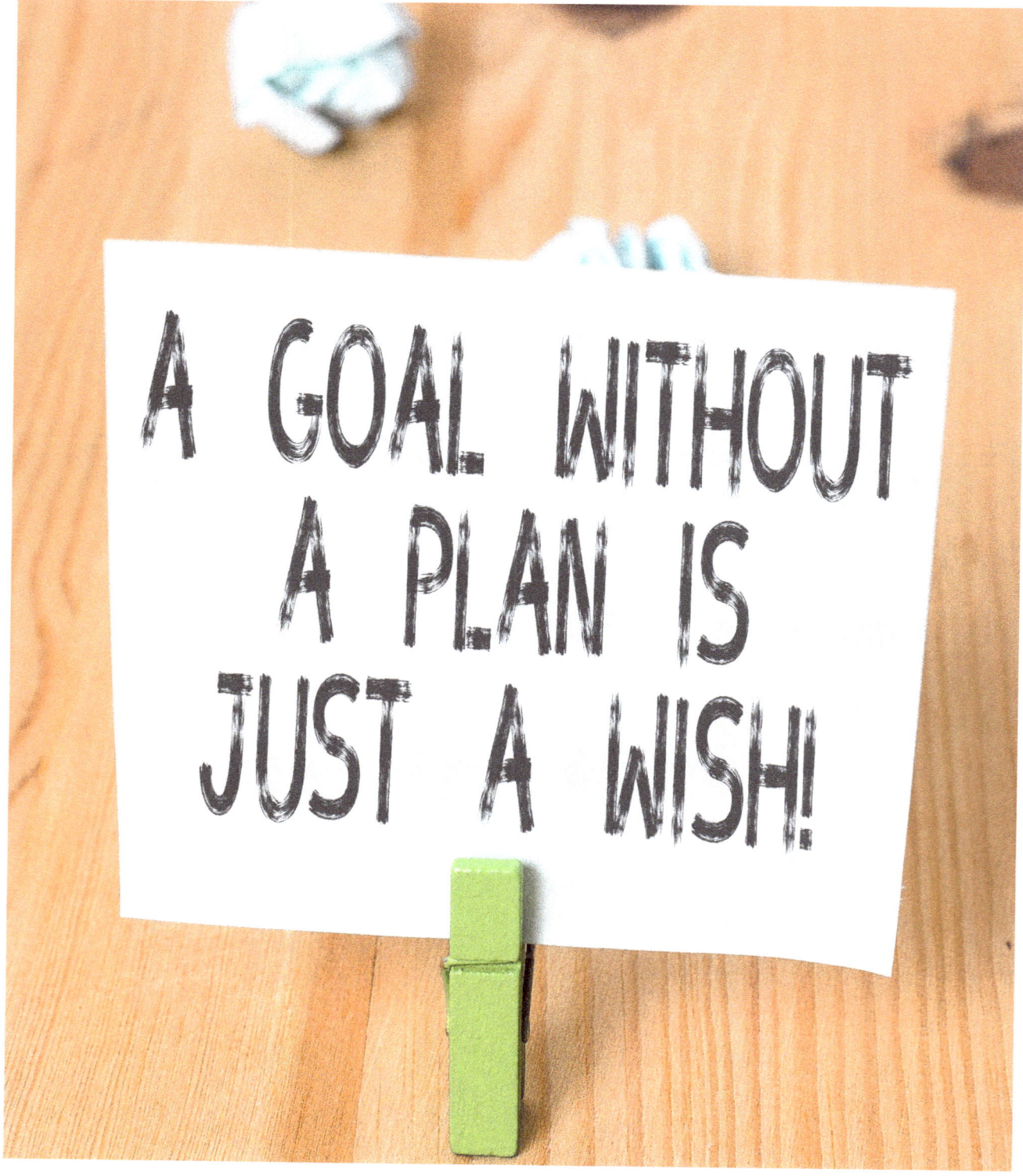

CHAPTER 6

SETTING QUANTITATIVE NUTRITIONAL GOALS

How do you set your own nutritional goals? What you decide to eat is influenced by your culture and personal history. Beyond that, perhaps you look to the experts, but it sure would be nice if they could all agree. With the vast amount of research that has gone into human nutrition and continues today, you would think that we'd have the "perfect diet" defined by now! Even so, there seems to be a plethora of recommended diets – or eating styles – out there in the world. Having studied well over 100 reports while researching the topic of nutrition and dietary guidelines, it has become clear that:

1. regional and cultural differences exist, and

2. nutrition is not an exact science – ranges and estimates are the reality.

When you study the various government-published guidelines – MyPlate by the USDA, The Food Pyramid in Europe (and there are differences in the pyramid as you move from country to country), the Chinese Food Pagoda, and the Japanese Food Pyramid – you find a significant amount of overlap. While the recommended ratios change as you move around the world, all are based on similar food groupings as shown below:

- Bread, cereal, rice, and pasta
- Vegetables
- Fruits
- Meat, poultry, fish, legumes (including soy products), eggs, and nuts
- Dairy
- Fats and oils

To calculate food requirements in later chapters of the book, we need to have a base case of dietary guidelines to work from. For our purposes, we will use the dietary guidance issued by the US government: "Dietary Guideline for Americans 2020-2025" (DGA)[7].

The DGA is a highly detailed nutritional reference based on decades of science[8]. It provides guidelines for "average" people (see below). Keep in mind that some health experts judge these nutritional guidelines to be inadequate at best or based on outdated science and influenced by special interest politics at worst. However, for many people, even coming close to meeting these guidelines would be a vast improvement over their current diets, so they serve as a useful starting point.

It is important to remember that the examples in this book are intended to illustrate the process, not dictate your nutritional objectives. It is up to you to determine the eating style that is best for you and then apply these techniques to accomplish your personal goals.

Figure 9 – Estimated Calorie Needs per Day (Moderate Activity) – DGA[7]

Males		Females	
Age	Calories/Day	Age	Calories/Day
2	1,000	2	1,000
3-5	1,400	3	1,200
6-8	1,600	4-6	1,400
9-10	1,800	7-9	1,600
11	2,000	10-11	1,800
12-13	2,200	12-18	2,000
14	2,400	19-25	2,200
15	2,600	26-50	2,000
15-25	2,800	50+	1,800
26-45	2,600		
46-65	2,400		
65+	2,200		

The DGA starts by estimating the daily calorie requirements for average individuals based on age, gender, and physical activity. Figure 9 on the previous page summarizes the estimated calories per day for males and females (over two years old) with a moderately active lifestyle. Appendix B shows tables with the estimated calorie levels, for higher and lower activity levels and a calculator for adults who are significantly different than average in height and/or weight.

Most of our example calculations will be based on quantitative guidelines for the USDA "Reference Man" and "Reference Woman" with a moderate activity level as described below. When you do these calculations for yourself and your family, you will start by estimating calorie levels for each individual. Remember that these are approximations and serve as a starting point to calculate the amount of Priority Foods to plan for.

Figure 10 – USDA Reference Woman and Man

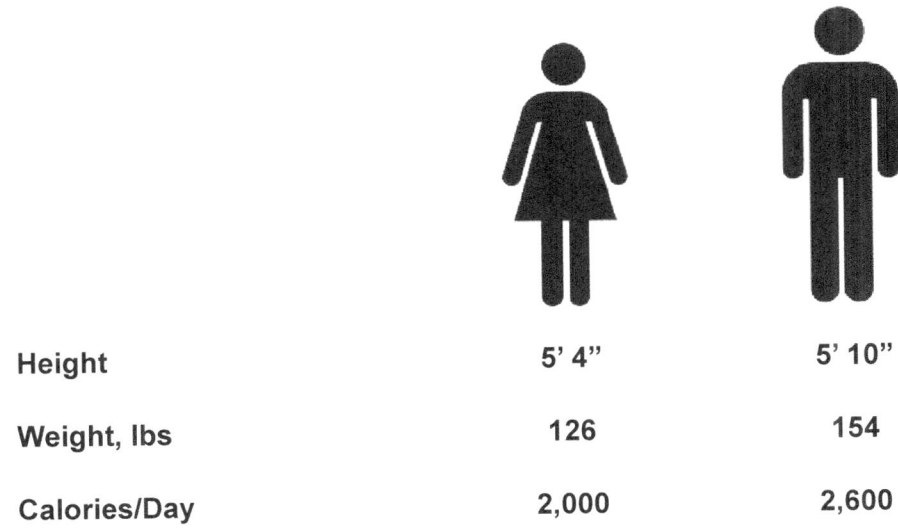

Height	**5' 4"**	**5' 10"**
Weight, lbs	**126**	**154**
Calories/Day	**2,000**	**2,600**

Source: USDA Dietary Guidelines for Americans 2020-2025

Macronutrient Ratios

Much of our dialog about food and nutrition is centered around the three key macronutrients (carbs, fats and protein) and what the perfect combination should be. However, gross macronutrients are only part of the picture. Simply put, food contains both macronutrients and micronutrients. Macronutrients are the bulk of our food and include carbohydrates, proteins, and fats. While fiber, a type of carbohydrate, is essential to health it is often only mentioned as an afterthought.

Micronutrients are the vitamins, minerals, antioxidants, etc. that our bodies need in small quantities to thrive. Most foods are complex, containing a range of both macronutrients and micronutrients. In general, the more refined a food is, the less nutritious it is. For example, whole-grain brown rice contains more micronutrients and fiber than refined white rice.

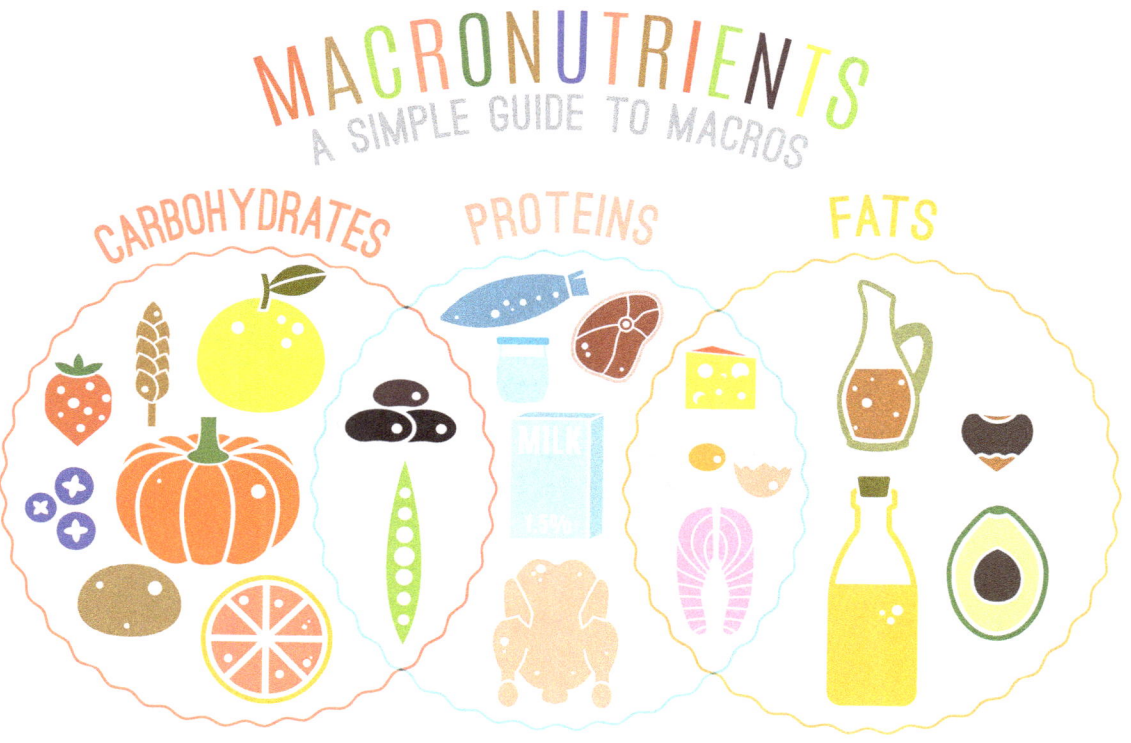

Many diets are based on target macronutrient ratios; specifying the ratio of calories obtained from carbs, proteins, and fats. Figure 11 on page 47 shows how several popular types of diets stack up against the average Acceptable Macronutrient Distribution Ranges[9] (AMDR) incorporated into the DGA. The Acceptable Macronutrient Distribution Ranges are:

- Carbohydrates: 45-65% of calories
- Fats: 20-35% of calories
- Protein: 10-35% of calories

Figure 11 – Typical Macronutrient Distribution by Type of Diet

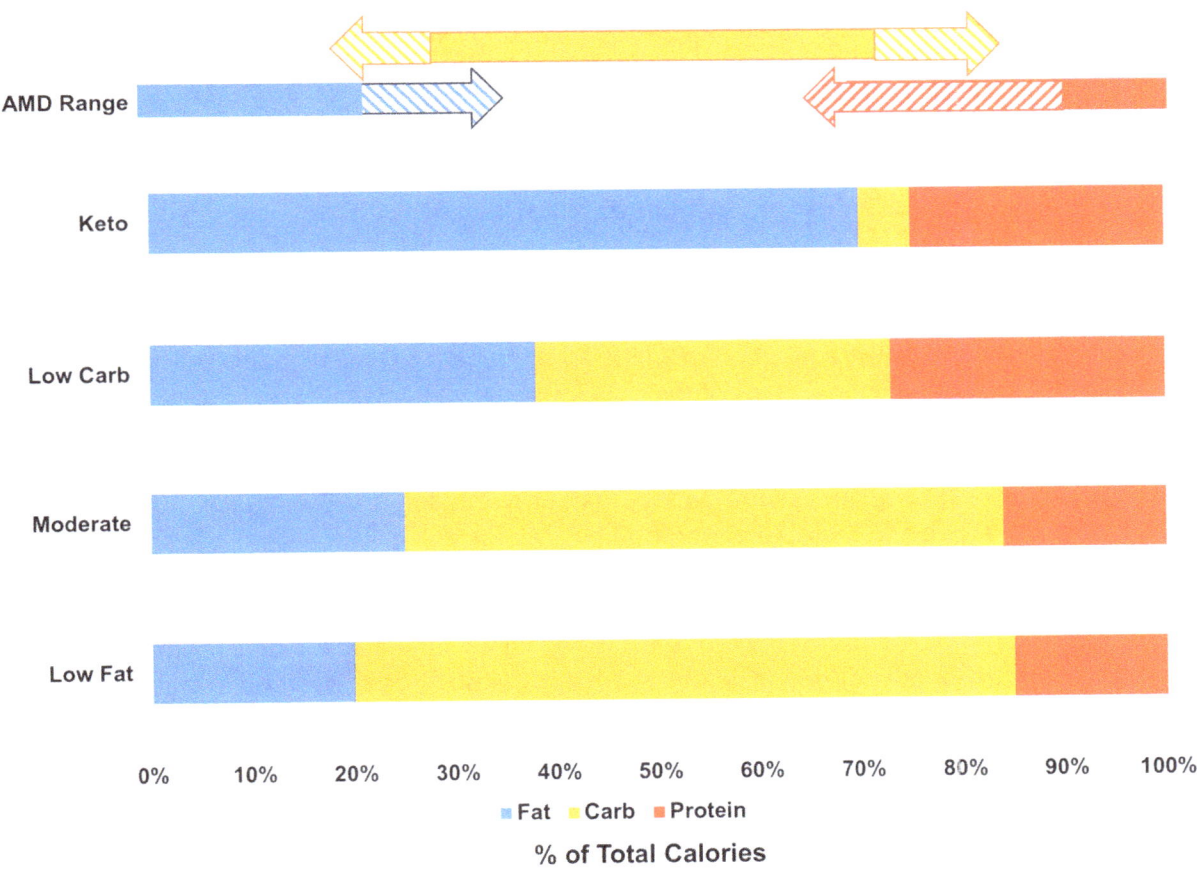

You might be surprised to hear that it is not hard to meet these recommended macronutrient ranges. For example, a diet of only McDonald's hamburgers meets these guidelines, providing 32% fat, 49% carbs and 19% protein. So, macronutrient ratios alone do not determine a nutritious diet. The quality of the macronutrients is important as well as the micronutrients and critical fiber.

Various populations around the world do just fine on differing ranges of macronutrient ratios. Perhaps managing the exact ratio of carbs, fats and protein in our diets is not at all what we should be focusing on. It is sort of like buying a house based on the ratio of cement, wood, and bricks: they may be important components, but it sort of misses the point of providing a home that meets all your needs.

So, what is the best macronutrient ratio or diet for you? That is up to you to decide. Maybe as an athlete, you have a higher protein requirement. Perhaps you are concerned about your blood glucose so are watching carbs. In any case, we will use the USDA guidelines as the starting point for our examples. You can adjust your calculations to meet your individual needs. No matter what eating style you choose, this book will help you plan, shop, and cook to meet your objectives.

All Diets "Work"

Have you noticed that it doesn't seem to matter which diet people go on? They seem to lose some weight and get a bit healthier (at least at first). Popular diets and eating styles can vary greatly: a lot of fat to a little fat, high carb to low, higher protein levels or lower, and even elimination of whole food groups. I've known people who have had success on Atkins, Weight Watchers, South Beach, keto, paleo, intermittent fasting, raw food, vegan and even the cabbage-soup diet, which you can only stand for a few days. People do well for as long as they can stay the course. Eventually, however, most people revert to their old eating habits.

While diets can be vastly different, the one thing they have in common is the exclusion of highly processed foods. I can't think of a single mainstream diet regime that encourages a lot of sugary drinks, commercially baked goods, fast food or packaged snacks. Maybe the best diet for you is the one you can manage to stay on for the longest time. Or maybe, the best diet starts with just eating Real Food.

Setting Quantitative Nutritional Goals – Key Points

USDA Dietary Guidance for Americans (DGA)
- » **Used for examples throughout the book**
- » **Defines reference people**
  - » **Woman – 2,000 calories/day**
  - » **Man – 2,600 calories/day**

Macronutrients – bulk of diet
- » **Carbohydrates, fats, and proteins**
- » **Ratios differ by diet**
- » **Fiber is essential**

Micronutrients – vitamins and minerals
- » **Small amounts needed for health**

Example calculations – use DGA recommendations
- » **Adjust for your preferred diet**

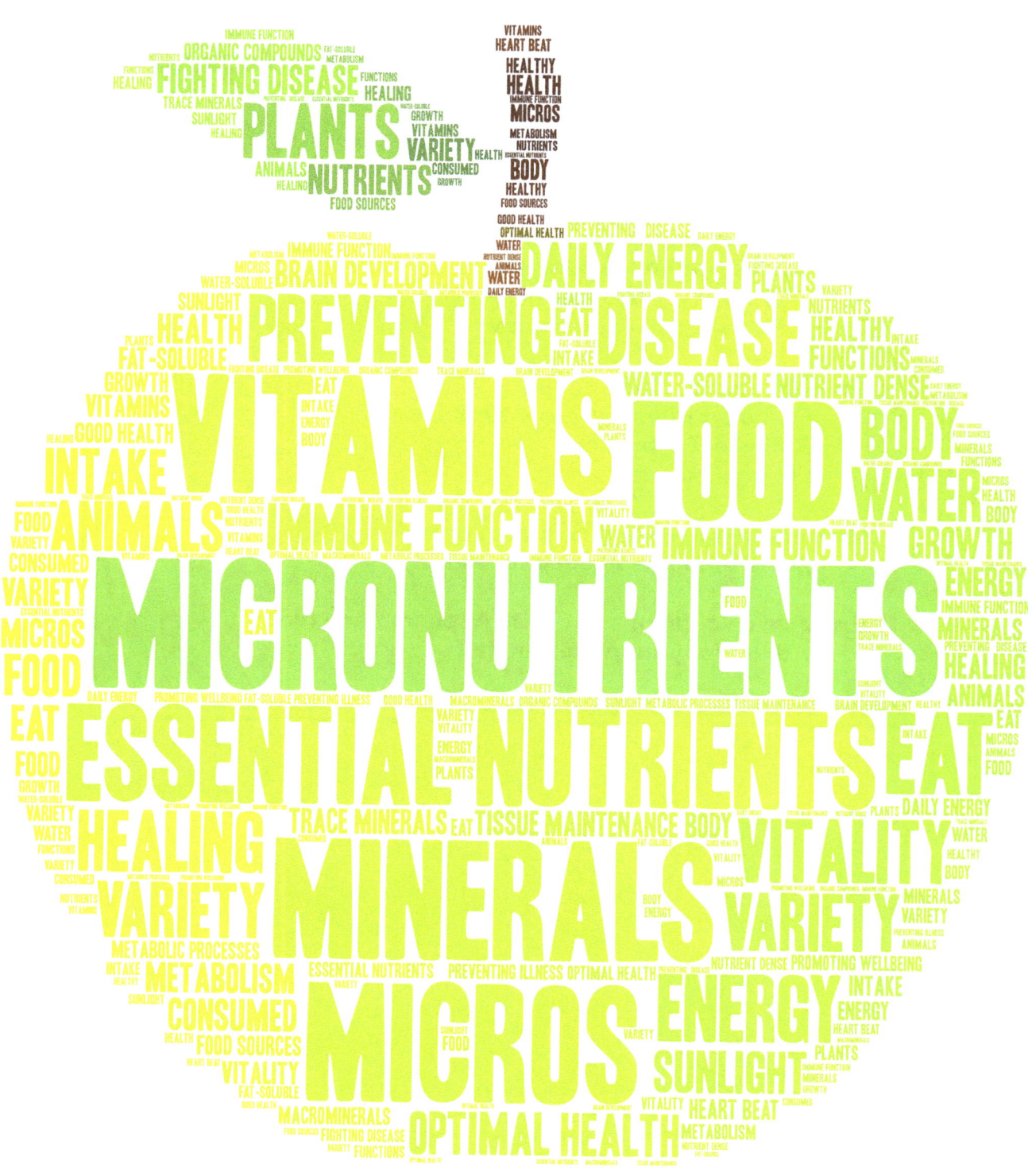

CHAPTER 7

MICRONUTRIENTS SIMPLIFIED

Micronutrients include the vitamins, minerals, antioxidants, flavonoids, fatty acids, amino acids, and probiotics needed in small quantities to perform certain functions in the body, and are vitally important to our health and wellbeing. When we say that junk food is "empty calories", it is primarily micronutrients that are missing.

Food labeling tends to focus on the Big Three: fats, carbs and protein, but if you read the small print, you might see information about vitamins and minerals included on packaged foods, especially on fortified foods.

However, produce, the biggest source of micronutrients, generally has no food label. Even in dietary recommendations, micronutrients are usually vaguely addressed with a blanket statement about eating a variety of whole foods with lots of fruits and vegetables. So, how do we make sure we get enough in our diet?

Today there are 13 vitamins and 14 minerals considered essential for health. In addition, there are essential fatty acids and essential amino acids. Then there is a plethora of beneficial micronutrients that are not considered "essential". This means you can survive without them, but your body may be much (much!) happier if they are available.

So, why does the subject of micronutrients seem confusing? Mostly because it's fairly complicated. There are thousands of combinations of compounds interacting with living systems; the variables are almost infinite. The foods eaten together can help or hinder the bioavailability of the micronutrients consumed. Micronutrients are an integral part of a multitude of complex hormonal signaling pathways controlling everything from metabolism to blood chemistry to mood to cellular function. Any signaling pathway can malfunction if one essential compound is lacking. Antioxidants are essential to prevent oxidation throughout the body involved in damaging processes such as atherosclerosis and cellular mutations. If you want to develop a better understanding of individual micronutrients, The Linus Pauling Institute's Micronutrient Information Center, which is associated with Oregon State University, is an excellent, free and scientifically substantiated source of information. (pi.oregonstate.edu).

But how many of us really want to delve into a complex biochemistry research project just to figure out what's for dinner? The good news is that you don't have to understand biochemistry to embrace micronutrients as the nutritional gold they truly are. Carbs, fats, and proteins might be the building blocks, but micronutrients are the magic keys that allow the intricate mechanisms of life to function properly.

Micronutrients = Nutritional gold

Nature = Best source of micronutrients

The better news is that those magical micronutrients are readily available in normal, whole foods. The following Food & Micronutrient Charts give you an idea of the key vitamins, minerals, phytochemicals, and other nutrients your body needs. While it is a summary and certainly not complete, it should provide a starting point in understanding that your body needs a lot more than simply protein, carbs, and fats. The foods listed in Figures 12-15 are simple whole foods, including our nutrient-dense Priority Foods.

The micronutrient charts were developed using data from the following sources:

U.S. Department of Agriculture – Food Data Central[9]

WebMD – Food Sources for Vitamins and Minerals[10]

U.S. Food & Drig Administration – Nutrition Facts Labeling Requirements[11]

Healthline – Micronutrients: Types, Functions, and Benefits[12]

WebMD – Vitamins & Minerals - How Much Should You Take?[13]

Mayo Clinic – Chart of High-Fiber Foods[14]

Linus Pauling Institute – Micronutrients for Health[15]

Figure 12 Phytochemicals	Carotenoids	Chlorophyll	Curcumin	Flavonoids	Garlic	Indole-4 Carbinole	Isothyocyanates	Lignans	Phytosterols	Resveratrol	Soy Isoflavones
Tofu				X							X
Whole Grains & Breads								X			
Oats	X			X							
Rice – White & Brown				X					X		
Quinoa									X		
Broccoli	X			X		X	X	X			
Brussels Sprouts	X					X	X	X	X		
Cauliflower						X	X				
Dark Green Leafy Vegetables	X	X				X	X	X			
Garlic					X						
Onion				X							
Orange Vegetables	X										
Peppers – Red & Green	X										
Tomatoes	X										
Apples				X							
Apricots	X			X				X			
Bananas									X		
Berries – All				X				X		X	
Citrus Fruits									X		
Grapes		X		X						X	
Kiwi		X									
Plums & Prunes				X							
Beans & Legumes									X		
Nuts & Seeds		X						X	X		
Tumeric			X								
Cinnamon				X							
Coffee								X			
Tea				X				X			
Red Wine				X	X			X		X	
Chocolate				X	X					X	

Figure 13
Vitamins

	A	Thiamine B1	Riboflavin B2	Niacin B3	Pantothenic Acid B5	Piridoxine B6	Biotin B7	Folic Acid (Folate) B9	Cobalamines B12	C	D	E	K
Milk	X	X	X		X		X		X		X		
Eggs	X	X	X		X		X	X	X		X		
Cheese	X		X				X		X		X		X
Yogurt			X		X		X						
Tofu			X	X				X					
Whole Grains & Breads	X	X	X	X		X		X				X	
Oats		X	X	X	X			X					
Rice – White & Brown		X	X	X	X			X					
Quinoa		X	X	X	X			X					
Avocado	X	X	X	X	X	X		X		X		X	X
Asparagus	X	X	X	X	X	X		X		X		X	X
Broccoli	X	X	X	X	X	X		X		X		X	X
Brussels Sprouts	X	X	X	X	X	X		X		X		X	X
Cauliflower		X		X	X	X		X		X			X
Dark Green Leafy Vegetables	X	X	X	X	X	X		X		X		X	X
Green Beans	X	X	X	X	X	X		X		X		X	X
Green Onions	X	X	X	X	X	X		X		X	X	X	X
Lettuce		X		X		X				X			
Mushrooms		X	X	X		X	X	X					
Onions		X	X	X	X	X		X		X			
Orange Vegetables	X	X	X	X		X		X		X		X	X
Peas	X	X	X	X	X	X		X		X		X	X
Peppers – Red & Green		X	X	X		X	X	X		X			
Potatoes		X		X		X				X	X		
Tomatoes	X	X		X		X	X			X			

Figure 13 Vitamins	Thiamine	Riboflavin	Niacin	Pantothenic Acid	Piridoxine	Biotin	Folic Acid (Folate)	Cobalamines				
A	**B1**	**B2**	**B3**	**B5**	**B6**	**B7**	**B9**	**B12**	**C**	**D**	**E**	**K**
Apples			X	X									
Apricots	X			X	X							X	
Bananas				X	X	X	X	X		X			
Berries – All	X							X		X			X
Cantelope	X	X		X				X		X			X
Citrus Fruits		X	X	X	X	X		X		X	X		
Figs	X			X		X		X					X
Grapes				X		X							X
Kiwi				X						X			X
Peaches	X			X				X					
Plums & Prunes				X				X					X
Pineapple		X		X		X				X			
Beef/Pork/Poultry			X	X	X		X		X				X
Organ Meats	X		X	X	X	X		X	X		X	X	X
Fatty Fish	X		X	X	X			X	X		X	X	
Non-Fatty Fish	X			X	X	X			X		X		
Shellfish	X	X	X	X	X	X		X	X	X		X	
Beans & Legumes			X	X	X	X		X					X
Nuts & Seeds		X	X	X		X		X				X	X

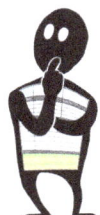

Did you know that the word "vitamin" was first used by the Polish chemist Kasimir Funk in 1912 and is a combination of the words "vital" and "amine".

Figure 14
Minerals

	Calcium	Chromium	Copper	Cobalt	Iodine	Magnesium	Manganese	Molybdenum	Phosphorus	Potassium	Selenium	Sodium Chloride	Zinc	Iron
	Ca	Cr	Cu	Co	I	Mg	Mn	Mo	P	K	Se	NaCl	Zn	Fe
Milk	X			X	X	X			X	X	X			
Eggs				X	X				X	X				
Cheese	X								X				X	
Yogurt	X							X	X	X			X	
Tofu	X					X			X	X	X		X	X
Whole Grains & Breads						X		X	X		X			X
Oats	X					X	X		X	X			X	X
Rice – White & Brown						X	X	X	X	X	X		X	X
Quinoa						X	X		X	X	X		X	X
Avocado	X		X			X	X		X	X	X		X	X
Asparagus	X		X			X	X	X	X	X	X		X	X
Broccoli	X		X			X	X		X	X	X		X	X
Brussels Sprouts	X		X			X	X		X	X	X		X	X
Cauliflower	X					X	X		X	X	X	X	X	X
Dark Green Leafy Vegetables	X			X		X			X	X		X		X
Green Beans	X		X			X	X	X	X	X	X		X	X
Green Onions	X		X			X	X		X	X	X	X	X	X
Lettuce	X		X			X	X		X	X			X	X
Mushrooms			X			X	X		X	X				
Onions	X		X			X	X		X	X	X	X	X	X
Orange Vegetables	X					X	X		X	X		X		X
Peas	X					X	X		X	X	X		X	X
Peppers – Red & Green	X		X			X	X		X	X			X	X
Potatoes	X	X	X		X	X	X	X	X	X	X	X	X	X
Tomatoes			X			X	X		X	X			X	

Figure 14 Minerals	Calcium (Ca)	Chromium (Cr)	Copper (Cu)	Cobalt (Co)	Iodine (I)	Magnesium (Mg)	Manganese (Mn)	Molybdenum (Mo)	Phosphorus (P)	Potassium (K)	Selenium (Se)	Sodium Chloride (NaCl)	Zinc (Zn)	Iron (Fe)
Apples	X					X			X	X				
Apricots			X	X		X		X	X	X				
Bananas		X				X			X	X				
Berries – All	X			X		X	X		X	X				
Cantelope	X		X			X							X	X
Citrus Fruits	X	X	X			X		X	X	X				
Figs	X					X			X	X				
Grapes		X				X			X	X				
Kiwi	X			X		X			X	X				
Peaches						X			X	X				
Plums & Prunes						X			X	X				
Pineapple			X			X	X		X	X				
Beef/Pork/Poultry		X		X					X		X		X	X
Organ Meats			X	X		X		X	X		X		X	X
Fatty Fish						X			X	X	X	X	X	X
Non-Fatty Fish						X			X	X	X	X	X	
Shellfish	X		X	X		X	X		X	X	X	X	X	X
Beans & Legumes	X		X	X		X	X			X			X	X
Nuts & Seeds	X		X	X		X			X	X	X		X	X

"You can trace every sickness, every disease, and every ailment to a mineral deficiency."

Linus Pauling

Figure 15 Other Nutrients and Dietary Factors	Other Nutrients				Dietary Factors		
	Choline	Omega-3 Fatty Acids	Omega-6 Fatty Acids	Fiber	L-Carnitine	CoEnzyme Q10	Lipoic Acid
Milk	X				X		
Eggs	X		X				
Cheese					X		
Yogurt							
Tofu			X				
Whole Grains & Breads		X		X			
Oats		X		X			
Rice – White & Brown		X					
Quinoa	X			X	X		
Avocado	X			X	X	X	
Asparagus	X			X	X		
Broccoli	X			X		X	X
Brussels Sprouts	X	X		X			X
Cauliflower	X			X			
Dark Green Leafy Vegetables	X			X			X
Green Beans				X			
Lettuce							
Mushrooms				X			
Onions							
Orange Vegetables	X			X			
Peas	X			X			
Peppers – Red & Green				X			
Potatoes	X			X			
Tomatoes				X			X

Figure 15 Other Nutrients and Dietary Factors	Other Nutrients				Dietary Factors		
	Choline	Omega-3 Fatty Acids	Omega-6 Fatty Acids	Fiber	L-Carnitine	CoEnzyme Q10	Lipoic Acid
Apples	X			X			
Apricots				X			
Bananas	X			X			
Berries – All	X			X			
Citrus Fruits	X			X			
Grapes				X			
Kiwi	X			X			
Peaches				X			
Plums & Prunes				X			
Pineapple	X			X			
Beef/Pork/Poultry	X				X	X	X
Organ Meats	X						X
Fatty Fish	X	X				X	
Non-Fatty Fish	X	X				X	
Shellfish	X	X					
Beans & Legumes	X			X			
Nuts & Seeds	X	X	X	X		X	

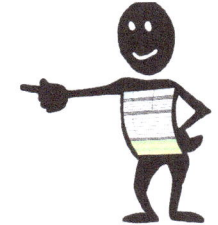

Little-known fact: Not all Omega-3 fats come from fish. We also consume plant Omega-3s from walnuts, flax seeds, some vegetable oils, algae, and seaweed.

Do you need supplements?

The typical Western diet is undoubtedly lacking in many micronutrients. If a large percentage of each day's calories come from sources with little to no nutritional value (sugar-sweetened drinks, for example), then it is almost impossible to consume enough nutritionally dense foods. Processed foods are nutritionally inferior to whole foods because processing typically removes or destroys many of the micronutrients. Many processed foods now are "fortified" or "enriched" with the addition of some critical micronutrients, e.g. vitamins and minerals added to breakfast cereal.

In addition, it is generally recognized that even whole foods contain less nutritional value now than historically, due to genetic manipulation (selective breeding, genetic modification and monoculture of both flora and fauna), production methods and soil depletion. It seems reasonable, maybe even likely, that many of us could be deficient in some micronutrients despite our best efforts to eat a healthy and well-balanced diet. For example, it is estimated that over 50% of infants and 35% of adults in the US have a vitamin D deficiency.[16] It makes you wonder about the other 26 essential vitamins and minerals.

The dietary supplement industry in the US is big business, with sales of about $50 billion in 2020. This translates to approximately $150 per year for each man, woman, and child in the country. They are successfully selling the idea that food alone is insufficient to meet one's nutritional needs. The ads for supplements in print, online and on TV are relentless. Every week it seems that there is a new "discovery" about a micronutrient that you have never heard of before but is (apparently) essential to maintaining one's health and vitality. If you are considering it, Appendix A provides some cautions and guidance about buying supplements.

To supplement or not, that is today's question.

The scientific community has successfully determined the negative health effects of critical shortages of key micronutrients, particularly vitamins and minerals. This has led to universally fortifying foods with some critical vitamins and minerals (e.g. iron, iodine), as well as routine supplement recommendations for certain populations (e.g. folic acid for pregnant women). However, studies have categorically failed to show clear improvement in clinical health outcomes of supplementing individual nutrients in otherwise healthy people. Is this because there really are no benefits?

Does the nutrient in question need to be consumed along with its thousands of companion compounds found naturally in food to reap the benefits? Or is it that the studies aren't long enough, or robust enough, to make the statistical determination? To sum it up, you can find studies showing (1) micronutrients are essential to health, (2) supplementation can treat a critical deficiency, and (3) supplementation generally does not produce a clinically significant difference in health outcomes. Hmmm... that's not very helpful, is it?

Most nutritional guidelines do not directly recommend supplements and, rather, advocate a healthy diet. Is that because there is a concern that people might deprioritize healthy foods if they think they can make up for it with a pill?

So, should you take supplements? Unfortunately, I can't give you an easy answer. (Please be sure to discuss your personal situation with your health care provider.) However, I do suggest that you embrace eating a wide range of whole, real foods with a new commitment, even if you do take supplements. When you add some grated carrots, red cabbage, seeds, and tomatoes to your salad, think of it as a sprinkling of magic nutritional fairy dust. Maybe the antioxidants in a handful of spinach are going to quench a critical free radical somewhere. Appreciate the nutritional complexity and contribution of an egg. When you eat real food, visualize your body saying, "Thanks, I needed that!"

Micronutrients – Key Points

Micronutrients: 13 Vitamins and 14 Minerals
 » **Essential fatty and amino acids**
 » **Antioxidants, flavonoids, etc.**
 » **Nature is the best source**

Should you supplement?
 » **Micronutrient deficiency is possible**
 » **Prioritize whole-food sources**

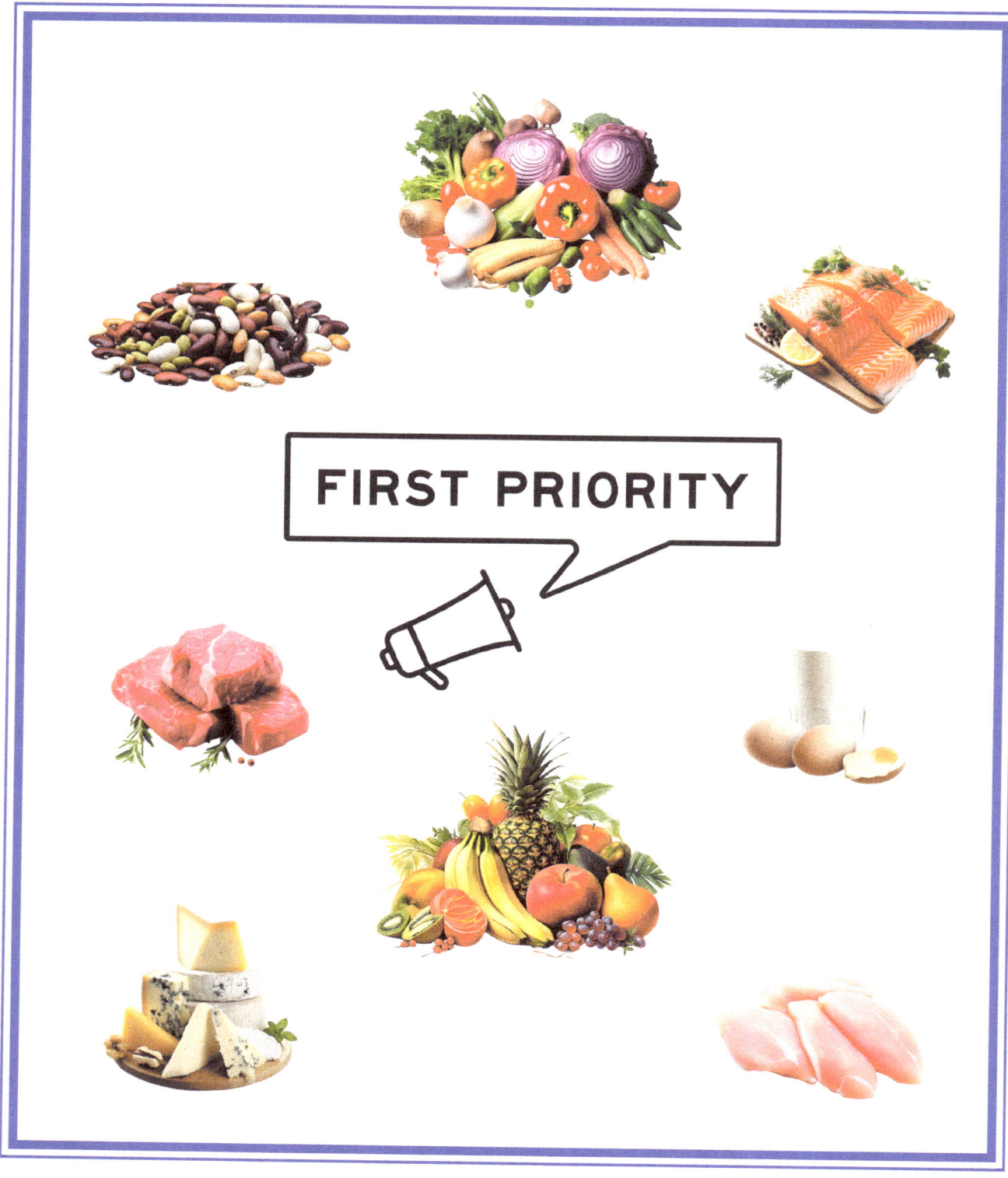

CHAPTER 8

DETERMINE PRIORITY FOOD TARGETS

We have all heard the story of the professor who filled a jar with marbles and asked the class if the jar was full. "Yes, of course!" the class answered. The professor then started pouring sand into the jar until it was full to the top. Again, he asked if the jar was full. The class affirmed that, yes, the jar was now full. Then the professor poured water into the jar until it was, again, full to the top. "Now," he said, "the jar is finally full and contains all three things: water, sand, and marbles!" The point being:

Priorities Matter

All three materials only fit if you put them into the jar in the right order. If you fill the jar with water and/or sand, there is no room for marbles. If marbles are the most important, they must go in first.

The marbles represent our Priority Foods, which are the nutritionally dense protein and produce we need to thrive. These are also the most challenging foods to get into our diet so we must make them the top priority in our Food Cycle planning process. To continue our analogy, sand represents the next nutritional priorities like healthy oils and whole grains. And lastly, the water represents the UPFs, including foods like refined flours, sugars, excess seed oils and other processed foods. These are the foods we want to minimize so we need to ensure there is little room left for them.

We know that we want to reduce the amount of UPFs in our diet, but the food industry won't make it easy. Engineered palatability, aggressive advertising, and relentless marketing make these highly profitable processed foods attractive and available everywhere you turn. This is a war being fought in every grocery, convenience store, fast-food outlet and cafeteria, with your family's food budget being the prize and your health simply collateral damage. To combat this, we need to set our priorities.

Setting Targets

We have defined our Priority Foods (PFs) as being vegetables, fruits, and high-quality proteins. We know these are important but how do we determine the right amount? We need to determine the amount of PFs we should eat to develop a plan. We need to do the math. Don't worry – we'll make it easy!

The Re-Engineered Food Cycle requires us to define our goals and put numbers to them. I am willing to bet that most people are not eating the amounts of these Priority Foods that they think they are. It may seem unfamiliar or even intimidating at first. Don't be put off because it is a new way of quantifying food (notice that we are quantifying food: not calories, carbs, protein, and fat). We will show you step-by-step how to figure out what quantity of food to buy to meet your goals and fit your lifestyle. After you have done it once, adjustments are easy.

There are innumerable nutritional guidelines available from governments, health institutions, universities, medical associations, as well as from a host of sources ranging from highly reputable to less-than-mainstream. However, most dietary recommendations have certain key elements in common:

- Whole vegetables and fruit = Good
- High-quality protein = Good
- Unprocessed, whole foods = Good.

We will use the Reference Man and Reference Woman defined in the DGA and discussed earlier as the basis for most of our example calculations. We will simplify the guidelines into weekly totals that are easy to use. We will also give you tables to make personal adjustments as necessary.

First, we will determine the target for vegetables and fruit, and then for protein.

Vegetables and Fruits – Targets

The DGA daily guidelines include weekly targets for five different categories of vegetables: dark-green, red/orange, legumes, starchy and other, and for fruits. Wait, what? Who can track six different targets just for veggies and fruit? We will simplify this dramatically by only using the total recommended quantity for the vegetable group and for the fruit group. We will further simplify this by correlating recommended calories by gender and age, assuming a moderate activity level (see Figures 16 and 17).

Using these charts, you can get an idea of how many cups of veggies and fruit each person in your family should be eating each day. Don't get too worried about exact measurements; these are just estimates to help us buy the right amount of our Priority Foods. We will be using cup equivalents, or c-eq, throughout the book to show required quantities of veggies and fruits.

Figure 16 – Daily Vegetable and Fruit Requirement – Male (DGA[7])

Male Age (Yr.)	Vegetables (c-eq)	Male Age (Yr.)	Fruit (c-eq)
2	1	2	1
3-5	1.5	3-10	1.5
6-8	2	11-15	2
9-11	2.5	16-25	2.5
12-14	3	26-76+	2
15-45	3.5		
46-76+	3		

Figure 17 – Daily Vegetable and Fruit Requirement – Female (DGA[7])

Female Age (Yr.)	Vegetables (c-eq)	Female Age (Yr.)	Fruit (c-eq)
2	1	2-3	1
3-6	1.5	4-11	1.5
7-9	2	12-50	2
10-18	2.5	51-76+	1.5
19-25	3		
26-76+	2.5		

While Figures 16 and 17 are convenient references we will perform our calculations of vegetable and fruit requirements based on calorie level as determined from Figure 7 or Appendix B. This accommodates higher and lower activity levels not shown in other tables.

To determine the weekly target for veggies and fruit, the daily numbers must now be multiplied by seven. For convenience, Figure 18 below shows the weekly vegetable and fruit requirements by calorie level. (Refer to Figure 9 on page 44 for estimated calorie levels by gender and age).

Figure 18 – Weekly Vegetable and Fruit Requirements (DGA[7])

Calorie Level	Vegetables (c-eq)	Fruit (c-eq)
1,000	7	7
1,200	10.5	7
1,400	10.5	10.5
1,600	14	10.5
1,800	17.5	10.5
2,000 (Ref Woman)	17.5	14
2,200	21	14
2,400	21	14
2,600 (Ref Man)	24.5	14
2,800	24.5	17.5
3,000	28	17.5
3,200	28	`7.5

Finally, to achieve a nutritional balance, aim to follow these guidelines:

- Include a wide variety of vegetables and fruits, including different types and colors.
- Aim for less than one-third of your vegetables to be "starchy". Starchy vegetables include corn, peas, beans, potatoes, and yucca.
- When eating fruit, choose mostly whole fruit and minimize fruit juices, which can be high in sugar and low in fiber.

Over time you will end up with a reasonable balance of fruits and vegetables. Using the table and our guidelines, we now have a goal for veggies and fruit each week.

What's wrong with "Servings"?

Nothing. Servings are an essential part of product labeling. Standard serving sizes have been developed for packaged products so that they may be easily compared against one another. However, while servings may provide a valuable standard framework for documenting nutritional data, they do not translate well to nutritional guidelines and actual quantities of food consumed.

Vegetable and Fruit recommendations are often expressed in "servings", especially in advertising and public service announcements. However, the DGA guidelines for fruits and vegetables are expressed in cup-equivalents (c-eq). One c-eq is often equal to two "servings". Confusing already! In addition, packages of prepared vegetables and fruit can define their own serving size – servings are not standard.

One c-eq is one measuring cup (1 C) for all uncooked fruits and veggies except for raw leafy greens, which take 2 cups to make 1 c-eq. We will only use cup-equivalents (c-eq) in this book as it directly translates to an actual measurement for most uncooked fruits and veggies.

Protein – Target

The DGA recommendations for protein are even more complicated. They include recommendations for the following:

- Meat, poultry, and eggs
- Seafood
- Nuts, seeds, and soy
- Dairy
- Beans and legumes

We have simplified this by adding up the total protein requirement associated with the recommended levels of all five high-protein foods. For example, the calculation for the weekly protein requirement for the Reference Woman is summarized in Figure 19 on the following page.

Figure 19 – Weekly Protein Requirements Example (DGA[7])

Protein Food Categories	Recommended Amounts	Approx. Protein (g/wk)
Dairy	3 c-eq/day	168
Meat, Poultry, and Eggs	26 oz-eq/week	156
Beans and Legumes	1.5 c-eq/week	21
Seafood	8 oz-eq/week	48
Nuts, Seeds, and Soy	5 oz-eq/week	192
	Weekly Total:	585

You will also be getting smaller amounts of protein from other foods such as grains and vegetables.

Individual protein requirements depend on variables such as age, gender, and level of activity, and are correlated with required calorie levels. Recommendations from different experts for optimal protein intake can range from 0.6 – 2.0 g/lb of lean body weight, and might be influenced by weight management goals, pregnancy, medical conditions, or physical activity level. We will be using the DGA recommendations for protein foods as the basis for our examples. However, I encourage you to come to your own conclusion about your target protein levels and speak with your health care provider regarding any specific concerns. All examples will simply use the total protein target by day and by week. This provides the flexibility to accommodate your dietary preferences and still manage total protein.

Figure 20 shows the total daily and weekly recommended protein from all sources of high-protein foods by calorie level based on the DGA recommended amounts of protein-rich foods. (Refer to Figure 9 in Chapter 6 for estimated calorie levels by gender and age.)

You can use this chart to estimate how much protein you should be eating every week. An adult at the 2,000 calories-per-day level should be getting about 585 g of protein-rich foods each week per the DGA. For our Reference Woman, this corresponds to 344 calories per day of protein (84g/day x 4.1 calories/g) or 17% of her 2,000 calories/day, well within the 10-35% Acceptable Macronutrient Distribution Range for protein.

Figure 20 – Daily & Weekly Protein Requirements (DGA[7])

Calorie Level	Daily Protein (g)	Weekly Protein (g)
1,000	38	269
1,200	50	361
1,400	63	441
1,600	80	560
1,800	81	567
2,000 (Ref Woman)	84	585
2,200	91	634
2,400	97	682
2,600 (Ref Man)	98	689
2,800	100	701
3,000	101	708
3,200	101	708

We will simplify our protein planning using the following guidelines:

- Choose minimally processed protein from a variety of sources.
- Aim for buying seafood at least 1-3 times per week (10% of your total).
- Aim for at least 5-10% of the total protein from legumes.

Throughout this book, there will be examples of simple calculations. There are charts of data and many example worksheets in the text. Blank worksheets are in Appendix B for your use. The blank worksheets are also available on the website www.ReEngineeringTheKitchen.com for book owners.

The Dietary Guidelines for Americans 2020-2025 is a good reference if you desire more information.

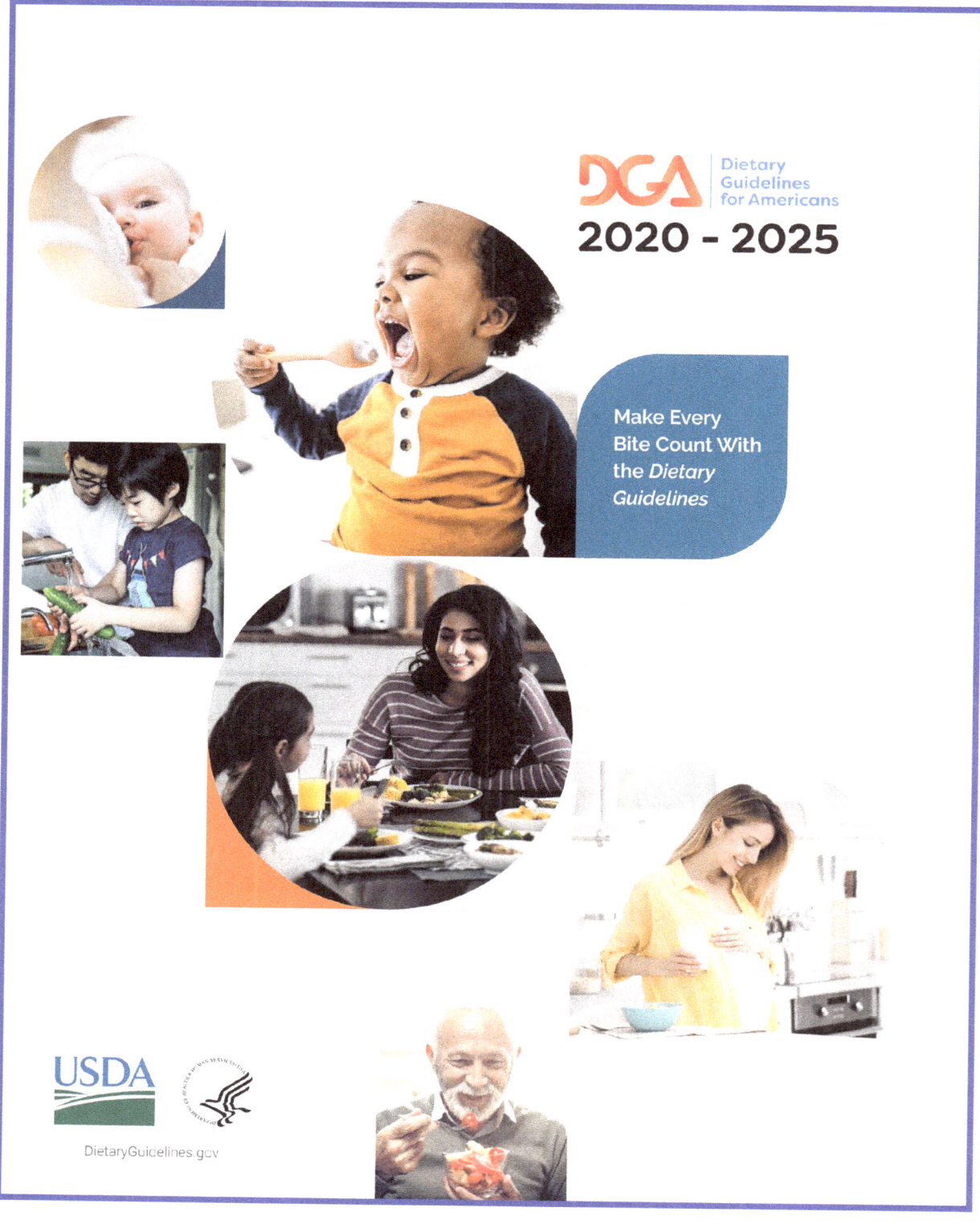

Priority Food Targets – Key Points

Priorities matter – vegetables, fruit, and protein first

Set weekly targets for vegetables, fruit, and protein

Calculate targets based on totals recommended in the Dietary Guidelines for Americans (DGA)

Weekly targets:

	Reference Woman 2,000 cal/day	Reference Man 2,600 cal/day
Vegetables	17.5 c-eq	24.5 c-eq
Fruits	14 c-eq	14 c-eq
Protein	585 g	689 g

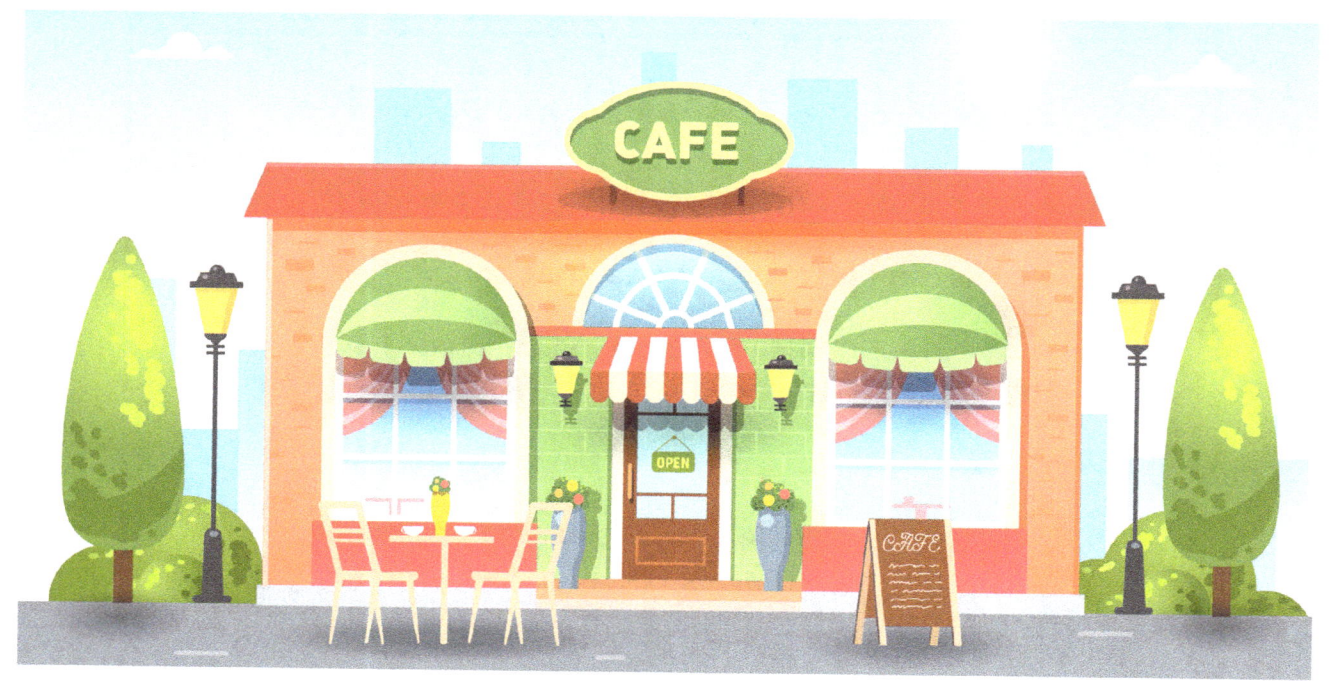

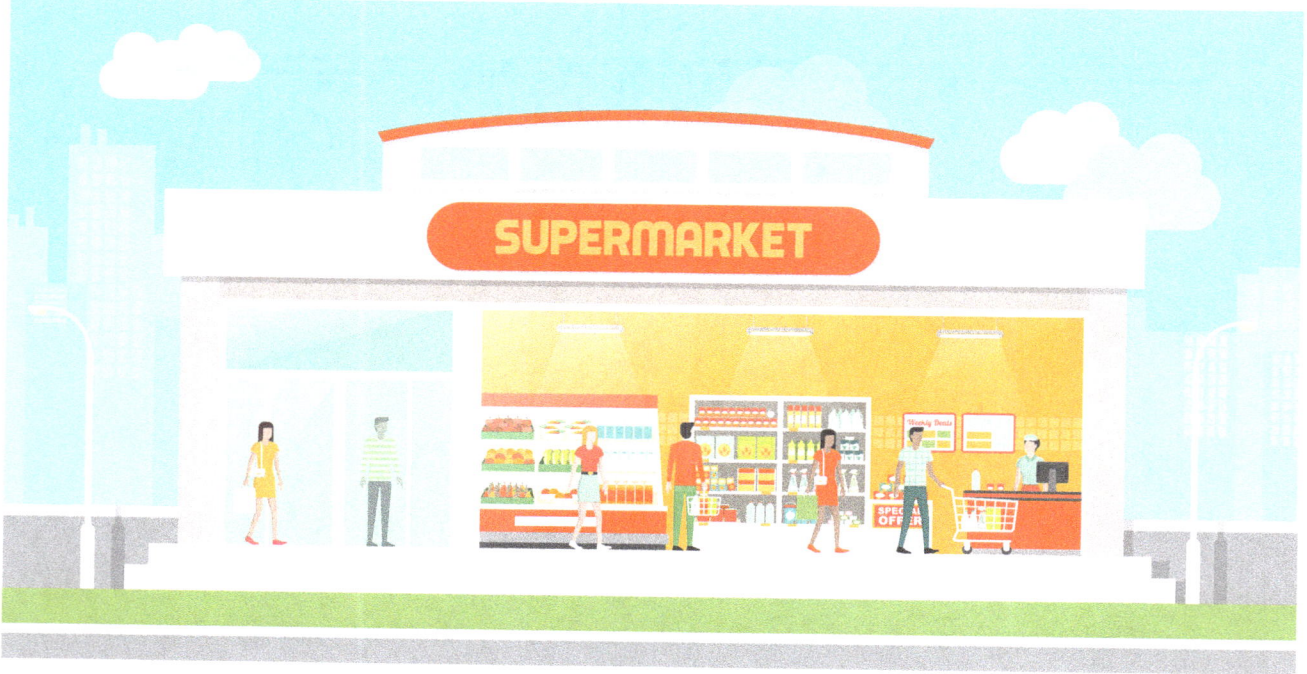

CHAPTER 9

DETERMINE PRIORITY FOOD SOURCES

Let's evaluate where your food typically comes from and how much of your required Priority Foods (PFs) come from each source. Our objective is to determine what PFs we need to buy at the market and what will come from other sources, such as fast food, cafeterias, and restaurants.

For most people, the answer is simple:

Almost all of your Priority Foods must come from the grocery store.

If you are diligent about ordering when eating out, the answer is:

Most of your Priority Foods still must come from the grocery store.

How can that be? The answer is that Priority Foods are generally not a significant component of cafeteria or convenience foods. When eating out, if veggies and fruit are available at all, they are served in small portions compared to your daily needs. Protein servings in institutions (schools, hospitals, etc.) are likely based on minimum recommended quantities, not optimum levels.[17] Protein servings in restaurants may be larger, but the nutrient value declines with the degree of processing, additives, flavorings, preservatives, tenderizers, breading, and frying. Vegetable-based protein, if available at all, is far more likely to be an ultra-processed industrial food product rather than something like a wholesome bean stew.

From the prior section, we know the total quantity of vegetables, fruit, and protein we need each week: Total Priority Foods (Total-PFs). The next question is "Where are those Priority Foods going to come from in a typical week?"

Evaluate your typical week

The easiest assumption is that 100% must be purchased at the grocery store or market and prepared at home (PF-Home). If you seldom eat out, this is probably close enough. However, if a significant amount of your food is coming from external sources, you will need to reduce the amount of PFs you purchase from the grocery store. The first step to estimate how much of your week's PFs are going to come from eating out: PF–Out. Then, the next step is to reduce the PFs you buy at the grocery store to prepare at home (PF–Home) accordingly.

PF-Home = Total PF – PF-Out

We can estimate the PF-Out by estimating how many meals you typically eat out, then the amount of PFs provided in each type of meal.

Figure 21 below shows the amount of money spent per U.S. household on food. You can see that on average almost 40% of food dollars are spent away from home.

Figure 21 – Average Annual U.S. Household Food Expenditures[18]

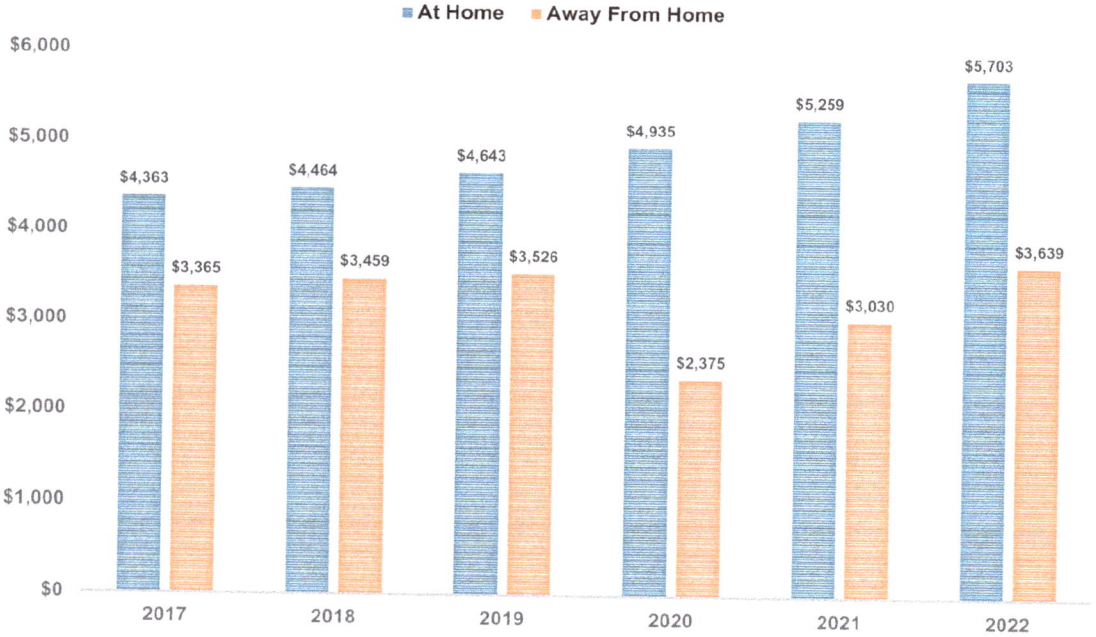

If you are like most people, your weekly eating pattern follows a fairly consistent routine. There are typical weeks where you follow a regular schedule, generally around work or school. Then there are non-typical weeks when you are maybe traveling or on vacation. We are first going to focus on a typical week, consider what meals will be eaten out and at home, and then we'll determine the average PFs associated with that meal distribution. The good news is that this is easier than it sounds. Once you have established your baseline, it generally won't change much week to week. As you get used to thinking of food this way, it will be easy to make adjustments when needed.

Plan for Vegetables and Fruit

Let's look at vegetables and fruits first. Figure 22 shows the Weekly Priority Food Targets for our Reference Man and Woman.

Figure 22 – Weekly PF Targets for Reference Man and Woman

	Reference Woman 2,000 cal/day	Reference Man 2,600 cal/day
Vegetables	17.5 c-eq	24.5 c-eq
Fruit	14 c-eq	14 c-eq
Protein	585 g	689 g

Figure 23 below is a list showing the estimated quantity of vegetables and fruit contained in commonly available menu items. These are estimates and your experience may vary. However, remember that using averages and estimates keep the process simple enough to be manageable.

Figure 23 – Typical Vegetable and Fruit Quantities in Common Menu Items

Menu Item	Vegetables, c-eq	Fruit, c-eq
Fruit Juice	0	½-1
Fruit Cup	0	¼-½
Veggie Omelette	¼-½	0
Entrée Salad	1-1 ½	0
Side Salad	½	0
Coleslaw	¼-½	0
Side Veggie	½	0
Stir Fry w/ Veggies	1-1 ½	0
Dish w/ Tomato Sauce or Incidental Veggies	¼-1	0
Vegetarian Entrée	2	0

As you can see, you would have to be very diligent in ordering to make a significant dent in the veggies and fruit you need to buy at the grocery store. You know what you normally eat. Do you order and eat enough fruit and veggies when you go out to make a difference? Do your kids actually eat any of the fruit or veggies they might get in a school cafeteria lunch? If the answer is no to these questions, and you are getting very few vegetables and fruits outside the home, then just assume that you need to buy 100% of your target Priority Foods at the grocery store.

Figure 24 – Fast Food vs. Home-Cooked Meal Comparison

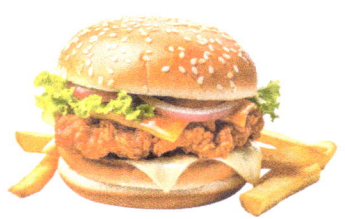 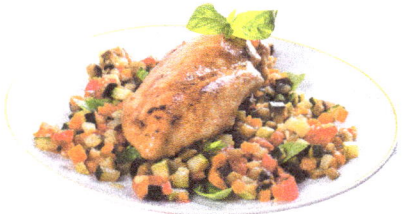

> » **Home-cooked meals typically have fewer carbohydrates, and less fat and sugar**
>
> » **Meals eaten out are often very high in processsed and ultra-processed foods**
>
> » **Approximatley 60% of meals eaten out of the home are fast food**
>
> » **Eating at home costs less than eating out**

If you are eating out often and getting significant veggies and fruits, you can adjust the Priority Foods you buy for home preparation to account for this. First, estimate the average amount of veggies and fruits that you typically get from eating out. For example, let's assume that you generally go out for two lunches and two dinners each week.

- Two Lunches: entrée salad (2 x 1 c-eq V)
- Two Dinners: a side salad (2 x ½ c-eq V) and a side vegetable (2 x ½ c-eq V).

Here is the calculation of your PF-Out for fruits and vegetables:

PF-Out Fruit = 0

PF-Out Veggies = 1 + 1 + ½ + ½ + ½ + ½ = 4 c-eq

If you are at the 2,000-calories-per-day level, your total vegetable requirement for the week is 17.5 c-eq. Reducing this by the 4 c-eq you are going to eat out means that you need to buy 13.5 c-eq at the grocery store.

Figure 25 – Weekly Veggie Requirement – Reference Female – 17.4 c-eq

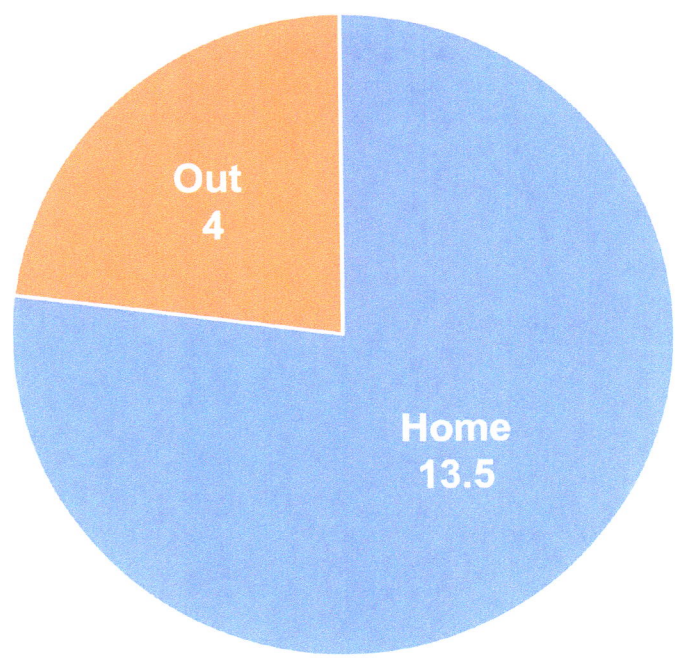

It is not easy to get a significant amount of vegetables and fruit from eating out. This has an important implication:

Home meals must be disproportionately loaded with veggies and fruit

If you are eating out a large percentage of the time, it becomes difficult to load enough veggies and fruit into the meals you do eat at home. However, don't let the default menu options dictate what you choose to eat. Many sit-down restaurants will substitute a veggie or salad for the French fries or potato if you ask (especially if you are willing to be flexible). In addition, consider ordering the extra vegetable side even if you must pay extra for it. As more people are asking for veggies, restaurants are making them more available.

Plan for Protein

Next, let's consider protein planning: what kind, how much, and where it is purchased. Again, we will look at the protein eaten out compared to at home. Below are estimated protein grams contained in commonly available restaurant items.

Figure 26 – Typical Protein Content of Common Menu Items

Menu Item	Typical Serving	Protein, g
Eggs	2	12
Milk	8 oz	8
Protein – Lunch Portion*	4 oz	28
Protein – Dinner Portion*	8 oz	56
Shellfish – Shrimp, Crab, Lobster	6 oz	36
Tofu	4 oz	12
Beans	1 C	14
Peanut Butter	2 Tbsp	7
Nuts and Seeds	1 oz	5
Cheese – Hard	1 oz	7
Cheese – Soft	½ C	14
Yogurt – Plain	6 oz	5
Yogurt – Greek	5 oz	15

* Beef, Poultry, Pork, Lamb, Fish

Let's assume that you generally go out for the same two lunches and two dinners each week. For lunch you get an entrée salad with grilled chicken and cheese (28 + 7 = 33 g). For dinner, you generally choose some sort of meat or fish (56 g).

- 2 Lunches: entrée salad chicken and cheese (2 x 33 g)
- 2 Dinners: meat or fish (2 x 56 g)

Here is the calculation of your weekly PF-Out for protein:

PF-Out = 33 + 33 + 56 + 56 = 178 g

If you are at the 2,000-calories-per-day level, your total weekly protein requirement is 585 g. Here is the calculation of your PF-Home for protein; how much protein you need to buy at the grocery store.

PF-Home = Total PF – PF-Out

PF-Home Protein = 585 grams –178 g

PF-Home Protein = 407 g

Figure 27 – Weekly Protein Food Requirement of 585 g

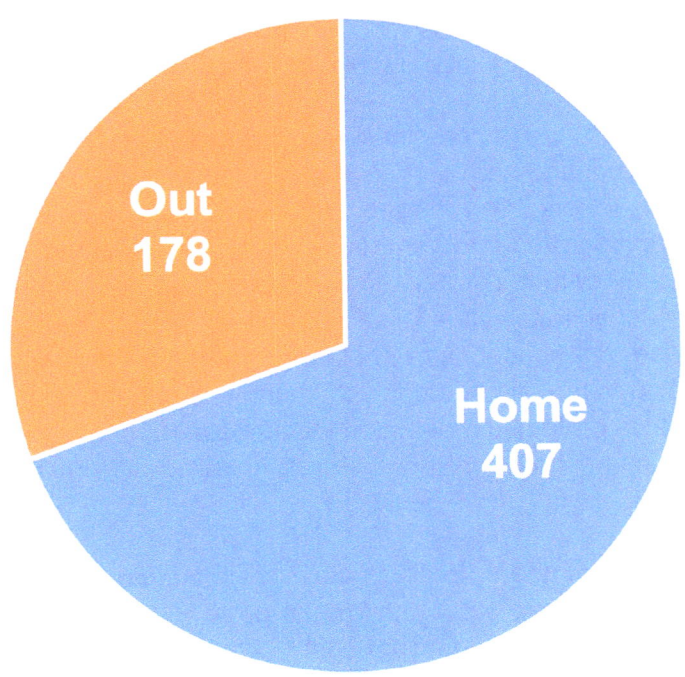

The Protein Minefield

Why is the topic of protein so...emotional? Long before the current popular drumbeat that consuming animal products is destroying the planet, protein has been a symbol of gluttony. Think of the image that comes to mind of a huge Henry VIII with a turkey leg in hand or the Hieronymus Bosch depiction of "gluttony" with several kinds of roast meats in his famous *Seven Deadly Sins* painting. Thinking back to your own childhood, which was judged more negatively: going for a second piece of chicken or another scoop of rice? Even as an adult, ordering an indulgent pasta alfredo or extra-large pizza is less likely to prompt a comment from your fellow diners than ordering a good-sized steak or two lobster tails. Meat, poultry, and fish have always been regarded as precious.

With this backdrop of emotion and moral judgement, the guidance from various health advisors can be less than helpful. From the *Dietary Reference Intakes: The Essential Guide to Nutrient Requirements* published by The Institute of Medicine, the Acceptable Macronutrient Distribution Range for protein is 10-35% of calories.[8] In practical terms, this means that 10% of calories is the minimum amount of protein to prevent most sedentary people from suffering a protein deficiency. It is absolutely not an optimum amount. Recommendations from various other nutrition organizations recommend protein levels two to three times this minimum, especially for physically active people.

In its food guidelines, the DGA recommends levels of protein-rich foods that would result in about 18-20% of calories coming from protein. But in another table in the DGA, the "Protein Goal" listed corresponds to just 10% of calories. Unfortunately, it is this minimum protein "goal" that has been incorporated into various health websites' protein calculators and is listed with titles such as "How much protein do you really need". Even more unfortunately, it is this minimum protein level that is often used in determining the standards for institutional food service. In the case of a school cafeteria lunch, if you start with one third of the daily minimum protein level and then assume each child drinks 8 ounces of milk, then the actual meal would need very little protein to meet the minimum standard: a budget win for the food manager. So, once again, most of your Priority Foods (in this case, protein) must come from home.

At the end of the day, humans need protein to grow, maintain muscle and thrive. The body can make energy out of anything, but it can't make protein out of carbs or fats. The real objective is to get the optimum amount and the best type of protein for you and your lifestyle.

From the estimates above, we now know how much vegetables, fruit, and protein we need to purchase at the grocery store for a typical week for this one person.

Figure 28 – PF-Home – Reference Woman at 2,000 cal/day

Priority Food Group	PF-Total	PF-Out	Weekly Req't – Home
Vegetables	17.5 c-eq	4 c-eq	13.5 c-eq
Fruit	15.5 c-eq	1.5 c-eq	14 c-eq
Protein	585 g	178 g	407 g

Priority Food Plan

We need to do this calculation for each person in the household and add it up to determine the food to be purchased at the grocery store. You can use the blank worksheets in Appendix B to do this calculation. Below is an example of a hypothetical family of four (two adults + two children). You will see the example calculations for this hypothetical family in Chapter 17.

Figure 29 – Example Weekly Priority Food Summary for Hypothetical Family

Person	Cal per Day	Vegetables (c-eq)			Fruit (c-eq)			Protein (g)		
		Weekly Req't	Eating Out	Home	Weekly Req't	Eating Out	Home	Weekly Req't	Eating Out	Home
Dad	2,600	24.5	2.5	22	14	0	14	689	175	514
Mom	2,000	17.5	2	15.5	14	0	14	585	70	515
Sister	2,400	21	0	21	14	2.5	11.5	682	110	572
Brother	1,800	17.5	0	17.5	10.5	2.5	8	567	110	457
Total:				76			47.5			2,058

The first time I did this calculation I thought: "Noooooo, this can't possibly be right. This means our example family needs to buy 123.5 c-eq (almost 8 gallons equivalent volume!) of veggies and fruit per week. Does anyone realize how much produce this is?" See figure 30 below.

And the sobering answer is a resounding "No". Our grocery stores would look very different if we all shopped this way.

Figure 30 - Eight Gallons of Veggies & Fruits

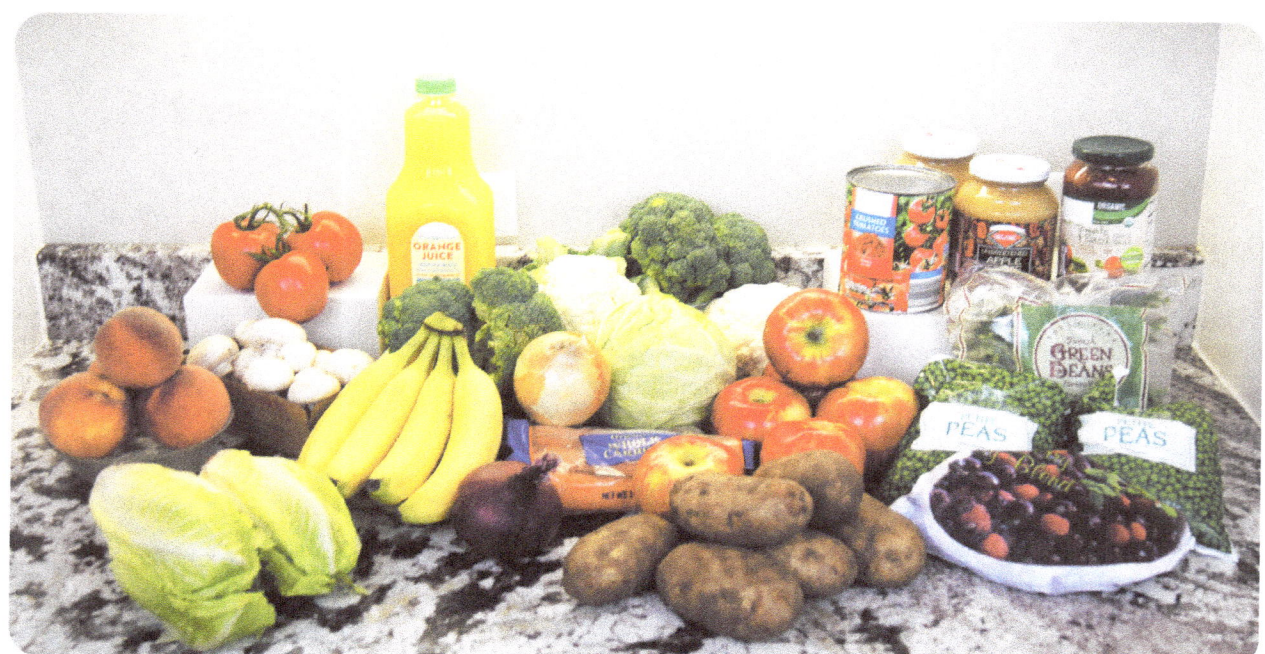

Since vegetables and fruits are so nutritious, we do all need to aim for this quantity, and in fact, these amounts should be considered minimums. Going a little over on fruit, veggies and high-quality protein is better than consuming more soda and cookies. It is important to remember that these are not precise calculations. Don't stress about the absolute accuracy of your inputs because the over/under averages out over time, and the simplifying assumptions are essential to make the process easy enough to be useful. The real value of this calculation is to develop a plan to reach your goals: if you truly want to eat better, here's how you do that.

In the next sections, we will take our weekly Priority Food requirements and turn that into a grocery shopping strategy.

Sources of Priority Foods – Key Points

Determine quantity of Priority Foods you get from eating out vs eating at home

Determine quantity of Priority Foods you need to buy at the grocery store for each person (PF–Home)
- » **Vegetables**
- » **Fruit**
- » **Protein**

Calculate total PF-Home for entire household

Note: Home meals generally need to be disproportionately loaded with vegetables and fruits.

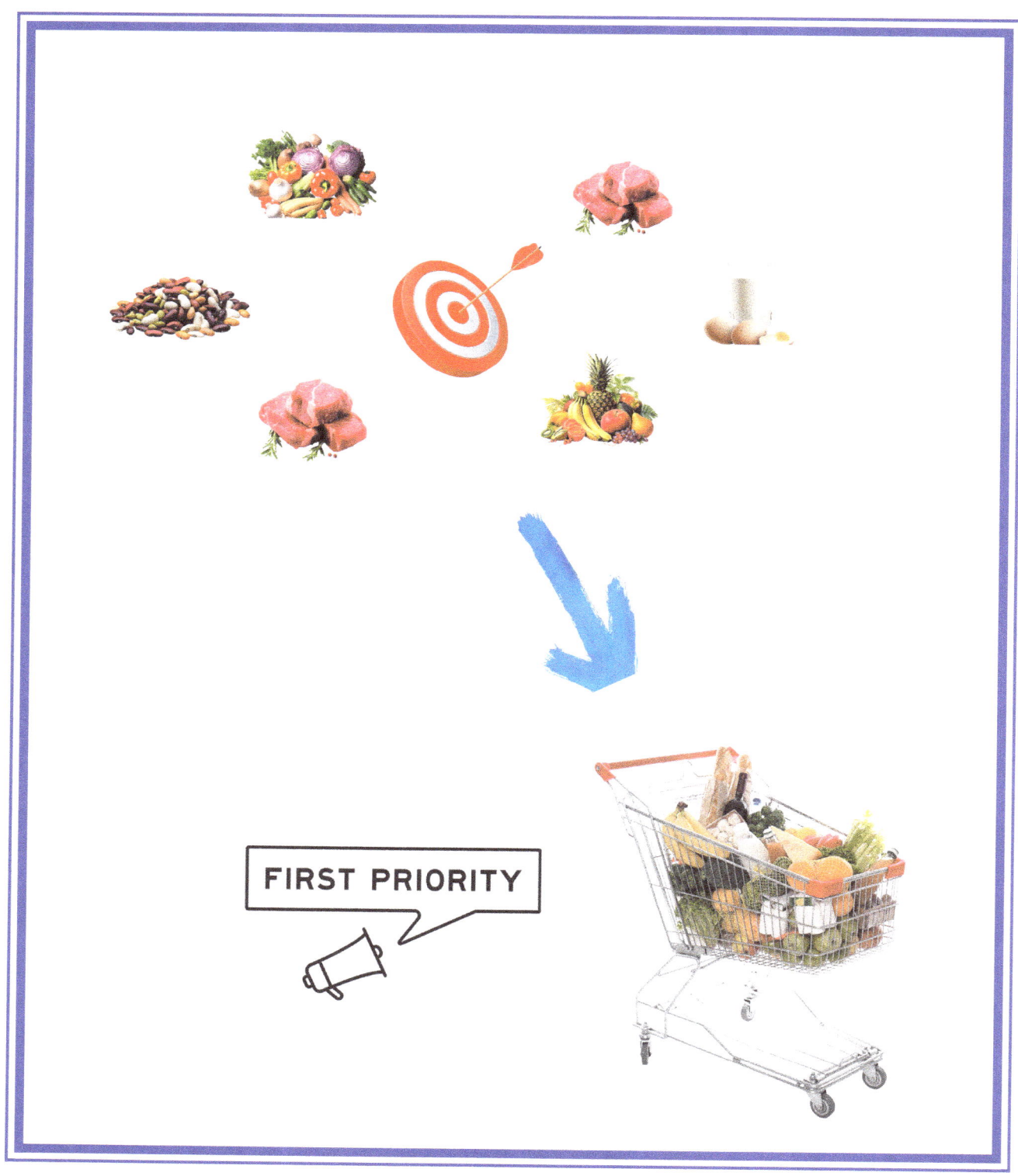

FIRST PRIORITY

CHAPTER 10

TRANSLATING PRIORITY FOOD TARGETS TO PURCHASES

So how do we know how much of what to buy? I've never seen a cantaloupe with the number of c-eq printed on it, or the grams of protein on a package of pork chops. I was surprised when I researched dietary references; I had assumed that there must be multiple references for anything to do with food. I found pictures showing what a serving of something looked like. I found lists of nutritional data on every conceivable food. On individually packaged foods, I found references to "servings" and cups and nutrition – so you could figure it out eventually. I found recipe equivalents. However, I could not find a single convenient reference listing what a typical grocery store item might yield in terms of nutritional requirements. If that exists somewhere, they do not make it easy to find.

The fact that this information is not readily available is revealing. It means that the translation of dietary recommendations to buying guidelines is not part of our normal conversation about food. It is not common knowledge that one package of fresh broccoli yields about 4 c-eq of prepared florets – which is less than two adults' daily veggies requirement. Did you know that an entire 15 oz can of beans (any type) provides less than one-third of an adult's daily protein requirement? We should all be able to look at food items in the store and have a good idea of how that relates to our dietary objectives.

So, I set out to create references showing how common grocery store items relate to nutritional requirements. The Fruit and Vegetable Buying Guide below provides the typically prepared yield per unit or package for many commonly available fruits and vegetables. To create this reference, I bought, prepared, and measured the fresh items. I did this for several packages and took the average. For items where size varies dramatically, I listed the weight of the item I purchased.

As you might imagine, the information for fresh food is not exact. It is influenced by size, packaging, and how I happen to prepare the food item. I may shred my cabbage finer than you do or discard more or less of the broccoli stems. However, it is tremendously useful to estimate the quantities you need to purchase to meet your objectives. I am certain you will find it as surprising as I have. For packaged foods (canned and frozen), I used the package information. For beans, I have used the average equivalents published on the Bean Institute's website (www.beaninstitute.com)[19].

Figure 31a – Fresh Vegetable and Fruit Buying Guide			
Produce as Purchased	**Type**	**Actual Weight**	**Approx. c-eq**
Acorn Squash, 1 gourd	Veggie-Orange/Red	1 lb 5 oz	1 ½
Apple	Fruit	8 oz	1 ½
Asparagus	Veggie-Other	1 lb	4
Avocado, 1 Haas	Veggie-Other	6 oz	1
Baby Bok Choy	Veggie-Dark Green	1 lb	4
Banana. 1 medium, 9 inch	Fruit	8 oz	1
Beets	Veggie-Other	1 lb 2 oz	4
Blackberries/Raspberries, ½ pint	Fruit	6 oz	1
Blueberries, 1 pint	Fruit	10 oz	2
Broccoli, 2 stalk package	Veggie-Dark Green	1 lb 10 oz	4
Brussels Sprouts	Veggie-Dark Green	1 ib 10 oz	5
Butternut Squash, 1 gourd	Veggie-Orange/Red	2 lb 10 oz	6
Cabbage, red/green, 1 head	Veggie-Other	3 lb 3 oz	8
Canteloupe, 1	Fruit	5 lb	8
Carrots, 6-8	Veggie-Orange/Red	1 lb	2
Cauliflower, 1 head	Veggie-Other	2 lb 8 oz	6
Collard Greens, 1 bunch	Veggie-Dark Green	12 oz	4 (8 actual)
Corn, small ear, 9 inch	Veggie- Starchy	-	⅔
Cucumber, mini	Veggie-Other	2 ¼ oz	½
Cucumber, English	Veggie-Other	14 oz	2
Grapes, 1 bunch	Fruit	13 oz	2
Green Beans	Veggie-Other	1 ib 4 oz	4

Figure 31a – Fresh Vegetable and Fruit Buying Guide			
Produce as Purchased	Type	Actual Weight	Approx. c-eq
Green Onions	Veggie-Other	5 ½ oz	1 ½
Green Peas	Veggie-Starchy	10 oz	2
Kale, 1 bunch	Veggie-Dark Green	9 oz	4 (8 actual)
Leafy Salad Greens	Veggie-Dark Green	3 oz	1 (2 actual)
Lettuce, Iceburg, 1 head	Veggie-Other	1 lb 12 oz	6 (12 actual)
Mushrooms	Veggie-Other	8 oz	2-3
Onion, 1 large, diced	Veggie-Other	10 oz	2
Orange, Naval, medium	Fruit	9 oz	¾
Oranges, 27 Mandarin bag	Fruit	3 lb	6 ¾
Peach	Fruit	7 ½ oz	1 ⅓
Peppers, 1 medium	Veggie-Orange/Red	7 oz	1 ¼
Pineapple	Fruit	3 lb 3 oz	4
Potato, 1 large, baker	Veggie-Starchy	12 oz	1 ¾
Potatoes	Veggie-Starchy	3 lb	6 ½
Romaine, 1 head	Veggie-Dark Green	7 oz	3.5 (7 actual)
Spaghetti Squash, 1 small	Veggie-Orange/Red	1 lb 10 oz	2 ½
Spinach	Veggie-Dark Green	8 oz	3 ¾
Strawberries, sliced	Fruit	16 oz	3 ½
Sweet Potato, 1 medium	Veggie-Orange/Red	13 oz	2 ¼
Tomatoes	Veggie-Orange/Red	10 oz	2
Zuchini, 1 small, 6 inch	Veggie-Other	4 oz	¾

Figure 31b – Dry, Canned and Frozen Vegetable and Fruit Buying Guide			
Vegetable	**Type**	**Package Weight**	**Approx. c-eq**
Canned			
Beans – all	Legumes	15 oz	1 ¾
Bean Sprouts	Veggie-Other	15 oz	2 ½
Beets, sliced	Veggie-Other	15 oz	1 ¾
Corn	Veggie-Starchy	15 oz	1 ¾
Green Beans	Veggie-Other	15 oz	1 ¾
Lima Beans, mature	Legumes	15 oz	1 ¾
Pumpkin	Veggie-Orange/Red	15 oz	1 ¾
Sweet Potatoes	Veggie-Orange/Red	15 oz	1 ¾
Tomatoes, diced	Veggie-Orange/Red	15 oz	1 ¾
Tomato Juice	Veggie-Orange/Red	46 oz	6
Tomato Paste	Veggie-Orange/Red	12 oz	1 ½
Tomato Sauce	Veggie-Orange/Red	15 oz	2
Dry			
Dry Beans – all*	Legumes	1 lb	6
Lima Beans, mature	Legumes	1 lb	3
Frozen			
Asparagus Spears	Veggie-Other	8 oz	2 ¼
Baby Lima Beans	Legumes	12 oz	2
Broccoli	Veggie-Dark Green	12 oz	4
Carrots, sliced	Veggie-Orange/Red	12 oz	3
Corn	Veggie-Starchy	12 oz	2 ½
Edamame	Legumes	10 oz	3
Green Beans	Veggie-Other	12 oz	2 ½
Green Peas	Veggie-Starchy	12 oz	2

* Bean information is from https://beaninstitute.com/bean-coucnting-the-bean-yield-chart/

Figure 31b – Dry, Canned and Frozen Vegetable and Fruit Buying Guide

Vegetable	Type	Package Weight	c-eq
Frozen			
Kale	Veggie-Dark Green	12 oz	4
Onions, chopped	Veggie-Other	10 oz	2 ½
Potatoes, shredded	Veggie-Starchy	26 oz	9
Sugar Snap Peas	Veggie-Other	10 oz	2 ¼
Spinach	Veggie-Dark Green	12 oz	4
Fruit*	**Type**	**Package Weight**	**c-eq**
Canned/Jarred			
Applesauce	Fruit	23 oz	5
Apple Juice**	Fruit	24 oz	16
Fruit Cups – 4 pack	Fruit	16 oz	4
Orange Juice**	Fruit	52 oz	13
Peaches	Fruit	15 oz	3 ½
Pineapple	Fruit	15 oz	4 ½
Frozen			
Berry Blend	Fruit	16 oz	3
Blueberries	Fruit	16 oz	3
Peaches	Fruit	16 oz	3
Pineapple, chunks	Fruit	16 oz	3
Strawberries, whole	Fruit	16 oz	3

* Choose unsweetened
** Limit fruit juice

The Protein Buying Guide

The Protein Buying Guide below shows the approximate grams of protein for commonly available packages of high-protein foods. For protein foods, the estimate of protein grams for a given package is based on weight and an average protein content. Obviously, this is not exact; there are minor variations in protein content between specific items within a group. However, it is intended to be a simple, handy reference to use in shopping. The estimate of meat protein is based on raw, lean content only. If the meat has appreciable fat content, reduce the protein content accordingly. For example, the protein content for a 1-lb package of 80/20 hamburger would be approximately 80 g. These guides will allow us to easily translate our target PFs' protein grams into specific items for purchase.

Figure 32 – Protein Buying Guide		
High-Protein Food	**Package**	**Approx. Protein (g)**
Cheese – hard	16 oz	112
Cheese – soft	16 oz	64
Cottage and Ricotta Cheese	16 oz	56
Eggs, large	12	74
Greek Yogurt	32 oz	85
Milk	½ gallon	64
Tofu – firm	16 oz	37
Yogurt	16 oz	20
Canned Tuna	5 oz	31
Meat, Fish, Poultry – Lean	16 oz	100
Dry Beans – all	16 oz	102
Canned Beans – all	15.5 oz	24
Almonds	16 oz	96
Cashews, Walnuts, Hazelnuts	16 oz	69
High-Protein Pasta	14.5 oz	80
Lentils	16 oz	100
Peanuts and Peanut Butter	16 oz	110
Pecans	16 oz	42
Pumpkin seeds	16 oz	136
Quinoa	16 oz	96
Wild rice	16 oz	60

Example: Translating PF-Home Requirements to grocery items

We have determined the amount of PFs to be acquired at the grocery store. We will continue to use the example of a person at the 2000-calories-per-day level. To recap from Chapter 9, the PF-Home requirements for a typical week are:

- Vegetables: 13.5 c-eq
- Fruit: 14 c-eq
- Protein: 407 g

Using the Fruit and Vegetable Buying Guide and the Protein Buying Guide, we can determine that the following items would fulfill these gross nutritional requirements:

Figure 33 – Grocery Items to Fulfill Nutritional Requirements

Item Requirement	Veggies 14 c-eq	Fruit 13.5 c-eq	Protein 407 g
Broccoli, Fresh, package	4		
Carrots, 1 lb	2		
Green Beans, fresh, 1 lb	4		
Mushrooms, 8 oz	2		
Lettuce, Romaine, 1 head	2		
Cantaloupe, 1		6	
Bananas, 2		2	
Strawberries, 1 lb		4	
Juice, two 8 oz singles		2	
Lean Ground Turkey, 1 lb			100
Fresh Fish w/ Skin, 1 lb			100
Cottage Cheese, 16 oz			56
Cheese, 12 oz			84
Eggs, 12			72
Total:	**14**	**14**	**412**

This list is a great starting point for meeting your weekly PF-Home targets. In the next section, we will fine-tune this shopping plan to best suit your lifestyle.

Translate Priority Food Targets to Purchases – Key Points

Nutritional goals $\longrightarrow$ Grocery list

Priority Foods reference for grocery items
- » **Fresh produce – vegetables and fruit**
- » **Packaged produce – vegetable and fruit**
- » **Protein**

Develop shopping plan

Is it a legume, a bean, or a pulse?

The three terms are often used interchangeably. Technically, the term **Legume** refers to the plant family Fabaceae that contains almost 16,000 species and includes all bean, pea, and pulse cultivars. A common characteristic is a seed-filled pod. Legumes are a great source of protein, fiber, complex carbohydrates, micronutrients, and have a low glycemic index. While not all legumes are edible, those that are tend to be the lowest cost source of protein as well. What's not to love?

Bean: A legume that has edible seed pods or individual seeds. Examples are fresh green beans, black beans, pinto beans, and kidney beans.

Pulse: The definition of a pulse is very specific. It is the seed of a legume pod that was grown and harvested as food – and then is dried. Examples are any dried beans, garbanzo beans, lentils, and dry peas.

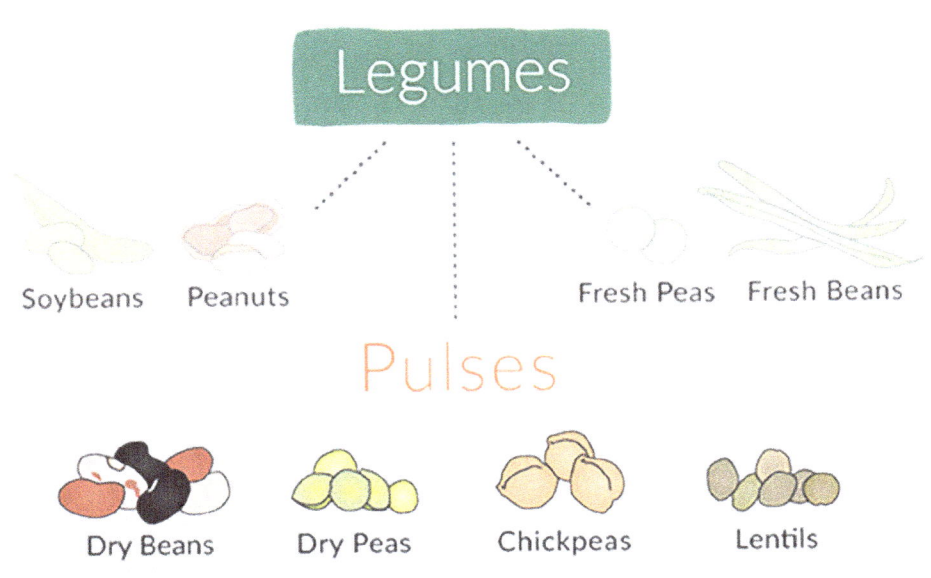

Source: USA Pulses[20]

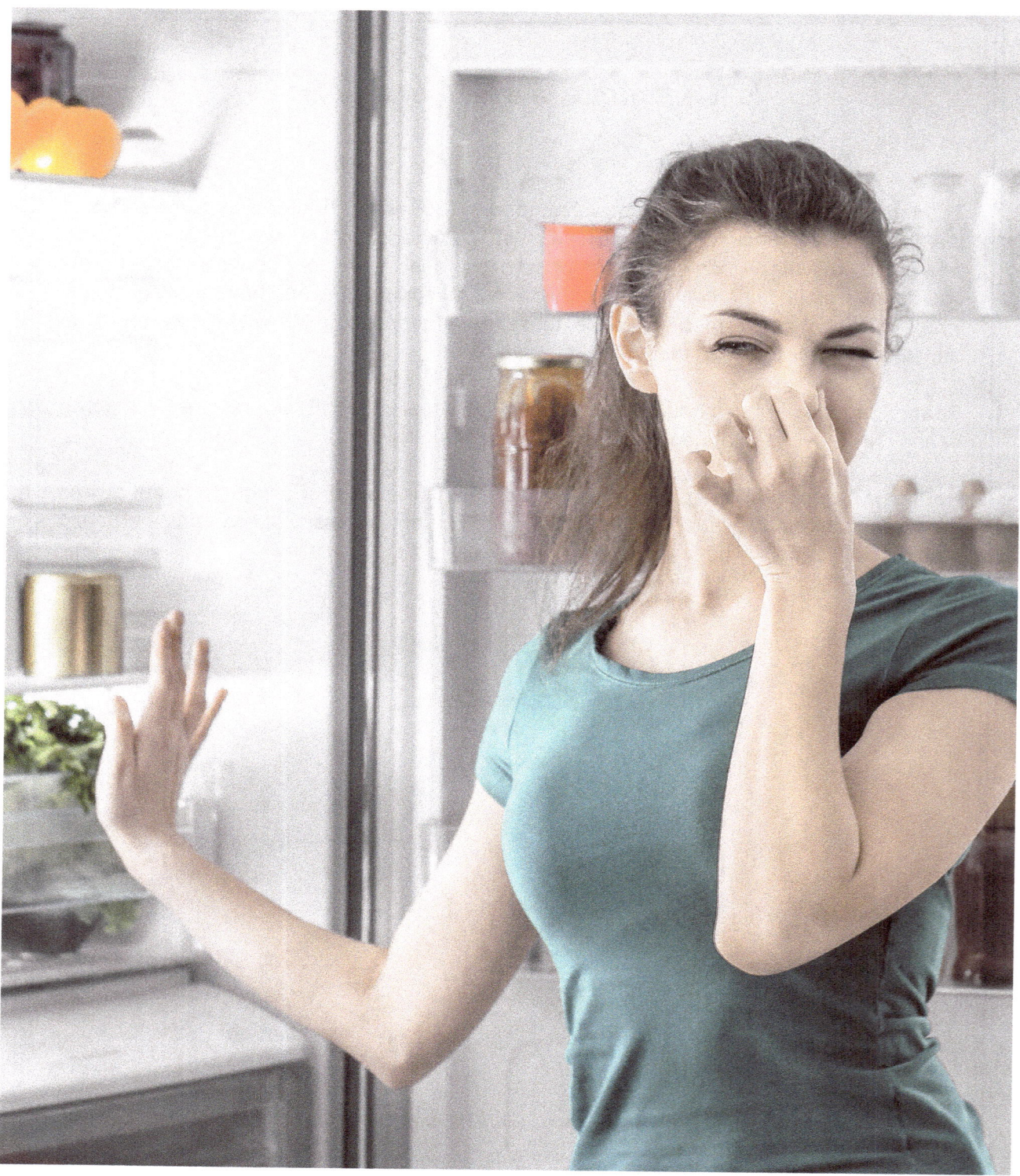

CHAPTER 11

FOOD LONGEVITY RATIOS

In developing our food shopping plan, we also need to consider how long the food will last compared to our schedule and the likelihood of preparing it. On one hand, we want to use everything that we buy before it goes bad. On the other hand, we want to have as much fresh unprocessed food as possible.

Food Longevity vs Shelf Life

Shelf life is a common, widely used term, so why are we introducing the concept of "food longevity"? Shelf life is how long a product, food in our case, will last before it becomes unfit for use. Long shelf life is a characteristic of processed foods that are engineered by removing readily degradable components, by processing them with heat, pressure, radiation and/or chemicals and by adding preservatives. Extending shelf life is a major reason why ultra-processed foods were created in the first place.

We will use the term "food longevity" to describe the characteristics of unprocessed and minimally processed foods. Food longevity is a native characteristic of food, influenced by storage methods, but not engineered. Food longevity describes how long a food will last before it becomes unfit for use, expressed as a range of time. The three food longevity category time ranges are:

- Fast-Fade (3 days) – foods like fragile produce (e.g. salad greens or very ripe berries), fresh fish, sliced deli meat, prepared deli salads, ground meats and foods at their buy-by dates.
- Fresh-Medium (3 days to 2 weeks) – includes sturdy produce like broccoli, peas, squash and cauliflower, packaged fresh meats, milk, root vegetables, cured packaged meats, yogurt, soft cheese.
- Long (2 weeks to 12 months) – includes foods such as dry beans, grains, spices, and dried fruits, canned and frozen vegetables, fruits and meats, hard cheese.

Since every food fits into one of these categories, it is simple to use as a food freshness management tool. Food Longevity is the better concept to use than shelf life when buying our Priority Foods. Examples of which foods fit where are shown on the following page.

Figure 34 – Food Longevity Food Category Examples

Fast-Fade (up to 3 days)

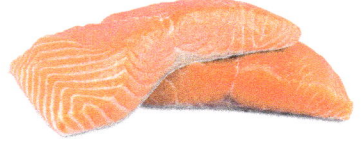 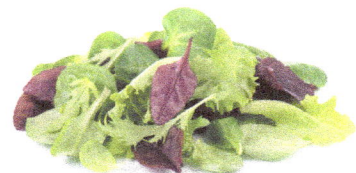 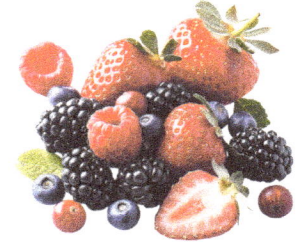

Fresh-Medium (3 days to 2 weeks)

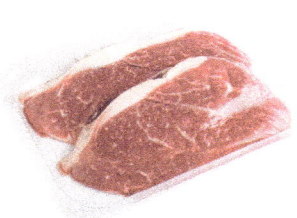 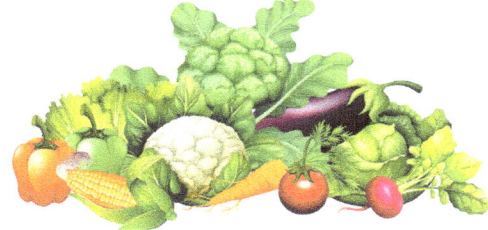 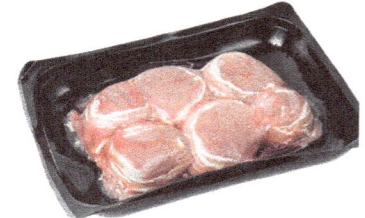

Long (2 weeks to 12 months)

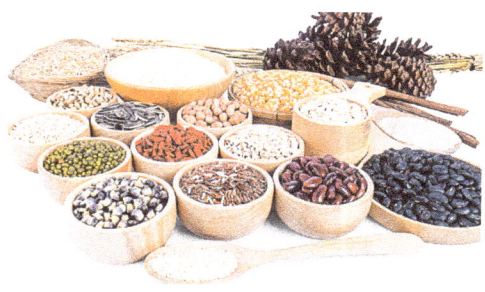 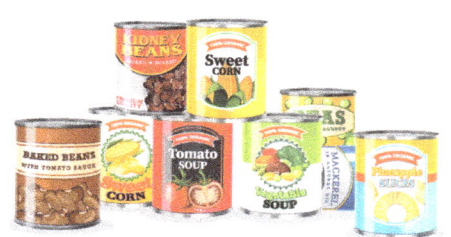 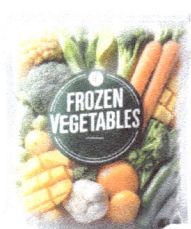

Using Food Longevity in our daily lives

It sounds simple, right? Be aware of the foods you buy and how long they last, in order to avoid food waste and maximize your nutrition. However, rather than trying to manage every food item, we will make it easier by simply buying the right proportion of food from each food longevity category; that is, the best food longevity ratio for you. Let's look at three different lifestyle categories and how these might affect the recommended food longevity ratios.

Figure 35 – Lifestyle 1 – Cook Daily

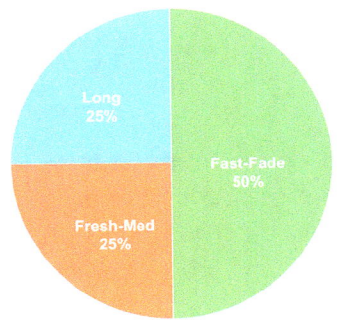

In this case, there is very good knowledge and control of the schedule. This household might choose to go out occasionally, but life seldom throws them a food schedule curve ball that they can't handle. They are committed to cooking every day and have allocated the time to do so. This may be by choice, or it may be influenced by a family member's dietary restriction. It makes sense, then, that they can buy a greater percentage of fresh food without the risk of wasting it. The recommended longevity ratio, in this case, would include up to 50% Fast-Fade, 25% Fresh-Medium, and 25% Long. While this lifestyle will tolerate up to 50% in the Fast-Fade category, there is no harm in shifting some of that to the Fresh-Medium category depending on availability and personal choice.

Figure 36 – Lifestyle 2 – Flexible

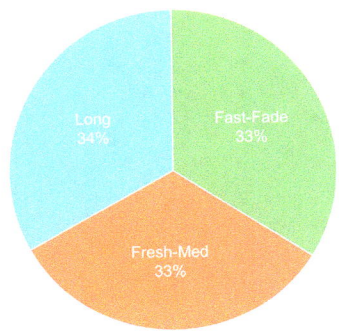

In this case, the household has a busy, but fairly stable schedule in terms of work, school, and outside commitments. However, flexibility is required as last-minute events can influence meal plans so this family might need a little extra time or resources to compensate. A late arrival home can preclude cooking the meal planned for that day. Any unexpected event can upset the apple cart when you have very limited time between arriving home and getting everybody in bed. This household needs to buy food so that meals can be shifted a day or two, or quantities can be increased or decreased as necessary. The recommended longevity ratio, in this case, would include 33% Fast-Fade, 33% Fresh-Medium, and 34% Long. While this lifestyle will tolerate up to 33% in the Fast-Fade category, you can shift some of that to the Fresh-Medium, or even Long, category.

Figure 37 – Lifestyle 3 – Unpredictable

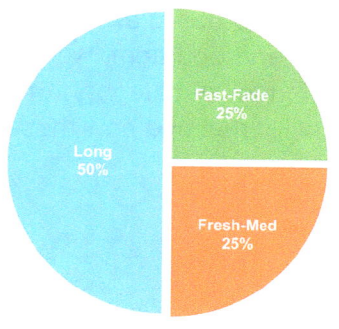

In this case, the household has a schedule that is both busy and highly unpredictable. This might include someone who travels extensively or has obligations that involve irregular hours. It could be a household where everyone is simply on their own schedule, and it is difficult to coordinate. This household has the greatest need for flexibility. (They also probably have the greatest need for some wholesome food in their lives!) The recommended longevity ratio, in this case, would include up to 25% Fast-Fade, 25% Fresh-Medium, and 50% Long. While we have a guideline of up to 25% for the Fast-Fade category, they should probably only buy as much as they can prepare in the 2-3 days following shopping.

Lifestyle 4 – Yours

How do you determine the best food longevity ratio for you? Pick the ratio above that you think is closest to your lifestyle and try it. You may find that it fits perfectly. You may decide that you need more flexibility or want more fresh food. You can always adjust as you go forward. The real value of these guidelines is that they provide an easy tool to guide food purchases based on the probability of preparing it. This will reduce waste and, consequently, reduce costs.

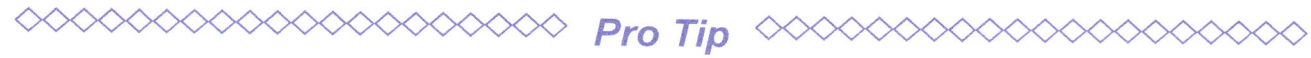

Pro Tip

First In First Out (FIFO) Inventory Control Process

Foods in the "Long" longevity category are often staples that are purchased in bulk for economy and convenience. However, they don't last forever, and dates still have to be managed. Anything in a package, can or bottle has a best-by date that is probably readable upon careful examination under a bright light. Do yourself a favor and buy a sheet of blank stickers to write dates on. Put a date sticker where it is clearly visible on each item before you put it away. This makes it easy, almost automatic, to organize foods by date and employ a FIFO process.

Food Longevity Ratios – Key Points

Three categories:
» **Fast-Fade: 3 days**
» **Fresh-Medium: 3 days to 2 weeks**
» **Long: 2 weeks to 12 months**

Lifestyle 1 – Cook Daily
» **Target ratios: 50% : 25% : 25%**

Lifestyle 2 – Flexible
» **Target ratios: 33% : 33% : 34%**

Lifestyle 3 – Unpredictable
» **Target ratios: 25% : 25% : 50%**

Lifestyle 4 – Yours – Pick the ratios that fit your life
» **Target ratios:**

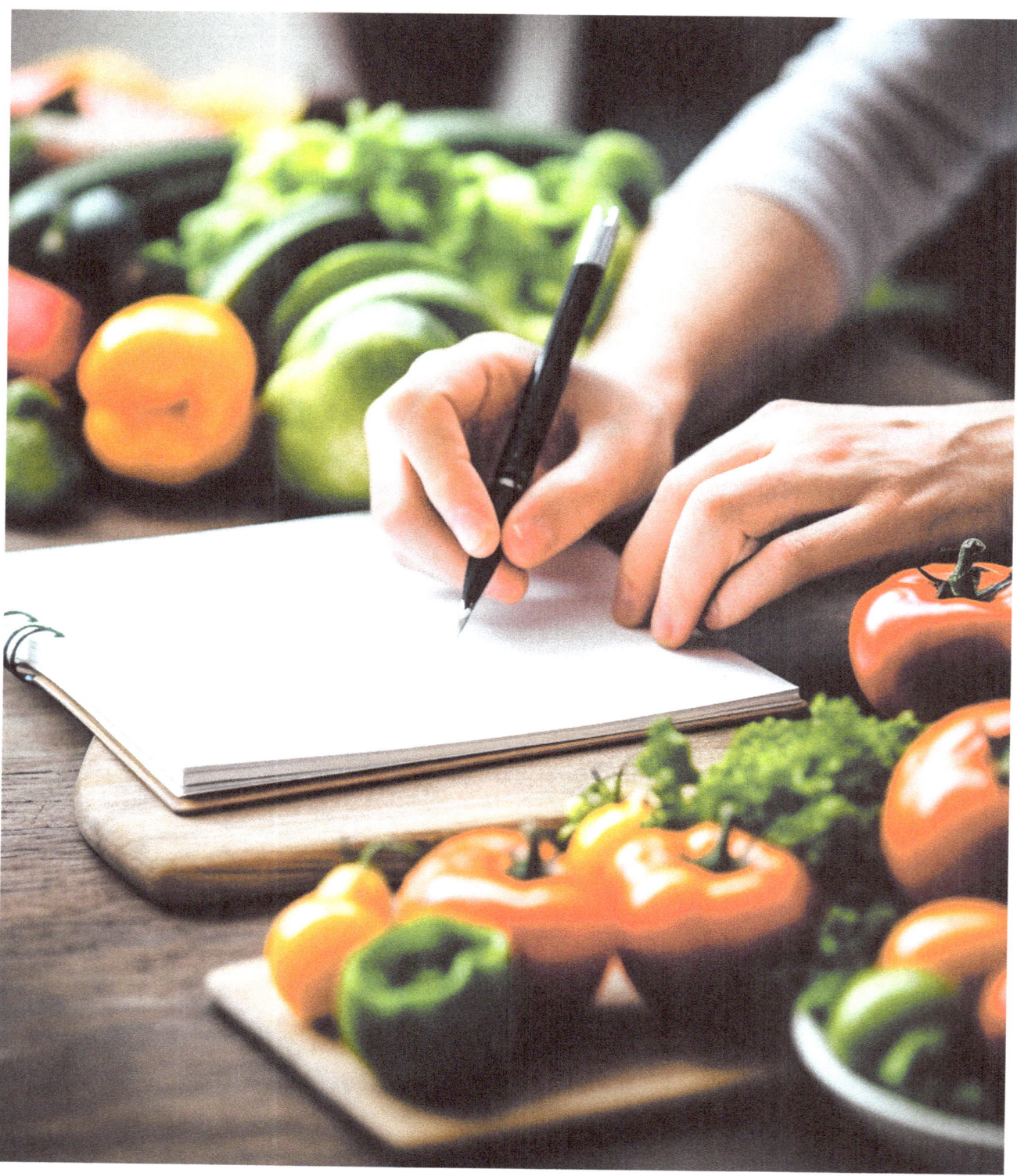

CHAPTER 12

BASELINE PRIORITY FOOD PLAN

We now have the tools to create a Baseline Priority Food Plan. This is the guide that you will take to the grocery store with you each week to ensure you purchase the right amount of Priority Foods. It might sound like a grocery list, but since it includes food groups rather than items, it is more useful and flexible. The idea of this plan is to guide you in buying foods that meet these criteria:

> » Meet your Priority Food targets.
> » Buy the right amounts of the right foods.
> » Buy foods that fit your best longevity ratio to minimize waste.

Example – Baseline Priority Food Plan

Our example is the woman from Chapter 8 who has a regular schedule but does occasionally work late or go out with friends after work. She generally eats out for two lunches and for two dinners per week. "Flexible" best describes this lifestyle, with a target food-longevity ratio of: 33%: 33%: 34%.

Figure 38 – Baseline Priority Food Guide – Longevity Distribution

Priority Foods	Total	Total Grocery	Longevity Distribution		
			Fast-Fade 33%	Fresh-Med 33%	Long 34%
Veggies, c-eq	17.5	14	4.6	4.6	4.7
Fruit, c-eq	14	13.5	4.5	4.5	4.5
Protein, g	585	407	134.3	134.3	138.4

Using the Baseline Priority Food Guide

The Baseline Priority Food Guide gives us target amounts of foods by both food type and food longevity. The food list we developed in Chapter 10 only considered Priority Food type. If we look at the initial distribution of food longevity for our PFs, we see that it needs to be refined to better match the target food longevity ratio.

Figure 39 – Longevity Distribution of Initial Food List

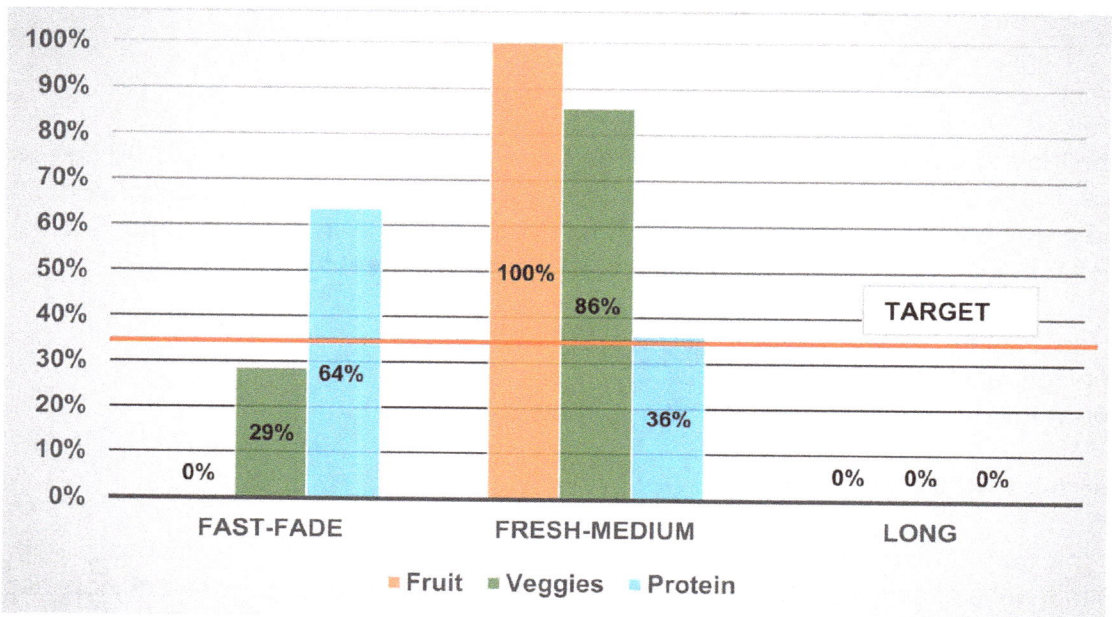

The key problem with this initial combination of foods is that everything falls into the two shorter food longevity categories, so we risk food wastage. For our example woman, we need to fine-tune our Baseline Priority Food Plan, and buy less of the Fast-Fade and Fresh-Medium foods or have a plan to extend their longevity by either cooking them promptly and/or freezing them. For example, immediately cooking spaghetti sauce using the mushrooms and ground beef and then freezing part of it, effectively moves most of these two items into the "Long" food longevity category. Speaking for myself, I always feel more ambitious about food prep while I am in the store than I do once I get home. It is often better to simply buy the more forgiving food longevity ratio of foods to start with.

The best way to buy the right combination of foods is to take your Baseline Priority Food Plan to the market with you as a guide. There are blank worksheets in Appendix B for you to develop your own Baseline Priority Food Plan. As you shop, you will choose items based on how they fit into your food plan. Initially, you can write each item down as shown in Figure 40 on the following page, but it will soon become more intuitive and automatic.

You may notice that the items don't necessarily add up perfectly to match the targets: this is fine. The Baseline Priority Food Plan is just a tool to increase the probability that enough Priority Foods are purchased and that those foods last long enough to be consumed. Compared to the initial selection of Priority Foods in Chapter 9, we made changes to better match our target food longevity ratio. Specifically, we decided to buy frozen green beans and berries instead of fresh and realized that the ground beef should be portioned and frozen right away. We also know that there will be eggs and cheese that carry over to the next week.

Figure 40 – Example Baseline Priority Food Shopping Guide

Weekly Target	Fast-Fade 4.6 c-eq	Fresh-Med 4.6 c-eq	Long 4.8 c-eq	Total 14 c-eq
Vegetables				
Broccoli, Fresh, Package		4		4
Carrots, 1 ib			2	2
Green Beans, Frozen, 16 oz			4	4
Mushrooms, 8 oz	2			2
Romaine Lettuce, 1 Head	2			2
Total:	4	4	6	14
Weekly Target	Fast-Fade 4.5 c-eq	Fresh-Med 4.5 c-eq	Long 4.5 c-eq	Total 13.5 c-eq
Fruit				
Cantaloupe		6		6
Bananas, 2	2			2
Juice, Two 8 oz Singles			2	2
Frozen Berries, 8 oz			4	4
Total:	2	6	6	14
Weekly Target	Fast-Fade 134.3 g	Fresh-Med 134.3 g	Long 138.4 g	Total 407 g
Protein				
Ground Beef, 1 lb (Freeze)			112	112
Fish Filet w/ Skin, 1 lb	91			91
Cottage Cheese, 16 oz		52		52
Eggs, 12		96		96
Cheese, 8 0z		56		56
Total:	91	204		407

Weekly Food Plan

The last step in developing our Baseline Priority Food Plan is to distribute the Priority Foods we've purchased by day. You will only need to do this for the first week or two. After that, you will get used to preparing the right amount of priority foods for each meal.

Below is how the food purchased above might be allocated by day. The daily Priority Foods targets for our example person are:

- » Vegetables: 2.5 c-eq
- » Fruit: 2.0 c-eq
- » Protein: 71 g

Figure 41 – Example Priority Food Allocation by Day

Day	Priority Foods Distribution		Requirements Check			
	Breakfast	Lunch	Dinner	Veg	Fruit	Protein
1	Banana Juice	Lunch Out Chicken Salad	5.3 oz Ground Beef ½ C Green Beans	2.5	2	70
2	2 C Cantaloupe	Lunch Out Chicken Salad	5.3 oz Ground Beef ½ C Green Beans	2.5	2	70
3	Banana Juice	½ C Cottage Cheese 8 oz Carrots ½ C Green Beans	Dinner Out Meat, Veg, Salad	2.5	2	69
4	2 C Berries	½ C Cottage Cheese 8 oz Carrots ½ C Green Beans	Dinner Out Meat, Veg, Salad	2.5	2	69
5	2 Eggs 4 oz Mushrooms	2 C Cantaloupe ½ C Cottage Cheese	8 oz Fish 2 C Broccoli	2.5	2	74
6	2 Eggs 4 oz Mushrooms	2 C Cantaloupe ½ C Cottage Cheese 8 oz Carrots	8 oz Fish 2 C Broccoli	2.5	2	74
7	2 C Berries 2 Eggs	2 c-eq Romaine 2 oz Cheese	5.3 oz Ground Beef ½ C Green Beans	2.5	2	67

Remember that this is only the Priority Foods: the foundation of what our example woman wants to ensure that she eats. These are just the "marbles". In addition to her Priority Foods, there will be bread, pasta, cereal, sauces, condiments, incidental ingredients, drinks, snacks, and desserts. However, as you can see, these Priority foods add up to a significant amount of food. If a person could manage to get all the Priority Foods into their diet, there is limited room left for junk. Armed with this treasure trove of nutrition, perhaps a body can better handle the impact of some less-healthy foods.

Phase I – Managing Priority Foods: Conclusion

The prospect of developing your Baseline Priority Food Plan can seem intimidating at first. However, once we define what we want to accomplish, we are one step closer to achieving it. Nutrition must start with planning what to eat – not by obsessing about what not to eat. By developing your own Baseline Priority Food Plan, you will be laying the foundation to reach your nutritional goals. It will become obvious where your current habits are misaligned with your objectives. For example, I believe that most people seriously overestimate the volume of vegetables they are eating. Until you try to eat a measured 2.5 to 3 c-eq of veggies every day, you are probably fooling yourself. Just use the blank worksheets in Appendix B and the steps shown in Figure 42 on the following page to develop your own Baseline Priority Food Plan. A detailed example of this process is given in Chapter 17.

Try using this for a week and see what you learn. It might not go perfectly but I assure you that it gets easier very quickly. Once you have done it a few times, it becomes second nature. In the next chapter, we will discuss how to use the Priority Foods Feedback loop to improve the process week over week.

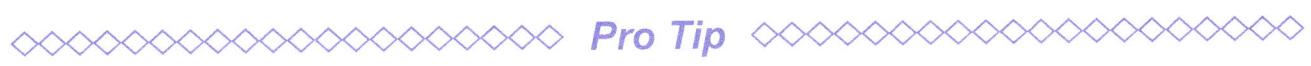

Pro Tip

For meat, protein is only in the lean, not in the fat.

For example, 80/20 ground beef has 20% less protein than 100% lean meat. It is important to keep this in mind when you are planning your Priority Food purchases.

Figure 42 – Household Priority Food Requirements Worksheet

	Person	1	2	3	4	5	6	Total
1	Name							
2	Age/Gender							
3	Activity Level							
4	Cal/Day (Figure 7 and Appendix II)							
	Veggies, c-eq							
5	Weekly Requirement (Figure 16)							
6	Weekly Veggies Out (Figure 20 est.)							
7	Weekly Veggies Home (Req't-Out)							
	Fruit, c-eq							
8	Weekly Requirement (Figure 16)							
9	Weekly Fruit Out (Figure 20 est.)							
10	Weekly Fruit Home (Req't-Out)							
	Protein, g							
11	Weekly Requirement (Figure 16)							
12	Weekly Protein Out (Figure 20 est.)							
13	Weekly Protein Home (Req't-Out)							

Figure 43 – Baseline Priority Food Plan Worksheet

	Priority Foods	Total	Out	Total-Home	Longevity Distribution		
					Fast-Fade	Fresh-Med	Long
1	Ratio						
2	Veggies, c-eq						
3	Fruit, c-eq						
4	Protein, g						

Baseline Priority Foods Plan – Key Points

Household Priority Foods requirements worksheet (Figure 29)
- » **Determine the Priority Foods requirements (veggie, fruit, protein) for each person**
- » **Estimate Priority Foods from eating out by person**
- » **Determine Priority Foods home (grocery store) by person**
- » **Add up the total Priority Foods home for household**

Baseline Priority Foods shopping guide worksheet (Figure 31)
- » **Enter the total Priority Foods home into the targets for veggies, fruit, and protein**
- » **Choose a food longevity ratio to fit your lifestyle**
- » **Allocate total targets by longevity category**
- » **Use this Baseline Priority Foods shopping guide at grocery store**

Daily Priority Foods allocation by day worksheet (Figure 35)
Allocate the Priority Foods purchased by day
- » **Check that target requirements are met (approximately)**
- » **This can be done by person or by household, depending on your situation**

Blank templates are in Appendix B

For more information about developing your own Baseline Pricrity Food Plan, visit www.ReEngineeringtheKitchen.com.

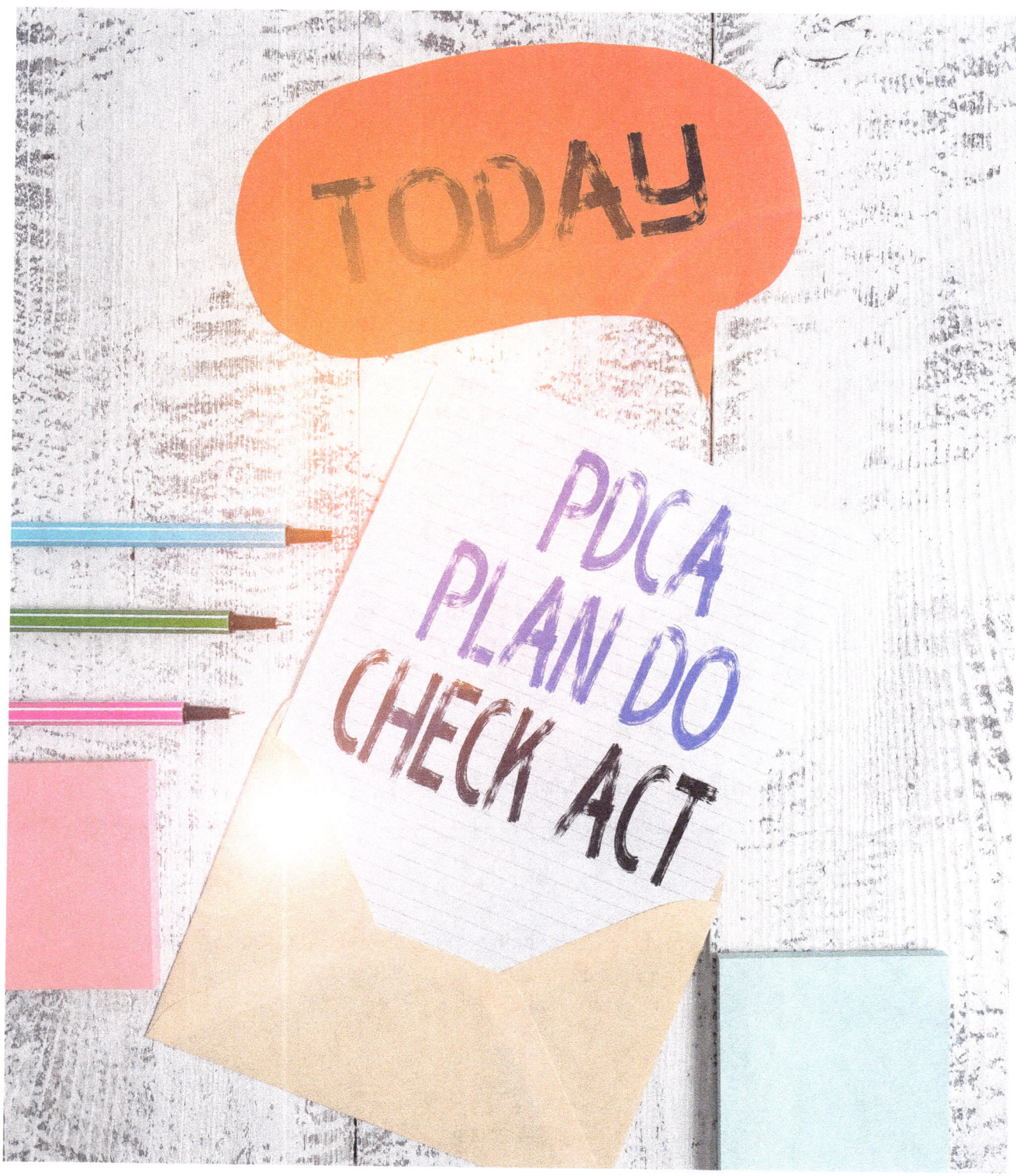

CHAPTER 13

THE PRIORITY FOODS FEEDBACK LOOP

I am sure you are familiar with giving and receiving feedback, perhaps at school or work. We can use it here to evaluate our efforts and improve our process going forward. At the end of each week, and prior to shopping for the coming week, we need to look at how we did. Our "control variable" is the amount of Priority Foods consumed. We will look at how much of the purchased Priority Foods were consumed; if everything was consumed, nothing was wasted, and there were no unplanned food purchases, then your Re-Engineered Food Cycle is working well. Your Baseline Priority Food Plan does not need any refinement.

However, it generally takes a while to fine-tune a process: that's what's called "continuous process improvement." There are lots of reasons why you may need to adjust your Priority Foods Plan to better accommodate your life and schedule. Let's see what went wrong, why, and how to fix it going forward.

Wasted Food

It is so disappointing to throw food away! First, determine what food is being discarded and why. If it is simply a matter of fresh food spoiling before you get a chance to cook it, this indicates that you need more flexibility. Consider shifting your Longevity Ratio to favor the Priority Foods that last longer. If you are discarding foods because you did not have time to prepare them, consider looking for time-saving preparation methods (See Agile Recipes™) or switch to less time-intensive foods.

If food is not eaten because people (including yourself) like other stuff better, you have to make a choice. The first option is to accept this and adjust your food targets accordingly. Maybe getting your teen to eat all those veggies is simply a bridge too far right now. The second option is to keep to your targets and try to increase consumption of these Priority Foods.

The strategies for increasing consumption include making other food less available (you eat what you buy), improving taste and presentation, cooperation, persistence, willpower, and various forms of persuasion. The Agile Recipes™ will give you some ideas for making the fruits and veggies more interesting and tastier. In the end, though, the entire family needs to be on board with the nutritional objectives. Children are inherently poor judges of what is good for them and, even if they know, need guidance to make good choices. This Re-Engineered Food Cycle can be a useful tool, providing a framework for on-going discussions about food and nutrition. Perhaps let children contribute ideas of how to meet the goals? The results may not be immediately evident, but the discussions could form a good foundation for understanding food and nutrition. Growing up is the ultimate "Process Improvement".

Unplanned Food Purchases

Plans change and we adapt. We want our food process to be efficient yet allow for flexibility. We need to know what caused the emergency trip to the grocery store, or the unplanned restaurant or takeout meal if we want to improve. If your family is simply eating more Priority Foods than included on your Baseline Priority Food Plan, then perhaps you need to increase your targets. This could happen because you have an active family that just eats more of the good stuff. It could also be because you are regularly feeding more than your own family. If this is a regular occurrence, consider adjusting your baseline targets to match what is typically consumed.

Most other unplanned food purchases can be addressed through kitchen management strategies (See Chapter 21 – A More Productive Kitchen). It is not unusual to need extra food due to a canceled dinner out or unexpected guests. Both cases can generally be accommodated with a few long-longevity foods in the cupboard or freezer. It is always a good idea to keep an easy "emergency" meal on hand for the day you had not planned to cook at all. Frozen spaghetti sauce, chili, and soup are all good options. For unexpected guests, you can often enlarge the planned meal by extending a dish (e.g., add chickpeas to the chicken curry) or add a substantial side dish to the planned meal. If you are not interested in feeding the neighborhood kids when they drop in after school, then you may have to specify what food is fair game and what is not. Other kitchen strategies like managing your staples and using Agile Recipes™ (showing substitutions) might save you from the emergency run to the grocery store for a missing item.

After you have evaluated the Priority Foods consumed for the past week, you can decide if you need to make changes to your Priority Foods Plan for the coming week. Maybe you need to adjust your targets or make other changes to the implementation. Over time you will fine-tune your management of Priority Foods. Don't worry if things are not perfect the first week. "Don't let perfection become the enemy of good," as the saying goes. The important thing is to make a bit of progress each week.

In Phase II, Improving Carbohydrates and Fats, we will add a layer of refinement to your grocery shopping by providing tools to work better carbohydrates and fats into your diet. In Phase III, Shopping and Cooking, we'll cover shopping strategies, introduce Agile Recipes™, and provide easy ways to cook what you buy. In Phase IV, Efficient Kitchen Management, we will give you kitchen-management strategies to make cooking fast, flexible, and efficient.

The Priority Foods Feedback Loop – Key Points

Feedback loop is essential to improve process
  » Priority Foods: quantity consumed vs quantity purchased

Wasted food: Spoils before being used
  » Shift longevity ratio to longer lasting foods
  » Choose less time-intensive foods and/or preparations

Wasted food: Food not eaten
  » Accept lesser nutritional goals and adjust targets accordingly
  » Keep goals and work towards acceptance
    » Improve desirability of Priority Foods
    » Reduce availability of less nutritious foods
    » Involve family in nutritional goals and planning

Unplanned food purchases
  » Consuming more Priority Foods
    » Increase targets if needed
  » Schedule changes
    » Kitchen strategies to provide flexibility

Focus on making progress each week

PHASE II

RE-ENGINEERING THE KITCHEN®

IMPROVING CARBOHYDRATES AND DIETARY FATS

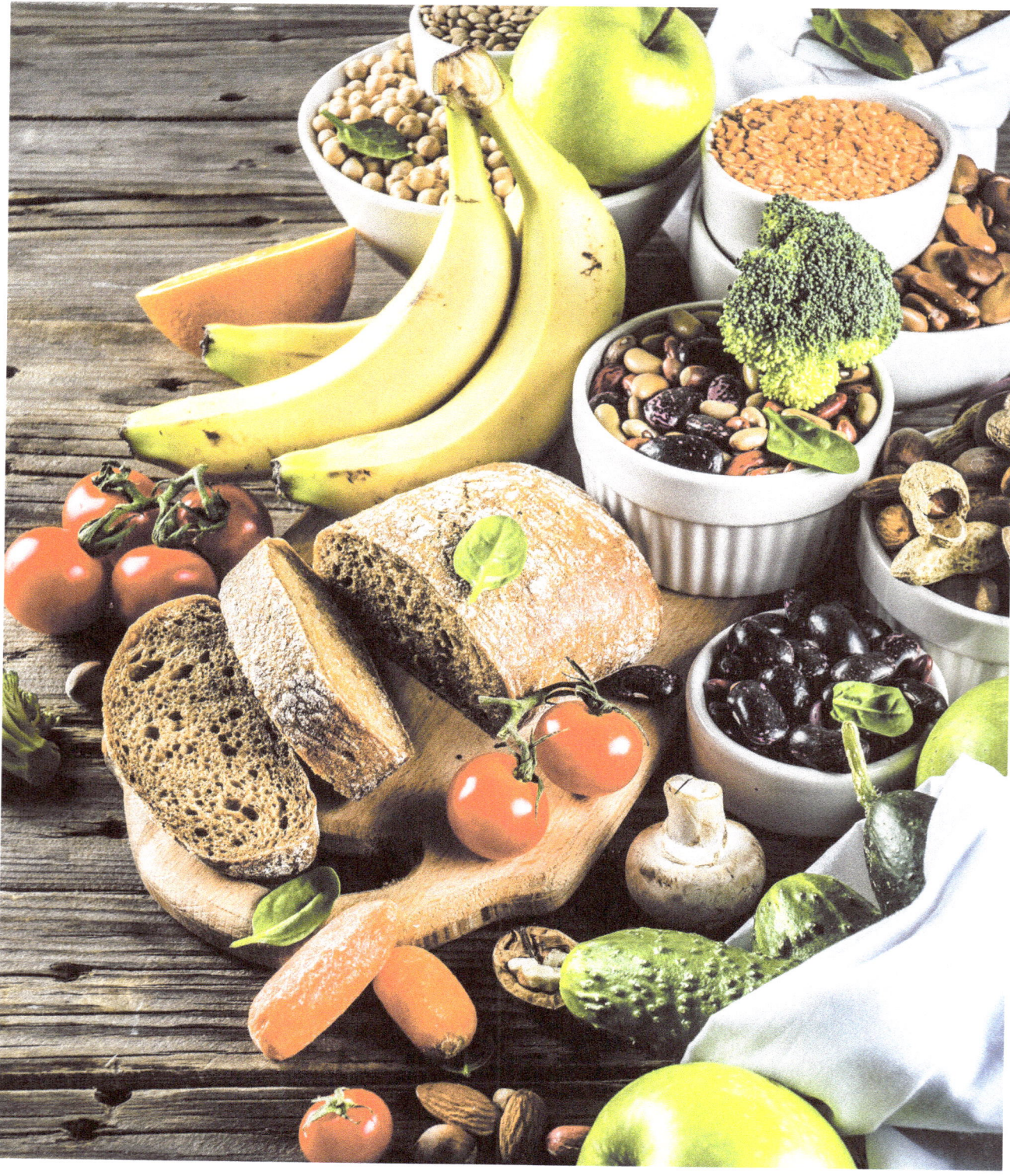

CHAPTER 14

CARBOHYDRATES

When we eat pizza, bread, pasta, rice or potatoes, we are fully conscious that we are eating carb-heavy foods. But did you know, we get carbohydrates from many sources, including grains, legumes, beans, pulses, vegetables, dairy products, and fruits? They all contribute significantly to our carb intake. However, even more carbs sneak into our diets through all manner of prepared foods, such as sugary drinks, desserts, snacks, and condiments.

Carbohydrates, one of the three macronutrients, generally comprise 45-65% of our calories consumed. Carbohydrates are often lumped together into one big category when talking about dietary guidelines. However, it may be more useful to divide them into three categories of: sugar, starch, and fiber as each of these is metabolized very differently.

Sugars

Sugars are made up of either one or two basic sugar molecules. These basic sugar molecules all have the same chemical composition of $C_6H_{12}O_6$, but the arrangement of atoms can vary to form one of the three basic sugar units: glucose, fructose, or galactose. Fructose is generally what gives food a sweet taste. When we talk about sugar, we are most often referring to sucrose, which contains both glucose and fructose. Refined cane and beet sugars and high-fructose corn syrup are major sources of glucose/fructose sweeteners in processed foods.

All carbohydrates are digested by breaking them down into their basic sugar units first. As glucose is metabolized and enters the bloodstream, insulin controls how much is needed to meet current energy demands, with the balance directed to either glycogen (liver starch) or fat for long-term storage. Fructose, on the other hand, does not affect blood glucose levels directly as it is largely metabolized in the liver in a process more like alcohol than glucose. Excess fructose can lead to a cascade of negative metabolic outcomes including visceral fat formation, liver insulin resistance, and uric acid production. Dr. Robert Lustig's YouTube video *Sugar: The Bitter Truth*[21] provides an excellent explanation of fructose metabolism and the associated health impacts. However, the takeaway message here is that glucose provides energy (perhaps too much and too quickly), but fructose is damaging to health. Does that mean even "natural" sugar is bad? No, not necessarily. If it is consumed in the form of a whole food like an apple, the fiber mitigates the negative effects of the small amount of sugar it contains.

Is sugar addictive?

We have all heard that too much sugar is terrible for our health, so why do we consume so much of it? Some experts posit that sugar is addictive in a clinical sense, just like nicotine, alcohol, or heroin. While one might quibble about the exact criteria to classify a substance as "addictive", the empirical data substantiates the reality that humans (in fact, most creatures) can't seem to resist sugar. If it is available, we will apparently eat it. With gusto. In the US, the average consumption is about 17 teaspoons per day (about 272 calories).[22] This includes everyone over 2 years old. John Yudkin first wrote **Pure, White and Deadly: How sugar is killing us and what we can do to stop it**, in 1972. So much has been written about the toxic effect of sugar in our modern diet in the ensuing 50+ years that we will simply stipulate here that limiting refined sugar consumption is (or should be) a critical dietary objective.

Starches

Starches are polysaccharides, meaning that they are formed by linking many smaller monosaccharides (simple sugars) together. If the molecule is a long straight chain, it is called an amylose, and if it is made of branched chains, it is an amylopectin. Starches are made by plants to store energy, and are found in grains, seeds, legumes, vegetables, and fruit.

Like sugars, starches are broken down in the digestive system into their smallest component: primarily glucose. Digestive enzymes help break the large molecules apart so that the glucose can be absorbed. Once absorbed, glucose from starch is metabolized the same way as glucose from sugar. The only difference is how quickly the starch goes from the bite of food to glucose ready for absorption. The more complex the starch and the less processed it is, the slower the glucose is absorbed. A gradual rise in blood glucose requires a moderate insulin response to bring it down. This is good: just how the process is supposed to work. A rapid rise in blood glucose, however, requires a rapid spike in insulin to bring it down. Eventually the delicate blood glucose/insulin feedback mechanism can't keep everything balanced. Sometimes too much insulin can bring the blood glucose too low leading to hypoglycemia (low blood glucose). I'm sure you have all experienced (or seen someone) who is on a "sugar high" after a carb-heavy meal (or birthday party) and then "crashes" a short time later, feeling tired, drowsy, headachey, and maybe even nauseated. For most of us, the aim is to balance our blood glucose levels and avoid going on this roller coaster too often.

Imagine if you routinely stomp on the gas in your car and then slam on the brakes, you will eventually need to press the brakes harder and harder to get the same stopping effect. Similarly, if you experience regular blood glucose spikes, it takes more and more insulin to control it. This is called insulin resistance and is a key factor in Type II diabetes (or metabolic syndrome).

Fiber

It is easy to forget about fiber, or not be exactly sure what it is. Fiber goes along for the ride in plant-based foods as it is used by plants to create the structure of cells, leaves, skins, and stems. Fiber may be included as a "carbohydrate" on a food packaging label. Fiber is also a polysaccharide made of many glucose molecules, but it is organized in a matrix-like structure that is indigestible for humans, and therefore doesn't contribute calories. Many animals do have the proper enzymes and digestive systems to thrive on fiber, such as cellulose found in hay and grasses.

There are two kinds of fiber: soluble and insoluble, each with an important job. Soluble fiber thickens our food, which slows gastric emptying (food moving out of the stomach). Soluble fiber allows the body to better manage glucose and fructose as the food is being digested and moderates the blood glucose/insulin roller coaster. This is why the sugar eaten in the form of a whole fruit has a low impact on blood glucose whereas the juice from that same fruit has a higher impact.

Soluble fiber is digested by the bacteria in the gut (microbiota): it is necessary to feed our essential gut biome. It is the original "prebiotic"! Insoluble fiber is the stringy stuff in plants that provides bulk and structure in the digestive system, keeping material moving through the bowel properly. So, let's think about this: We pay to buy food with the fiber removed (e.g. white rice or fruit juice) and then pay to buy it back as a supplement (which, by the way, does not provide the same benefit as fiber in whole foods). Hmmmm.

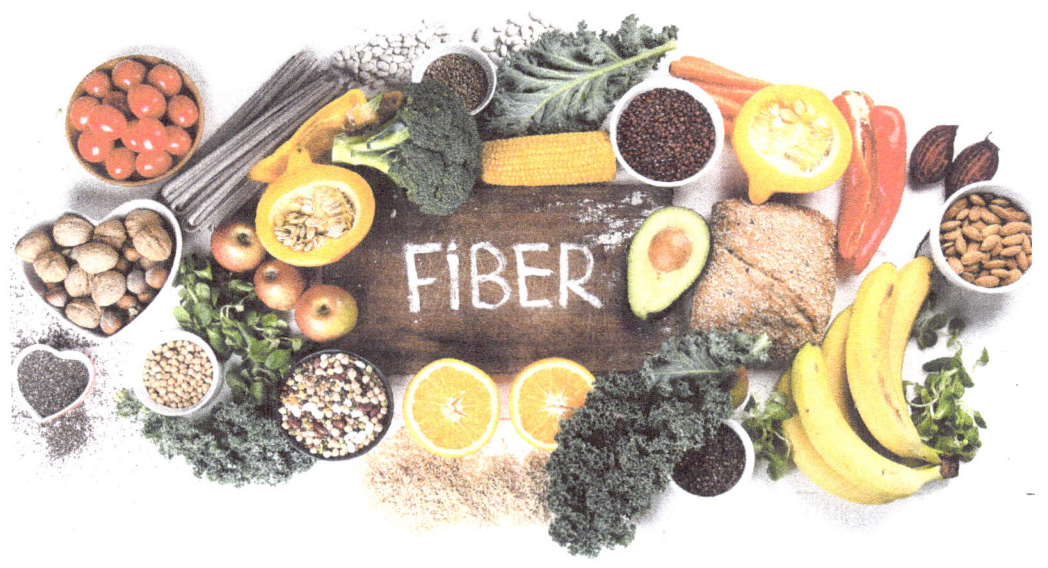

Does it even make sense to refer to sugar, starch, and fiber in the same breath, let alone try to manage them as a single macronutrient called carbs?

Sugar = damaging to health

Starch = energy

Fiber = essential for gut health and to moderate sugar metabolism

Again, maybe we should focus on eating whole foods instead of trying to manage our diet by labels and macronutrients.

Given the popularity of "low carb" diets and products, one might think that carbs are inherently evil. Not necessarily. However, the average American is probably eating too many in total and certainly too many in the form of refined grain products and added sugars. In Chapter 2 we talked about the dire consequences of eating too many ultra-processed foods. The bulk of prepared foods include refined grain-derived ingredients and sugars as these are economical and tasty, particularly when combined with highly processed oils and salt. There are many mechanisms that explain why highly processed foods are less than healthy. Let's look at these now.

Effect of Processing

It is interesting to note that even simple mechanical processing changes how our bodies metabolize food. Oatmeal is a good example, because it is available in many forms, including instant, quick, rolled, and steel cut. All oats are first cleaned, dehulled, steamed and then kilned (heat dried) to produce oat groats ready for further processing. Steel-cut oats are produced by cutting the oat groats into smaller pieces. For quicker cooking oats, the groat is first softened with steam and then smashed through rollers to create flakes; rolled oats. The thickness of the oat flakes determines their cooking time: traditional are thicker, quick oats are thinner, and instant oats are the thinnest. Each of these is a whole-grain product that includes the same nutritional components. However, our bodies react differently to each of them.

The Glycemic Index

The Glycemic Index (GI) is a ranking of foods on a scale of zero to 100 based on how that food affects blood glucose over time. High GI foods raise blood sugar very quickly, followed by a fast decline, and low GI foods raise blood sugar more slowly and hold it steady for longer.[23] As we discuss in the section about sugar, the roller coaster of blood sugar levels caused by high GI foods is damaging to our health. Glycemic Index is a useful indicator of how processing influences food metabolism. Figure 44 on the next page illustrates how the GI of oatmeal increases with the degree of processing.

Mechanical Processing Matters

A study from the *British Journal of Nutrition*[24] on mice highlights the tremendous potential impact of even minor food processing. In over-simplified terms, the study investigated the impact of feeding mice more calorie-dense foods compared to their standard pellet chow to see if diet could induce the same metabolic impacts (obesity, fatty liver, etc.) as it does in humans. Unsurprisingly, the short answer is "yes". However, they also tested the same three diets again but ground each into a powder form: mechanical processing. The surprising result was that the standard chow now resulted in approximately the same weight gain and other negative health effects as the "poor" diets. The title of the study gives away the conclusion: Diet-induced obesity in ad libitum-fed mice: **Food texture overrides the effect of macronutrient composition** (emphasis added). We are not mice, and we do not eat standardized pellets of food. Nonetheless, assuming that there is some correlation between mice and humans, a reasonable conclusion is that even simple mechanical processing can have a great impact on how we metabolize food.

Figure 44 – Illustration of Processing Effect on Glycemic Index

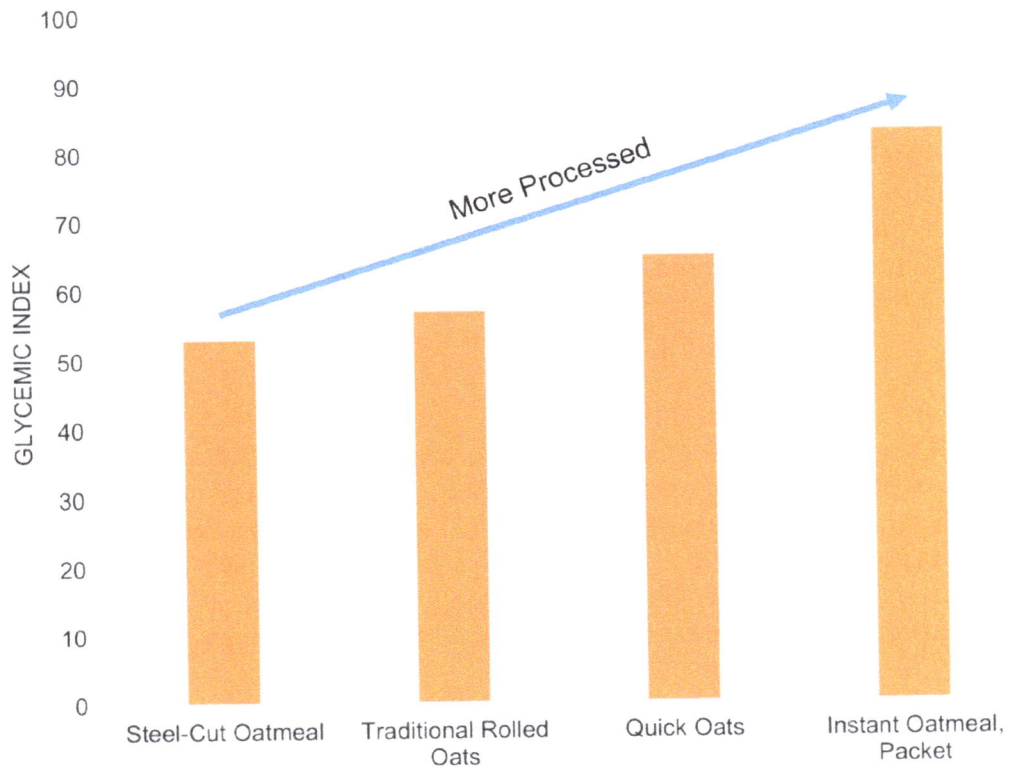

Does this mean that unsweetened instant oats are "bad"? Not necessarily, they are undoubtedly better than many other breakfast choices. It just means that rolled oats would be better for you, and steel cut better yet. You can envision a similar graph for many other foods with a range of processing options: e.g. whole apple=>applesauce=>apple juice.

Wheat Overload

In 2019, the annual per-person grain consumption in the US was about 131 pounds of wheat products, 36.5 pounds of corn grain products, and only 6.1 pounds of all other grains.[25] While there may be a lot of buzz about quinoa, whole oats, teff, and "ancient" grains, the data says we are eating a preponderance of wheat. I suspect that very little of that wheat is in a whole-grain form.

Refined wheat flour and derivative products are everywhere: bread, pizza, noodles, cookies, crackers, snacks, breading on fried foods, and more. You will also find it hiding in sauces, gravies, and some condiments. For people with Celiac disease, who react violently to the smallest trace of wheat gluten, this presents a constant challenge. It makes me wonder about the recent explosion of people becoming gluten sensitive. Could part of this increase in gluten sensitivity simply be a result of eating so much highly refined wheat? Perhaps some of these bodies are saying "Enough, already! Can you please eat some other stuff for a change?"

There are plenty of other grains, but they are more expensive than wheat. Any commercially prepared food is going to utilize the most economic and efficient ingredient to serve the purpose. This is generally refined, wheat flour – or a wheat flour-derived starch. Any whole-grain flour will have a shorter shelf life than its more refined counterpart. This is due to the presence of a small amount of unsaturated oil in the germ, which will oxidize with time and exposure to air, becoming rancid. Prepared foods with alternate grains (marketed as gluten-free) or with whole grains are generally more expensive. When preparing foods at home, you can both control your cost and opt to use a variety of grains and carb-dense vegetables, always choosing the less processed alternatives.

Added Sugars

According to the American Heart Association[27], the average American adult consumes 77 g of sugar per day (over 300 calories) and children consume 81 g. About 47% is in the form of sweetened beverages and another 31% is from snacks and sweets. Besides the extra, empty calories, the metabolic impact of this mountain of sugar is a terrible burden on bodies young and old. While the country is struggling with the burden of epidemic obesity, heart disease and type-2 diabetes, it is beyond ironic that sugar production (including high-fructose corn syrup) is supported by agricultural subsidies.

It is easy to say: Just Stop! But it's hard, isn't it? Every food package seems to have added sugar. Added sugars can go by many names on an ingredient list. Besides the obvious names like sugar, high-fructose corn syrup, molasses, and honey, watch for any word ending in -ose, any type of syrup, and fruit juice concentrates. The Hypoglycemia Support Foundation maintains the "Added Sugar Repository" which currently lists 262 names for added sugar on ingredient labels (https://hypoglycemia. org/added-sugar-repository/[26]). New labeling in 2021 requires that added sugars be listed separately in the nutritional data, which should help consumers understand what sweeteners have been added no matter what they are called.

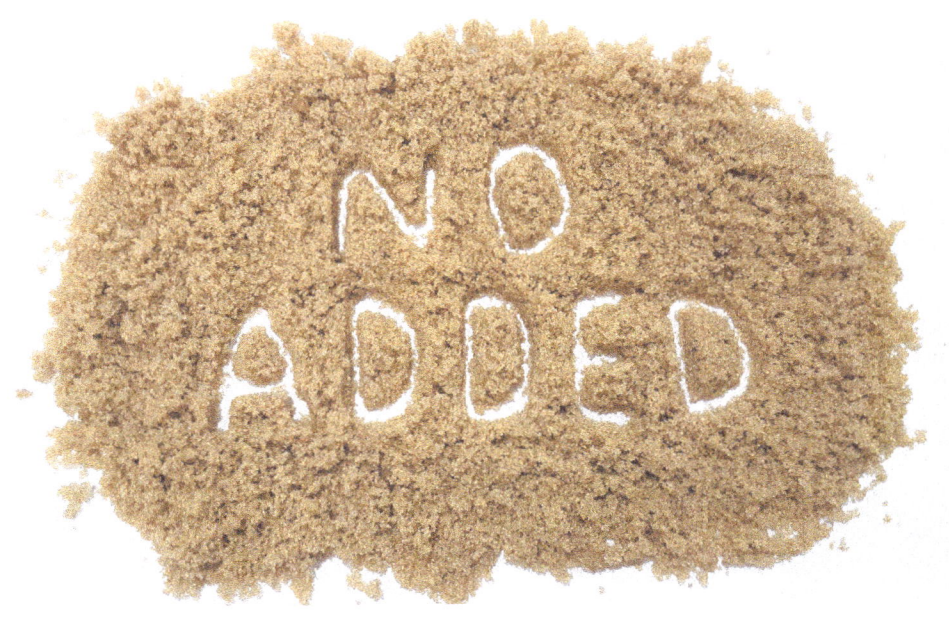

We have become used to everything tasting extremely sweet. We expect every drink to be a treat as opposed to, well, a drink. Part of the challenge is to shift our expectations of taste – and those of our children. The first step is to believe that it is possible. The next step is to believe that it is worth the effort.

Improving Carbs

There is a growing legion of health advisors who recommend minimizing grain intake and eliminating sugar completely. However, most of us get approximately 50% of our calories from carbohydrates. For our Reference Woman who consumes 2,000 calories per day, about 1,000 calories will come from carbohydrates. At 4 calories per gram of carbs, that means about 250 g of carbs per day (our Reference Man would be about 300 g). That sounds like plenty if you look at normal foods like bread (20-40 g per piece), a banana (20 g) or a potato (40 g). However, if you grab the wrong muffin and latte for breakfast, you could consume 125 g of carbs (mostly sugar) before you even get to work!

In nature, delicious carbohydrates generally carry a nutritional payload of added nutrients in the form of fiber and phytonutrients. Think of a sweet, juicy apple, complete with fiber and vitamins. In commercially prepared foods, carbs are frequently the trojan horse carrying an added-sugar-and-processed-fat bomb.

Carbs are typically the least expensive and most accessible part of our diets. Refined carbs are also the easiest to manage as they require no refrigeration and can happily sit in our cupboards (or desk drawer) for a very long time. The challenge is often choosing the best carbs as opposed to simply getting enough of them.

The guidelines for choosing carbs are simple:

- Choose a variety of whole-food sources of carbs: fruit, veggies, dairy, beans, as well as whole grains.
- Always choose unsweetened products – cereal, creamer, yogurt, milk, drinks.
    - You can add sweetener later, but you can't take it out.
    - You will probably add less sugar than the pre-sweetened alternative.
    - The unsweetened version is more flexible, suitable for multiple uses.
- Avoid added sugars in drinks, condiments, baked goods, and snacks.
- Choose the least processed option.
- Try to make as many foods at home as possible:
    - You will use less sugar
    - You will use less processed ingredients.

If you have pre-loaded your diet with whole veggies, fruits, and proteins including dairy and legumes, there is less room for grain-based carbs and added sugars. If you are making food at home, you have a better chance to control the ingredients. For example, when making your own desserts you can often cut the sugar by 50% in a recipe before anyone notices.

Added Sugar Targets

Ideally, we should just eliminate all refined sugar from our diets. I'm certain that many of society's health problems would evaporate almost overnight. While that may seem unattainable to many, there is a growing number of researchers and clinicians who are leading the charge in beating sugar and its deleterious health impacts (for further information, see www.quitsugarsummit.com).

For our examples, however, we are using the DGA recommendations as a starting point. The DGA recommends limiting added sugar to 10% of daily calories.

Added Sugar Limits per DGA[8]:

	Calories	Grams Sugar	Teaspoons Sugar
Reference Woman	200	48	12 ½
Reference Man	240	57	15

This includes sugar added to cereal, condiments, bread, desserts and other processed foods in your diet. Fruit juice often flies under the sugar radar as it is fruit and therefore considered "natural". Just remember, it is really sweet too. It should be included in the "added sugar" category. An 8-ounce serving of apple juice, fancy coffee drink, or soda each have about 25 g of sugar. Studies have shown that while sweet drinks deliver a lot of calories, they do not provide much satiety. After drinking your calories, you still eat just as much food. It is not much of an exaggeration to suggest that these sweetened drinks are going to be the death of us.

The Substitution Solution

A factor working in our favor is that we can make substitutions that greatly improve the nutritional profile of our diets, without compromising on flavor. Commercially prepared foods and beverages contain such a huge amount of sugar that we can slash it with minimal impact. For example, a 20-ounce Coca-Cola contains 65 grams of sugar: equivalent to one-third cup of granulated sugar. (I'm not picking on Coke: Pepsi and Mountain Dew are even higher.) It would be ridiculous for anyone to add that much sugar to a drink at home; I doubt it would all dissolve. A very sweet, iced tea might have 2 or 3 teaspoons of sugar: a small fraction of the sugar in a soda.

Keep this handy conversion in mind:

4.2 g of sugar = 1 tsp of granulated sugar

When you read a food label, look at the grams of sugar (listed under carbohydrates). Do the math in your head: each 4 grams of sugar is approximately a teaspoon of sugar. Then ask yourself if you would have added that much sweetener to the item. For example, if a ½ C serving of sweetened cereal (who eats just a half cup?) has 13 grams of added sugar, that is about 3 teaspoons of granulated sugar. Would you have added that much?

Making switches requires forethought and some effort. It may require gradual shifts over time to reach your goal of shifting taste expectations. A family I know with two young children wants to shift from white rice to brown rice, which the children think they don't like. Their strategy is to start by mixing the two types of rice and then gradually shift the ratio as everyone gets used to the taste and texture. It is these incremental steps that are so powerful. Whatever you make at home is almost always better than something that is commercially prepared.

Carbohydrates – Key Points

Three types of carbohydrates:
- » **Sugar – Damaging to health**
- » **Starch – Energy**
- » **Fiber – Essential for health**

Choose the least processed carbohydrate
- » **Processing increases Glycemic Index**

Choose a variety of whole foods containing carbohydrates
- » **Vegetables and fruits**
- » **Dairy**
- » **Legumes and pulses**
- » **Whole, minimally processed grains**

Limit added sugar

Avoid sweetened drinks and limit fruit juices

What Happened to Tea?

I grew up drinking tea, always with a teaspoon of sugar and a splash of milk. This undoubtedly came courtesy of my Latvian heritage. As a child, I remember that none of my friends were allowed this "grown up" beverage and adults freely showed their disapproval with raised eyebrows. In my Metro-Detroit neighborhood, beverage choices were limited for children: milk, maybe orange juice (or Tang) at breakfast, and Kool-Aid. Faygo pop, with its myriad of flavors, was a special treat. When I was very young, briefly steeped tea was an occasional option – perhaps a Sunday breakfast or with a celebratory dessert. By the time I could make it myself, it was an acceptable option for any breakfast, whenever we went out to a Chinese restaurant, and the comforting hot beverage of choice. How is it that tea is no longer considered a suitable beverage for children while soda and other totally artificial, hyper-sweetened and even "energy" drinks are perfectly acceptable? Trust me – a lot of money was spent to make that happen.

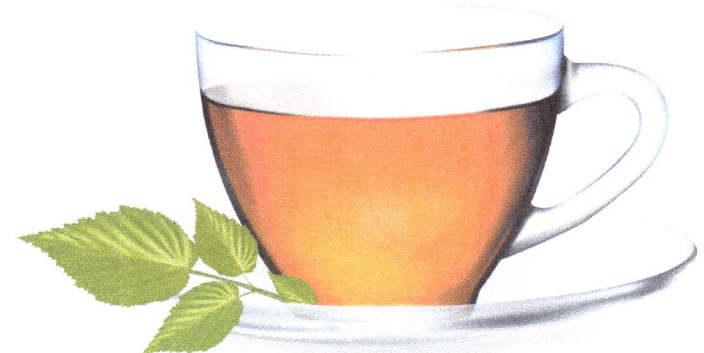

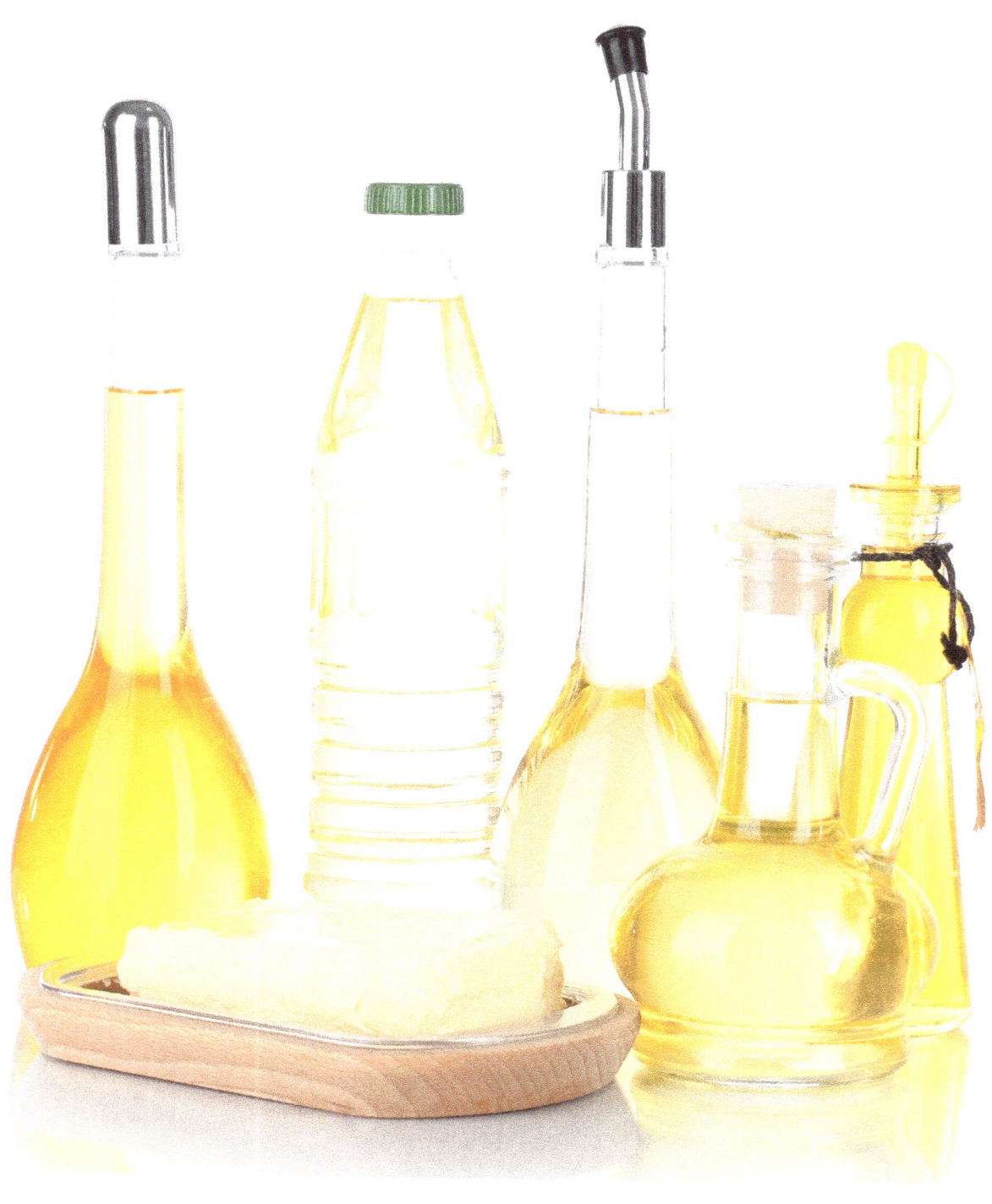

CHAPTER 15

DIETARY FATS AND OILS

So far, we have focused on veggies, fruit, protein, and carbs. We are now going to look at fats and oils; what you spread on your bread, the salad dressings, what you cook with, and what comes in your processed foods. As with all foods, the nutritional quality of fats can vary considerably depending on the source and the degree of processing. Your biggest opportunity to shift your intake to healthier choices will be the grocery store and avoiding highly processed food products.

Importance of Dietary Fats and Oils

For decades, we were advised to lower our total intake of fats and oils (we will use the term "fat" or "oil" interchangeably to include all dietary fats and oils). There was a proliferation of low-fat diets and products, many of which replaced fats with refined carbs and sugars to maintain palatability. Our understanding of the health effects of dietary fats and oils has evolved; it is now widely recognized that fats play an essential role in health and nutrition. Besides being a high-density energy source, fats perform many critical functions, including:

- Fats are required to carry oil-soluble Vitamins A, D, E, and K.
- Fats are the building blocks of the hormones that regulate bodily functions.
- Your brain is mostly fat and every cell in your body is surrounded by a lipid (fat) layer.
- Body fat cushions organs and stores readily accessible energy.
- Dietary fat stimulates feelings of satiety, helping you to feel full and satisfied.

Good Fats and Bad Fats?

It has become common to refer to dietary fats and oils as being "healthy" or "unhealthy" or even "good" or "bad". According to recent conventional wisdom, unsaturated vegetable oils were considered healthy fats, regardless of their source or processing, while naturally occurring saturated fats were villainized. Since the 1960-70s, saturated fat was blamed for elevated cholesterol levels and, by extension, increases in cardiovascular disease. Since then, innumerable studies have countered this theory[27], but you wouldn't know it. Public opinion, policies, food manufacturers, and the medical establishment are slow to change, largely due to the inertia of vested interests. The book *Eat Rich Live Long* by Ivor Cummins and Jeffery Gerber MD, provides an excellent summary of the science and history around the ill-fated war on fat.

Since the early 1960s, a great deal of advertising money has been spent to convince America that animal-based fats are "bad", and all vegetable-based fats are "good". It's been money well spent: the amount of butter and lard consumed has decreased while the amount of shortening (primarily hydrogenated vegetable oil) and salad/cooking oils has exploded. The graph below shows the historical food availability data for certain added fats and oils from 1909 to 2010 (when the government stopped tracking this data this way).

Figure 45 – Food Availability of Certain Added Fats per Capita

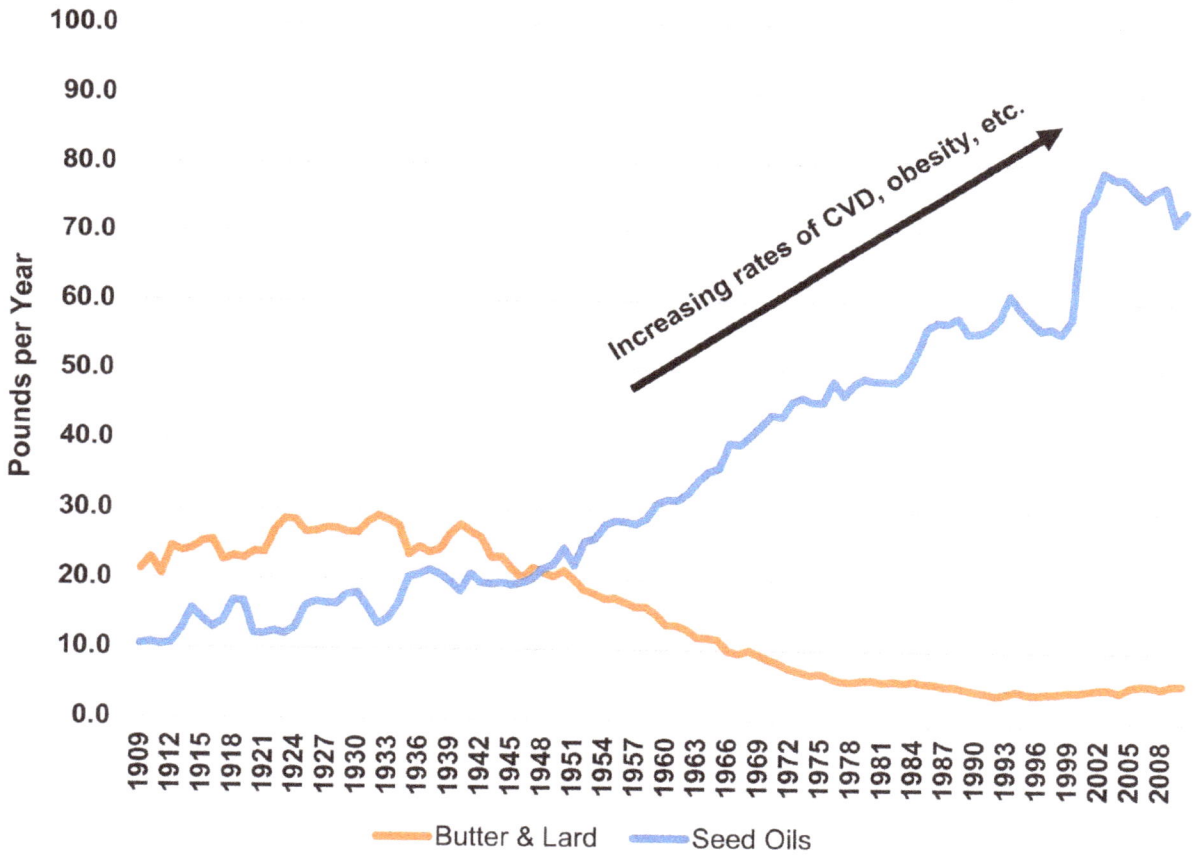

Source: USDA Economic Research Service and US Census Bureau 2019

Based on this graph, it would be tempting to conclude that there is a correlation between the rise in vegetable/seed oil consumption and the increase in chronic disease. However, correlation does not mean causation. Perhaps these industrial seed oils are perfectly safe (in these quantities) but just happen to be part of processed foods, which are unhealthy for other reasons. Or perhaps the problem is that they are combined with refined carbs and sugars in processed foods? Regardless, based on the graph I think it is safe to say that a dollop of butter on our peas never was the problem.

While we have been obsessing over air-frying and buying skim milk and lean meat to reduce our saturated fat intake, our consumption of processed seed oils continues to climb. It is the elephant in the room that no one is talking about. In 2023 the United States per capita consumption of just palm, palm kernel, and soy oils was 95.3 lbs per year or over 1,000 calories per day. These oils are used almost exclusively in making processed and restaurant foods. This does not include the many oils that are used both in processed foods and in home kitchens, nor the fats naturally contained in whole foods such as milk, cheese, peanut butter, yogurt, eggs, meat, avocados, and nuts.

Industrial seed oils including soy, palm, peanut, cottonseed, canola (rapeseed oil), corn, sunflower, safflower, and coconut oils are often highly processed to make them shelf stable in a bottle and useful in making inexpensive and palatable processed foods. If a food comes in a bag, box or bottle, it probably includes at least one of these oils. It is interesting to note that in 2023, approximately 83% of the US consumption of these oils came from soy, palm and canola, while the much-touted olive oil contributed only about 2%[28].

Just a little chemistry

Dietary fat molecules are made up of a glycerin backbone attached to three fatty acids (hence the term triglyceride). The fatty acids are long carbon and hydrogen chains with a carboxyl group (CO-OH) at one end making it an acid. Dietary fats are categorized based on how they are hydrogenated; that is, whether they are "saturated" with hydrogen atoms in every possible position. If hydrogen atoms are missing (unsaturated), then the carbons atoms form a double bond with one another. The single bonds between carbon form a regular, straight chain. Wherever there is a double bond between carbon atoms, the molecule will bend, as illustrated on page 130.

Figure 46 – Fat Chemistry Simplified

Saturated Fat	Monounsaturated Fat	Polyunsaturated Fat
Every carbon atom holds the maximum number of hydrogen atoms possible, only single carbon-carbon bonds.	The carbon chain contains two fewer hydrogens, allowing for one double carbon-carbon bond.	There are four or more missing hydrogen atoms, allowing two or more double carbon-carbon bonds.
Stable	Less stable	
Solid at room temperatire	Liquid at room temperature	

Saturated fats tend to be unreactive (stable) with high melting points. The long straight geometry of saturated fats allows the molecules to pack together densely, forming solids at room temperature. The irregular shape of the unsaturated fat molecules means that they tend to pack together less densely and are commonly liquids at room temperature. The double bonds in unsaturated fats mean that they are more reactive. They readily oxidize, becoming rancid on the shelf and bioactive in the body. There are over 40 naturally occurring fatty acids and these are found in various proportions in naturally occurring foods. Industrial food processing changes the composition of fats, for example through filtration, distillation, fractionation, interesterification, and hydrogenation (adding hydrogen where there was a double bond)[29].

Figure 47 on the next page shows the relative fatty acid profiles of common types of dietary fats and oils[30].

Figure 47 – Fatty Acid Profile of Common Dietary Fats and Oils

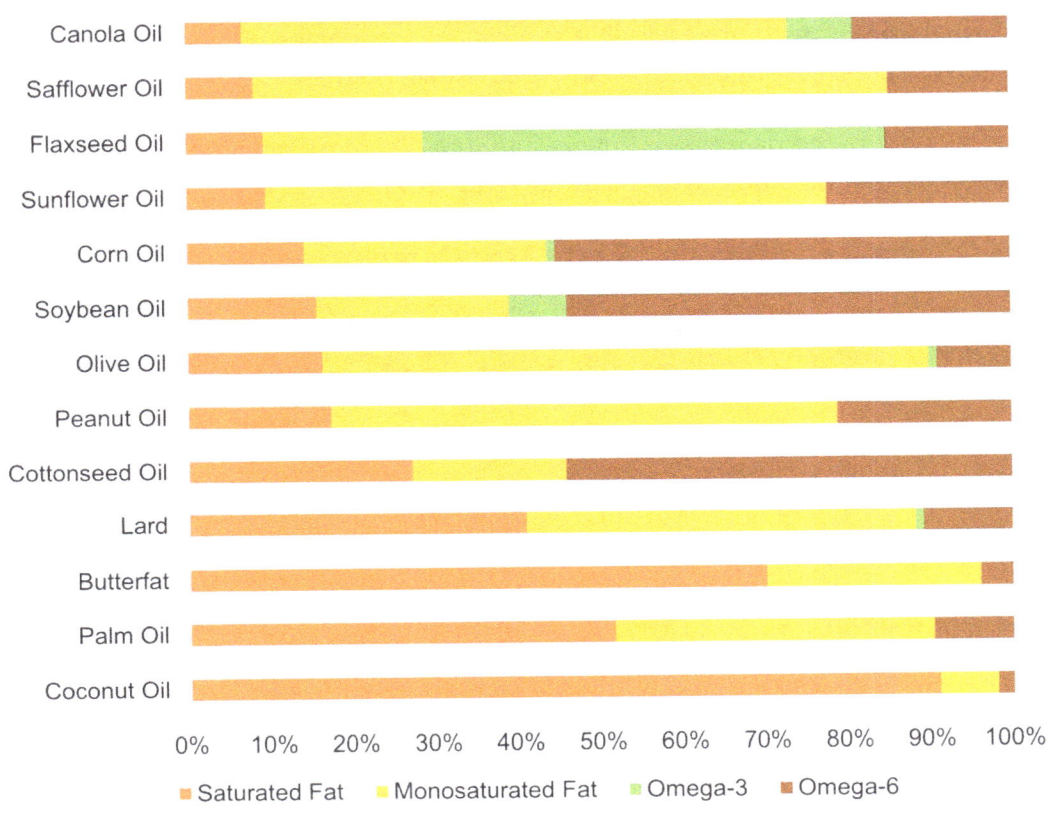

Fatty Acid Composition (Percent of Total)

Source: USDA Food Data Central (https://fdc.nal.usda.gov/fdc-app)

The nutritional value of fats is more complicated than just saturated vs unsaturated. The most consumed vegetable oils are highly processed; manufacturers use heat, mechanical, and chemical processing to create a stable, uniform product. While many institutions (including the USDA and American Heart Association) continue to advise choosing unsaturated fats despite their degree of processing, a growing number of health advisors are sounding the alarm in favor of less processed fats. Maybe the real issue is not saturated vs unsaturated, but rather, the tidal wave of highly processed vegetable/seed oils that have crept into our diets along with the ultra-processed foods.

The Omegas

You have undoubtedly heard about the omega-6 and omega-3 polyunsaturated fatty acids (PUFAs) and that they are "essential" for human health. Essential means that the human body cannot synthesize these required molecules; they must come from food. While both are essential, the total amount your body requires is very little; on the order of 20-40 calories per day. You have probably heard that we are not getting enough of the omega-3s, but beyond that, the story becomes very complicated, very quickly. However, here are the basics to understanding how the omegas fit in your diet and why.

Figure 48 – Omega-3 and Omega-6 Fatty Acid Comparison

	Omega-6	Omega-3
Fatty Acid in Food	Linoleic Acid (LA)	Alpha-Linolenic Acid (ALA)
Created in Plants	Seeds	Leaves
Primary Food Source	Nuts, Seed/Grain Oils	Greens – Land & Sea
Secondary Food Source	Tissue of Animals That Eat Grains/Seeds	Tissue of Animals That Eat Green Leaves
Stability	Moderately Stable	Prone to Oxidation

Looking at the chart, you can see why grass-fed beef has a higher omega-3 to omega-6 ratio than grain-fed beef. No wonder fish, which eat plankton or algae (or eat other fish that did), are a good source of omega-3s.

Omega-3 and omega-6 are the yin-and-yang of PUFAs. Both are essential and they are linked metabolically. In the body, omega-6 linoleic acid is converted to arachidonic acid, which supports a complex symphony of inflammatory signaling. The simplest omega-3, ALA, is converted into eicosapentaenoic acid (EPA) and docosahexaenoic acid (DHA), which are essential for the eyes, nerves, and brain, in addition to moderating inflammation. To spotlight the importance of omega-3s, consider that about 15% of your brain is made up of DHA.

However, when it comes to the omegas, it is not enough to simply get enough: they need to be in balance. Linoleic acid and alpha linolenic acid compete for the same enzyme in their metabolic pathways. If there is too much of one, it inhibits the conversion of the other. In our Western diet, omega-6 (LA) is far more prevalent due to the extremely high quantity of very high linoleic acid content in the seed oils in our food supply: soy and corn, for example. Since omega-3 (ALA) is more prone to oxidation (becoming rancid), it is not compatible with processed foods, and has been systematically eliminated.[31] *The Queen of Fats* by Susan Allport provides the fascinating history of omega-3 research and how this essential fat is disappearing from our foods. www.susanallport.com.

Historically, the omega-6 to omega-3 ratio in the human diet is estimated to have been close to 2:1. The ratio in the current Western diet is estimated to be 15:1 or even higher (some estimates range up to 30:1). The illustration below is very simplified but may help visualize how this imbalance plays out in the human body.

Figure 49 – Metabolic Dynamics of Omega-3 and Omega-6 Imbalance – Illustration

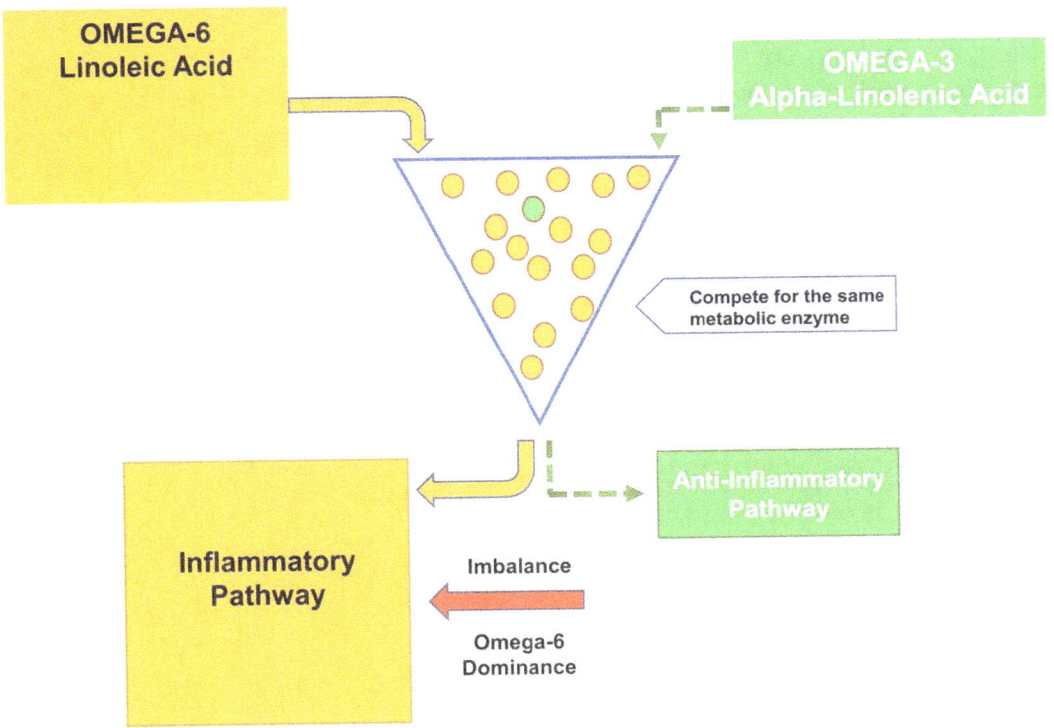

Adequate omega-3 intake is suspected to reduce the risk for a vast array of chronic diseases including:

- Coronary heart disease
- Rheumatoid arthritis
- Age-related macular degeneration
- Cognitive decline (such as Alzheimer's)
- Some cancers[32]

While ensuring adequate omega-3 intake is vital, it is equally important to limit the intake of omega-6 as well, i.e. soy and corn oil.

You may be thinking, "This doesn't apply to me: I don't use much corn oil, and I've never bought soy oil in my life!" Actually, you do, and you have: both are ubiquitous components in many processed foods. These processed vegetable oils are used in everything from salad dressings to frying oil to commercially baked goods, including bread.

Figure 50 below shows the omega-3 and omega-6 content of some selected foods to illustrate the relative amount of both omegas in a typical serving. Very few natural foods have more omega-3 than omega-6: these are primarily fish, green plants and flaxseed. For nearly everything else, the balance shifts to favor omega-6, particularly as the seed and grain oil content of the food increases.

Besides demonstrating that soy and corn oil are really high in omega-6, the other takeaway is that prepared foods are a wild card. You really can't judge the omega-3/omega-6 content since you don't know how much of what combination of oils were used. At least when you make things at home, you know what you put in it.

Figure 50 – Omega-3 and Omega-6 Content of Selected Foods per Serving (mg)

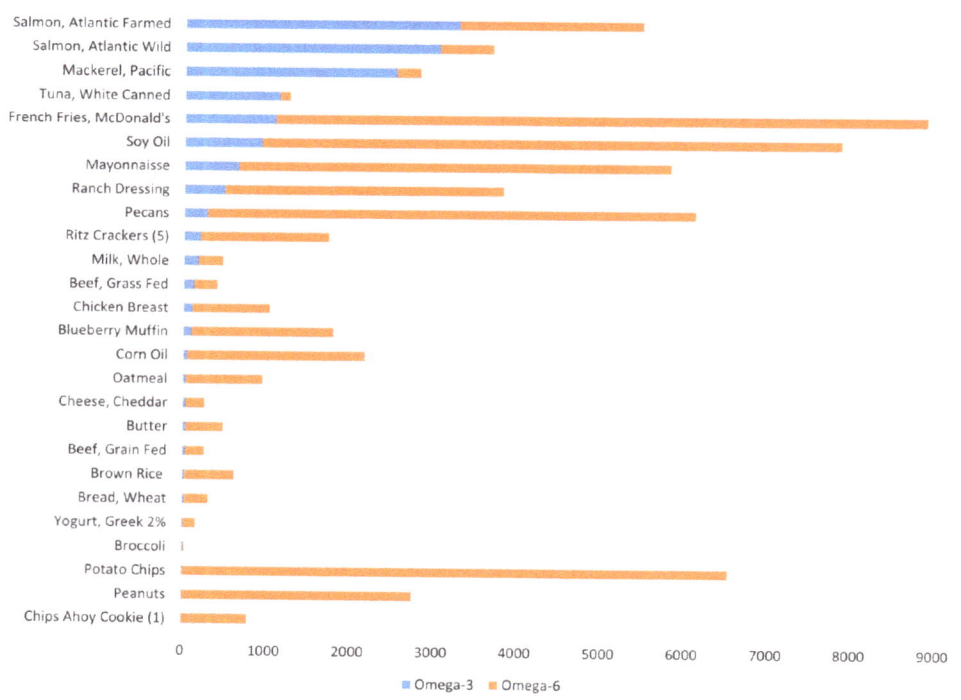

Source: USDA Food Data Central (https://fdc.nal.usda.gov/fdc-app)

The omega-6 content in many commercially prepared foods is simply huge, primarily due to the soy and corn oil content. The average American diet is swimming in omega-6, making it almost impossible to achieve a reasonable omega-6 to omega-3 ratio. For example, look at the graph and compare salmon to the ranch salad dressing. If you wanted to "balance" out the high omega-6 salad dressing with a very high omega-3 food like wild salmon, you would need to eat over three servings of wild salmon to achieve a 1:1 ratio. Practically speaking, this means that you need to limit the high omega-6 foods, else you simply can't eat enough high omega-3 foods to compensate.

In a typical Western diet, where highly processed foods are estimated to comprise 60%, it is easy to see how a state of constant omega-6 dominance would exist. To address this chronic imbalance, manufacturers are making more and more products fortified with omega-3s (frequently in the form of EPA and DHA). You can also buy omega-3 supplements, primarily from marine sources. The inescapable conclusion is: if you want to achieve a better omega-6 to omega-3 ratio, you will need to work at it, very diligently.

Figure 51 – Sources of Omega-3 Fatty Acids

Omega-3 Fatty Acids	Key Sources
ALA – Alpha Linolenic Acid EPA – Eicosapentaenoic Acid DHA – Docosahexaenoic Acid	Vegetable Sources: Flaxseed oil, chia seeds, hemp seeds and oil, navy beans, lingonberries, algae and seaweed. Seafood Sources: Salmon, tuna, bass, sardines, herring, whitefish, anchovies, trout, swordfish, pollock, snapper, clams, grouper, mussels, oysters, calamari. Supplementary Sources: Eggs (hens are fed EPA and DHA), fortified dairy products, and fish oil or algal-based supplements.

Managing Dietary Fats and Oils

To say that there is no consensus on the issue of dietary fats is a gross understatement. Highly respected scientists, doctors and institutions are still giving wildly contradictory advice. The DGA guidelines suggest that total lipids (fats and oils) make up 20-35% of an adult's total daily calories, with saturated less than 10%. Other dietary guides may differ. For example, The American Heart Association[27] recommends that saturated fats be limited to about 5-6% of total calories and specifically recommends eating more of the polyunsaturated oils such as soy, corn and sunflower (which we have learned, are very high in omega-6).

At the other end of the spectrum, "high natural fat" diets (paleo and keto, for instance) recommend that total fat comprise up to 80% of calories, but only include natural, unprocessed fats and oils. This would include whole-food sources such as nuts, olives, and avocados. It would also include animal sources such as meat, fish, and full-fat dairy products. Bottled oils would be limited and only include those which were simply expressed, with no heat or chemicals (i.e. cold pressed) and protected from oxidation. The natural fats approach has a certain "common sense" appeal. Why would we assume that highly processed, unsaturated vegetable oils made from genetically modified commodity crops are nutritionally superior to the whole-food and animal-sourced fats that humans have been consuming for thousands of years?

So how do we wade through all the conflicting advice? It is up to you to decide where you are on the spectrum based on your own analysis and medical guidance. Personally, I believe that unprocessed and whole-food sources of fats are inherently better than those found in highly processed foods. Remember that ultra processed foods are a major source of highly processed fats making it easy to consume much more of them than we ever intended. By choosing to prepare food at home you can choose the amount, type, and quality of your fats.

Making nutritious choices

For our examples, however, we will use the DGA guidelines. As always, these are an excellent starting point to create a baseline plan. You can always adjust to meet your own objectives. For our reference man and woman, the USDA-recommended fat amounts are:

- Woman – 49 g (443 calories) total fats, less than half saturated
- Man – 62 g (566 calories) total fats, less than half saturated

With fats, there are four key nutritional objectives to consider, when planning your diet:

1. Balance unsaturated and saturated fats
2. Minimize the degree of processing
3. Balance the ratio of omega-6/omega-3 fatty acids
4. Watch for hidden fats to avoid going over your intended levels

Fats make foods taste delicious and craveable. You can assume that commercially prepared foods contain plenty of highly processed fats and oils. While getting healthier fats in prepared foods may seem impossible, here are actions you can take to get more of the better fats and less of the others:

- Avoid ultra-processed foods – switch to home-prepared where possible.
  - Make your own salad dressings, sauces, and baked goods.
  - Read the labels on packaged foods, to identify the fat content and type of fat.
- Ensure that you get regular sources of omega-3 fatty acids.
- Eat whole-food sources of fats like nuts, dairy, seeds, fish, avocados, eggs and meat.
- When buying bottled oils choose minimally processed (choose cold pressed/expressed)
- Avoid deep-fried foods – everywhere.

The bottom line is to strive for balance – in fats as in everything else. With data, you can set priorities and make informed choices. For example, you can choose olive oil for a quick salad dressing rather than the soy oil in a bottled dressing or you can choose a small amount of canola to pan-fry chicken rather than the deep-fried takeout alternative. When you make food at home, you can choose which fats you use and how much. Home-prepared salad dressings, sauces, and baked goods are easier than you've been led to believe, as you will see when we get to the recipe section of this book.

Figure 52 on the next page shows the different types of fats and oils, how they might be labeled and what foods they are primarily found in. Use this chart to guide you in making better choices.

What about trans fats?

Trans fats are formed when a fatty acid is converted from its cis isomer to its trans isomer; it is the same molecule except just one bond is twisted a different orientation. Trans fats are found in nature but in small quantities. More commonly trans fats are a byproduct of oil processing and became ubiquitous in our food supply with the advent of hydrogenated fats for margarine, shortening, and processed foods. In the 1990s studies indicated that trans fats were a significant cause of coronary heart disease and pressure mounted to remove these from the food supply. By 2015 an FDA ruling went into effect that trans fats were no longer GRAS (generally recognized as safe), which effectively required the near total phase-out of trans fats in processed foods after 2019.

Figure 52 – Dietary Fats and Oils: Labeling and Food Source

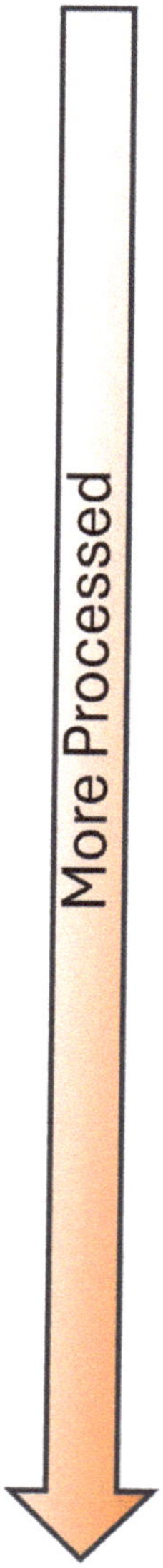

Type of Oil	Key Sources
Whole Foods	• Nuts and seeds • Avocados • Meat and fish • Eggs • Dairy
Unrefined/Natural	• Avocado oil • Coconut oil • EVOO and VOO • Butter • Rendered or leaf lard • Natural nut butters

Refined Unsaturated Oils	• Refined bottled vegetable oils
	   • Canola
	   • Corn
	   • Regular olive oil
	   • Peanut
	   • Soy
	• Salad dressings
	• Peanut and soy butter spreads
	• Some baked goods
	• Some dips and spreads

Refined Saturated Oils: Tropical vegetable, palm, palm kernal, hydrogenated vegetable	• Commercially baked goods • Packaged prepared foods • Crackers, chips, cookies • Lunchmeat, pepperoni • Fried and deep-fried foods • Dips and spreads • Margarine • Salad dressings

More Processed →

Dietary Fats and Oils – Key Points

Dietary fats are important for health

Processed seed oils:
- » **Consumption has increased threefold since 1950**
- » **Processed foods contain a lot of hidden fats**
- » **High omega-6 to omega-3 ratio in most foods**

Omega-3 is essential but difficult to get enough

Shift to a healthier fat profile by:
- » **Avoiding ultra-processed foods – make food at home**
- » **Read label on packaged foods**
- » **Eat whole-food sources of fats**
- » **Ensure you get regular source of omega-3s**
- » **Choose minimally processed fats and oils when possible**
- » **Avoid deep-fried foods**

Palm Oils – Health and Environment

Palm Oils deserve special mention due to their prevalence in foods and environmental impacts. Palm trees produce both palm kernel oil and palm oil. While these are generally referred to as vegetable oils, they are highly saturated fats that are solid or semi-solid at room temperature. Palm oil is incredibly versatile and is used in soaps, cosmetics, animal feed, biofuel, as well as in foods. In fact, it is estimated that one-half of the products in a typical grocery store contain palm oil in some form. In foods, palm oil and its derivatives may be labeled as Vegetable Oil, Vegetable Fat, Palm Kernel, Palm Kernel Oil, Palm Fruit Oil, Palmate, Palmitate, Palmolein, Glyceryl, Stearate, Stearic Acid, Elaeis Guineensis, Palmitic Acid, Palm Stearine, Palmitoyl Oxostearamide, Palmitoyl Tetrapeptide-3, Sodium Laureth Sulfate, Sodium Lauryl Sulfate, Sodium Kernelate, Sodium Palm Kernelate, Sodium Lauryl Lactylate/Sulphate, Hydrated Palm Glycerides, Ethyl Palmitate, Octyl Palmitate, Palmityl Alcohol.[21]

As trans fats are being phased out, palm oils are increasingly being used in the processed food industry. Between 2000 and 2022, the US consumption of palm oils (palm oil and palm kernel oil) increased from about 2.3 lb/year to 13.8 lb/year per person, with no indication of leveling off any time soon. Obviously, palm oils are edible and safe in reasonable quantities. How much is reasonable? I guess we will find out in about 20 years.

Demand is growing steadily and, with its high yield per acre, palm oil is very profitable to produce. It is no surprise, then, that cultivation of oil palms is expanding in tropical areas. Indonesia and Malaysia produce 85% of the world's supply. Expansion of palm oil production is driving slash-and-burn deforestation of massive areas of virgin forest, draining of peat bogs, as well as water and air pollution. The devastating environmental impacts include destroying critical habitat for many endangered species and increased greenhouse gas emissions.

This World Wildlife Federation website (https://www.worldwildlife.org/industries/palm-oil) gives you more information about the environmental impact of palm oils and steps you can take to support more sustainably sourced palm oil[33]. For a more in-depth discussion of the critical health, environmental and social issues around the palm oil industry, read "The palm oil industry and noncommunicable diseases" published in the *Bulletin of the World Health Organization* (https://www.ncbi.nlm.nih.gov/pmc/articles/PMC6357563/)[34].

Dietary Oil FAQs

Are Rapeseed Oil and Canola Oil the Same?

While rapeseed oil and canola oil come from the same "rapeseed" plant family, canola is a cultivar developed to produce food-grade (or culinary) rapeseed oil. Canola oil has a much lower level of erucic acid than industrial rapeseed oil, making it safe for human consumption. Canola oil is low in saturated fat, has vitamin E, and has an omega-6 to omega-3 ratio of about 2:1. It has a high smoke point (about 400°F) making it a popular choice for cooking.[35] Canola oil is third in global vegetable oil production, behind only palm oil and soybean oil.

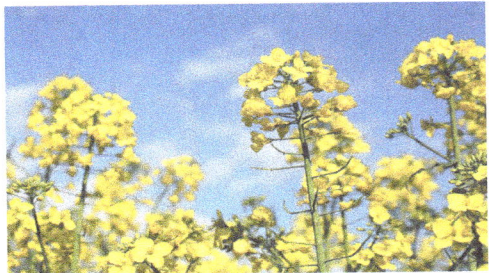

Rapeseed Plant

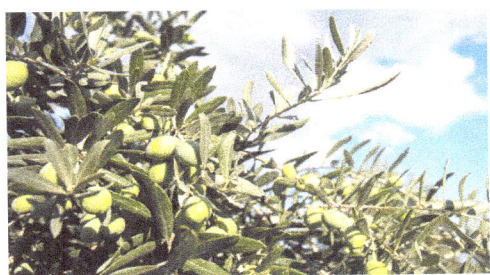

Olive Tree

Is Olive Oil a Seed Oil?

The oil in olives comes from the fleshy fruit of the olive, so olive oil is a fruit oil, not a seed oil. During production, whole ripe olives are ground into a paste and then the oil is extracted using sequentially more robust methods. The initial, mechanically produced oils are quality tested and graded as "extra virgin" and "virgin" olive oils. Regular olive oil and light olive oil are produced from oils extracted and refined using mechanical as well as heat and chemical methods. Lastly, olive pomace oil is made by extracting oil from dried, residual olive pomace paste with solvents, then the crude pomace oil is refined to produce a food grade oil.

Olive oil, especially virgin and extra virgin, is high in monosaturated fat content with potential cardiovascular benefits. The smoke point for olive oil varies between about 350°F and 470°F, with the more processed grades having the higher smoke point.[36]

PHASE III

RE-ENGINEERING THE KITCHEN®

SHOPPING AND COOKING

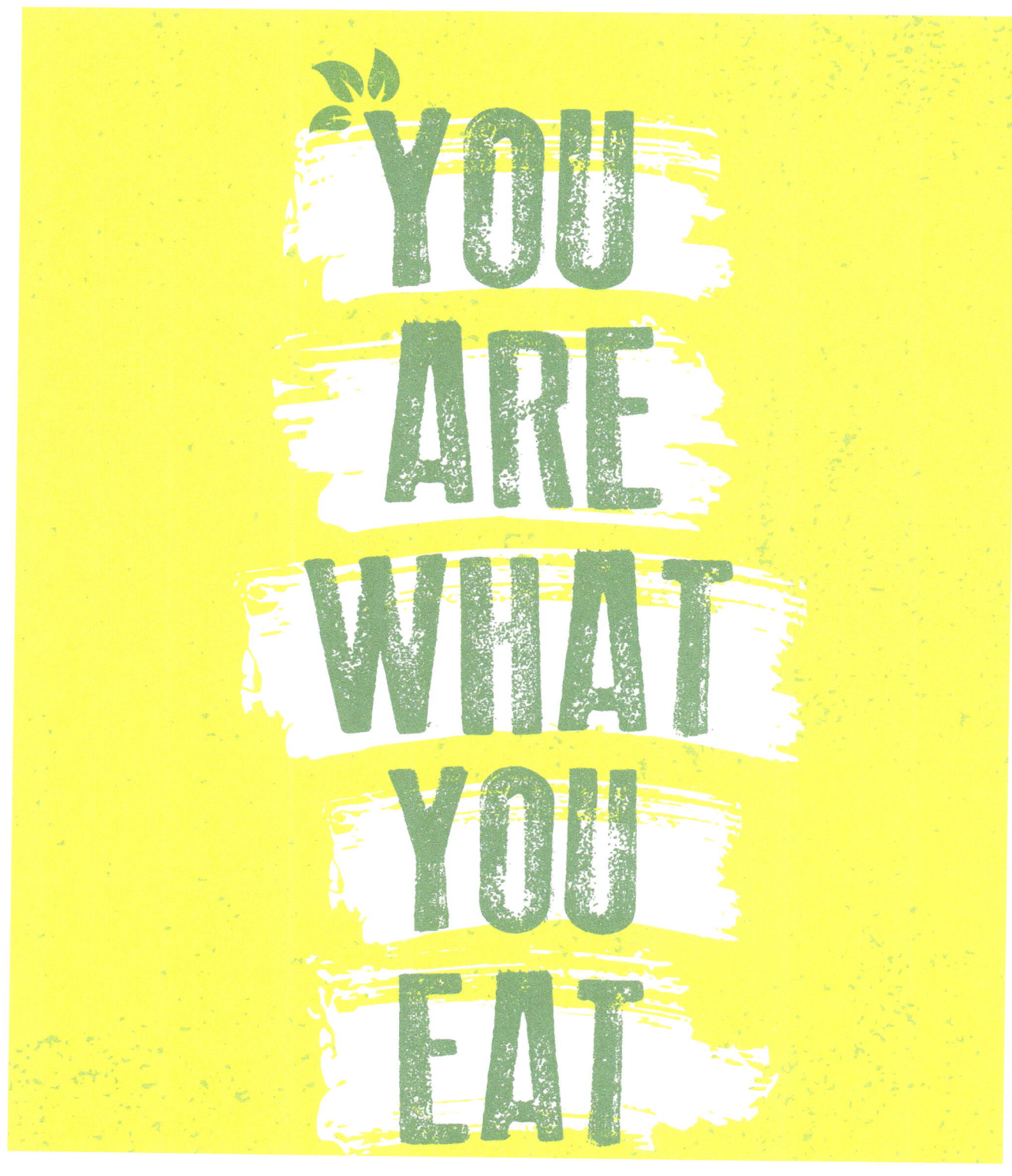

CHAPTER 16

GROCERY STORE STRATEGIES

When we go grocery shopping, we have many potential constraints:

- We are short on time
- We don't have unlimited money
- We only have so much mental bandwidth to spend on shopping
- The store may offer a limited range of choices

Prioritize Priority Foods

The solution to this is to spend our focus and attention on Priority Foods first, then everything else second. Once we know we have all the veggies, fruit, and protein that we need in the cart, then we may make different decisions about the packaged foods.

Buying Veggies and Fruit

With the Baseline Priority Foods Plan and the Vegetable and Fruit Buying Guides, Figures 31a and 31b, we are ready to shop for produce.

Starting in the fresh produce aisle, seek out the items that look the best and are at a good price: i.e., what is "in season". In addition, we are striving to meet our target food longevity distribution. For example, even if berries and bib lettuce are in season and look wonderful, we can only buy a couple of days' worth as they won't last all week. A few other points to keep in mind:

- Do you need to buy organic? The highest priority is to ensure that you buy the right quantity of produce you'll make and eat. The next priority is to select the best quality, time and cost combination for you. Don't let the organic/non-organic question distract you from getting the right amount of your Priority Foods.

- While you are looking at produce, remember that you may want to substitute starchy veggies for some of the processed grains you'd normally eat in order to diversify your sources of carbohydrates.
- Buy what fresh produce makes sense and then plan on filling in the rest with frozen or canned/jarred. Besides being convenient, frozen veggies and fruit can offer high quality and nutrition on par with (or even exceeding) fresh.
- items like onions, garlic and mushrooms may not specifically count toward the veggie goal if you plan to use small amounts in a prepared dish.

Buying Protein

Protein can be expensive and will take up as much of your budget as you let it. Because it does tend to be costly, buying the right amount is important. An informal survey of grocery prices for several basic high-protein foods in early 2024 yielded the data shown in Figure 53 below where each vertical bar shows the price range from low to high. For each protein type, the low end of the price range represents a generic store brand, and the high end is a premium brand-named product. The meat, poultry and fish shown in the graph represent the lower end of the cost spectrum and include fresh and frozen items. Higher end products, not included here, such as fish fillets, shellfish, steaks and roasts tend to be even more expensive, and the cost can vary greatly depending on cut and quality. Of course, costs will also vary with location and access to regional products.

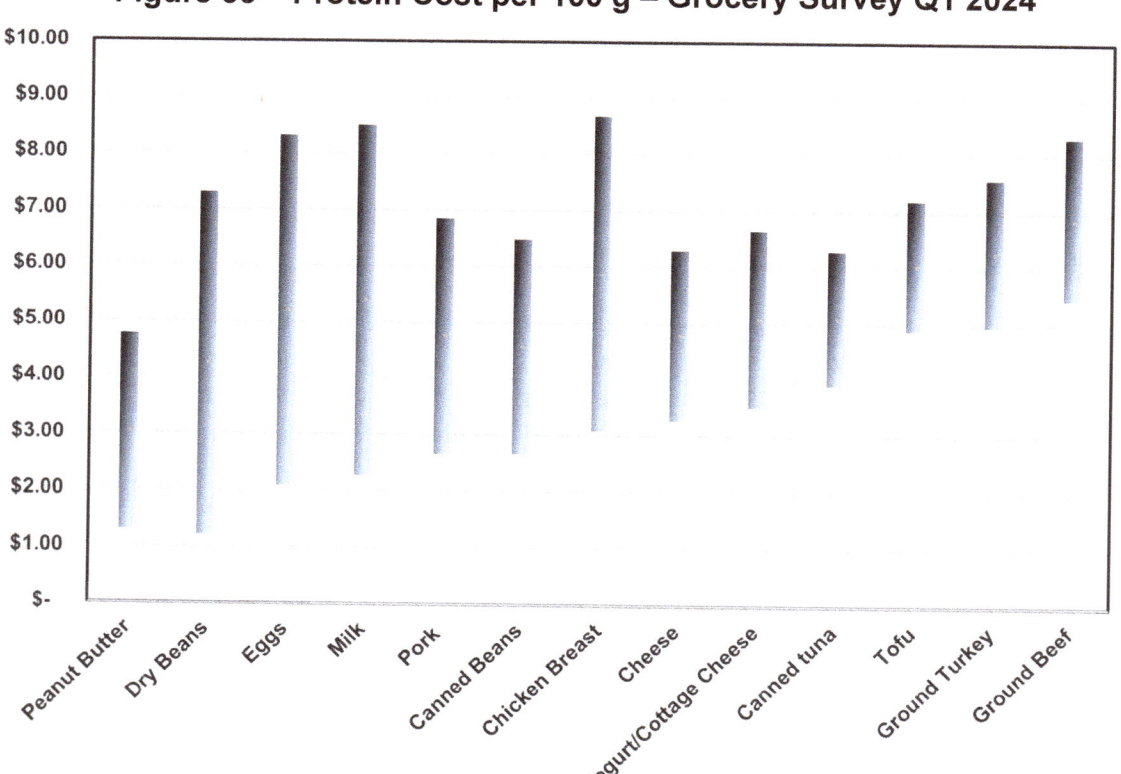

Figure 53 – Protein Cost per 100 g – Grocery Survey Q1 2024

As you can see, there is a range of prices for each type of protein. A couple of conclusions become apparent:

- The low-cost "store-brand" products can be a fraction of the cost compared to brand-named, more exclusive products.
- Legumes (including peanut butter, chickpeas, lentils and all beans) are often the least expensive source of protein.

Even the most careful, cost-conscious consumer will likely pay an average of $3-4 per 100 g of protein for a range of beans, eggs, dairy products, and meat. For the hypothetical family of four from Chapter 9 (Mom, Dad and two kids), the total weekly protein target for high-protein foods is about 2,523 g. Assuming they eat at home for every meal, the protein alone will cost at least $75-100 for a week. Obviously, these costs can escalate dramatically if organic products, and more expensive meats and seafoods are chosen.

Remember our protein guidelines from the DGA recommend at least 5-10% of our protein comes from legumes. Considering these are so nutritious, providing complex carbohydrates, fiber and micronutrients, it makes sense to make them a significant part of our protein plan.

Protein Quality when Eating Out

The cost of a fast-food hamburger is over twice the cost of a homemade one made with high-quality ground beef. The economic and nutritional value of the fast-food meal declines even further when you consider the overall quality and include the inevitable fries and soda.

An important issue about protein purchased in a restaurant is that the nutritional quality is difficult to evaluate. Some restaurants do an excellent job publishing information about their food quality, sources, and degree of processing. Ultra-processed foods like chicken nuggets and pepperoni are easy to identify ourselves. However, most of the time, the quality of protein being served is not obvious. Meat raised with antibiotics and treated with tenderizers, salt and sugar solutions, flavorings, and preservatives is hard to avoid at a restaurant, cafeteria, or fast-food outlet.

Another issue about protein from restaurants is that there is a limited variety to choose from. The most common protein sources in the US are dairy, beef, chicken, and pork. Fish, beans/legumes, tofu, shellfish, nuts and seeds are less common. If seafood is available, it is likely to be deep fried. Protein touted as "plant based" is often an ultra-processed GMO soy product.

Bioengineered: The food formerly known as GMO[37]

Starting in 2022, the USDA requires foods that had previously been labeled as a Genetically Modified Organism (GMO) will now be labeled as "Bioengineered" or "Derived from Bioengineering". There is even a pretty logo showing an idealized countryside to go on the label!

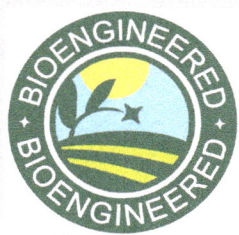

Crops are often bioengineered to be herbicide resistant, pest and disease resistant or to slow spoilage. AquAdvantage Salmon has been bioengineered to grow faster and GalSafe pork is free of a certain compound some people are allergic to. Bioengineered foods are hard to avoid in the US food system. In 2020, the most common commodity crops were nearly exclusively bioengineered:

> » Sugar beet 99.9%
> » Canola 95%
> » Corn 92%
> » Soy 94%.

In addition, 95% of animals used for meat and dairy are fed GMO feed.

The USDA has determined that these bioengineered foods are safe for consumption by humans and animals. However, if you prefer to avoid bioengineered foods, you may need to rely on buying organic.

Shopping for Quality Protein

There are many additional factors about the protein you purchase, particularly the animal-based products, which describe some aspects of production. How do you wade through all of the information? You might see any of the following on the packaging (or not):

- FDA grade
- Antibiotics or growth hormones
- Organic
- Non-GMO (Non-Bioengineered)
- Wild-caught vs farmed seafood
- The animal's diet (grass-fed, grain-fed, corn-fed...)
- Sustainability
- Free-range
- Country where it was produced
- Preservatives/additives.

These factors may be indicators of quality and may infer a higher or lower nutritional benefit. Or maybe not. Is a wild-caught shrimp from the Gulf of Mexico healthier than farmed-raised from Thailand? These labeled factors often indicate a more environmentally friendly production method. You will have to choose which factors are important to you and include these in your overall prioritization. However, keep in mind:

1. Better quality might be the better buy for you. Look at all factors carefully and review them frequently. The price premium for the "better" option may be minor and, as a trend is more widely adopted, the price premium will likely decrease. By way of example, a certain "expensive" organic milk is ultra-pasteurized. If your household rate of consumption is slow, this may be a better value for you since it lasts longer than regular milk.
2. Look for low-cost opportunities to upgrade. For example, you might not be ready to pay for organic, brand-named meat, which can be two to three times more expensive than the regular option. However, there may be an antibiotic-free, hormone-free, preservative-free, or minimally processed option available at a very small premium.
3. Since animal-based protein can be such a big part of the budget, buying in bulk and freezing/storing portions can be very worthwhile. Frozen meat and fish can often be available at a lower price than fresh.
4. Minimize processed meat products like bacon, lunchmeat, and pepperoni. If you do buy them occasionally, look for the least processed option with the least salt and preservatives.
5. You have more control over food quality from the grocery store. Grocery food labeling may be imperfect but at least it is there. This type of information is not readily available at all for food from restaurants, cafeterias, and fast-food outlets.

We have the greatest control over the protein we prepare at home. Therefore, this is the protein that is needed to provide the highest quality and greatest variety. We will judge protein on two criteria: degree of processing and variety. Here is a simple guide to protein selection for home preparation:

Figure 54 – Protein Selection Guide

Buy and Eat Less	Buy and Eat More
Chicken nuggets, pepperoni, lunchmeat, bacon, sausage, hot dogs, processed hamburgers, frozen meals, processed cheese food, processed yogurt.	Unsweetened dairy, tofu, whole nuts and seeds, beans/legumes, unprocessed fresh or frozen meat, poultry, and fish, minimally processed peanut and nut butters.

Then, Buy Everything Else

Once we have selected all the produce and protein we need, we might notice that the cart is pretty full, and we haven't gone down most of the aisles yet. The remaining items to be purchased fall into two categories: ultra-processed and not ultra-processed. The line between the two is not always clear. Look at the labels carefully – it is amazing how much stuff is added to what looks like a simple product. Preservatives added to processed meat. "Peanut butter" with added low-grade oils and sugars. Bread with 20 ingredients. Butter substitutes that are just processed seed oils and chemicals.

For each processed, packaged item that you pick up, ask yourself the following questions:

> » Do I need to buy this, or can I easily make it?
> » If I do need to buy it, is it the least processed option?

OK, so we can't spend the whole day in the grocery store evaluating every single item. However, we can work through our commonly purchased items week by week. Maybe we will do a deep dive on peanut butter this week and settle on a preferred brand. Then next week we'll consider marinara sauce, and so on. Over time we'll have our list of routine items by brand that we think offer the best taste, nutrition, and value. Gradually we will also develop our skills and confidence to make more of the typically ultra-processed foods at home.

It may seem ideal to try and make everything at home from locally sourced, premium ingredients. That's a lovely thought, romanticized in the media – social and otherwise. However, I believe that most people need to make trade-offs. Using minimally processed, but not ultra-processed, sauces (marinara, Indian curry, Asian, etc.) and ingredients (canned beans, peanut butter, cheese, yogurt, etc.) can leverage our cooking efforts to make more home-prepared meals containing more Priority Foods a reality.

In the next chapter we will pull together the Re-Engineered Food Cycle by walking through an example step-by-step for a hypothetical family of four.

Grocery Store Strategies – Key Points

Prioritize Priority Foods
» **Shop for protein and produce first**
» **Use Baseline Priority Foods Plan**

Produce – Vegetables and Fruit
» **Select fresh first then fill in with frozen or canned**

Protein
» **All protein is relatively expensive**
» **Be strategic about quality and cost**
» **Remember to buy a variety of protein-rich foods**
» **Choose minimally processed**

Everything Else (Non-Priority Foods)
» **It is either an ultra-processed food or it is not**
» **For every packaged item:**
   » **Do I need it, or can I make it?**
   » **Is this the least processed option?**
» **Use minimally processed sauces and ingredients to leverage your cooking efforts**

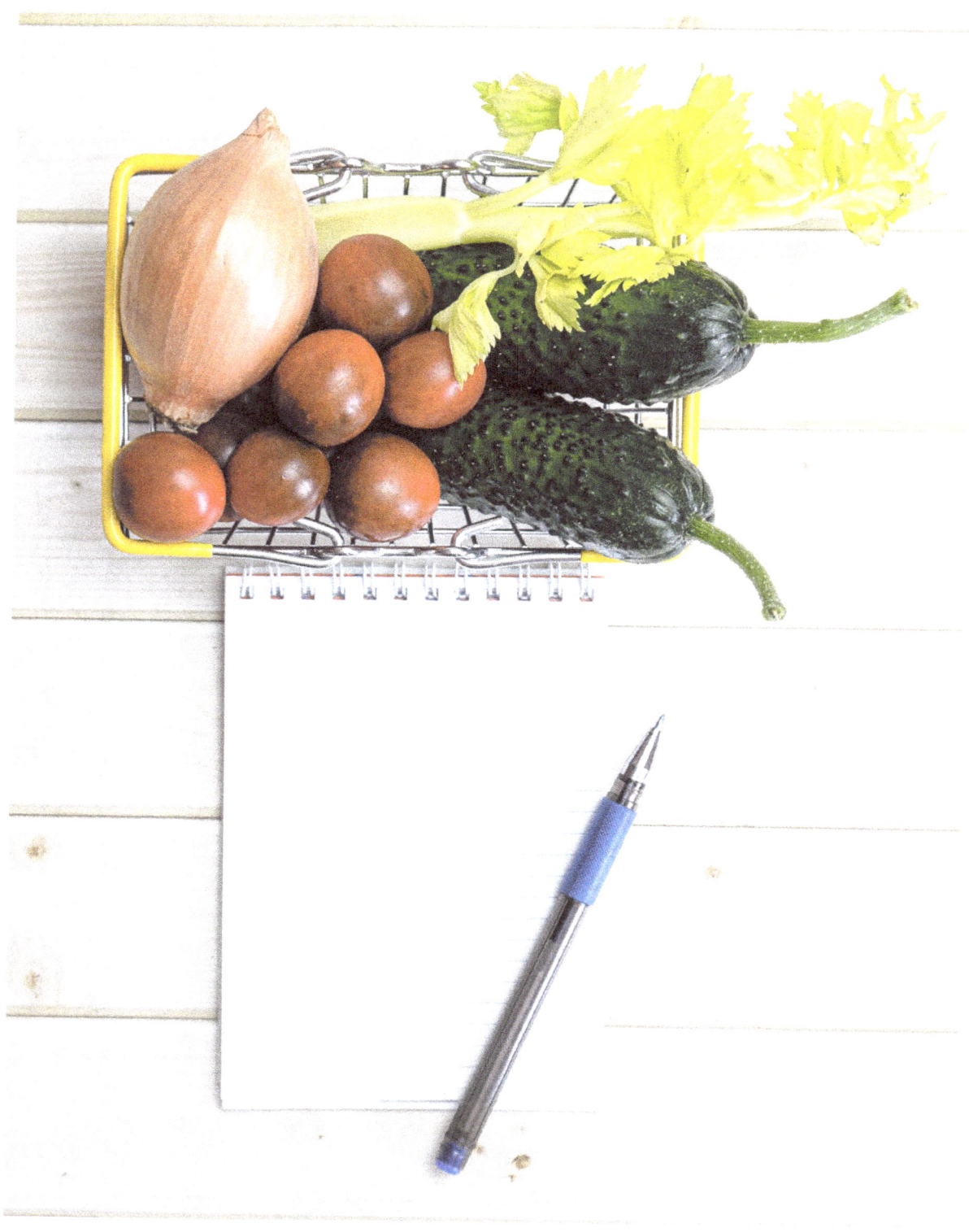

CHAPTER 17

THE RE-ENGINEERED KITCHEN EXAMPLE

We have covered a lot of ground in explaining the Re-Engineered Food Cycle. Let's pull it all together and walk through an example of a hypothetical family of four. Our fantasy family includes Mom (age 38), Dad (age 38), Sister (age 12) and Brother (age 9). All are close to average size and all fall into the "moderate" activity level except the daughter, who is a competitive (but not elite) athlete, falls into the "Active" level. Remember that these are all estimates, and we can make adjustments next week and the week after to better meet our needs and goals.

Step 1: Estimate the Priority Foods targets for each family member for the week using a blank Household Priority Foods Requirements Worksheet, Figure 55 on page 154 (all blank worksheets and referenced tables are available in Appendix B). We will start by recording age, gender and activity level in the first three rows of the worksheet on page 154 for each person. Next, we will look up the estimated calorie level per person in Figure 9 or Figures 65, 66, or 67 in Appendix B using these parameters and enter that value on the next line, Row 4.

Using the calorie level, we can look up the estimated weekly Priority Foods targets for each family member. We'll use Figure 18 for the target c-e for veggies and fruit and enter these numbers on Rows 5 and 8. Then we will use Figure 18 to look up the estimated weekly grams of protein from high-protein foods for each person and enter this on Row 11. Now we have the total weekly Priority Foods targets for veggies, fruit and protein.

The next step requires that we now consider how much of the Priority Foods each person is likely to obtain from outside sources like restaurants or school cafeterias. Let's start with Mom who generally eats two lunches out per week. She almost always orders a salad that has some sort of protein and cheese. Using Figure 26 we can estimate that the Priority Foods she will eat out in those two lunches are two c-eq veggies, zero c-eq fruit, and 70 g of protein, which we will enter on Rows 6, 9 and 12. Dad generally eats lunch out 5 days per week and gets a sandwich or entrée with meat, some cheese and maybe a small serving of a veggie. We can estimate that for each of five lunches he will be getting about 35 g of protein, a half c-eq of veggies and no fruit. We can put the weekly totals in Rows 6, 9 and 12, around 35 g of protein. Both of the kids eat lunch at school and have milk every day. School lunches tend to have on the order of two oz of meat or cheese for a total of about 22 g of protein including the milk. The kids don't generally eat the veggies at lunch but do eat the fruit, estimated to be a half cup per day. The weekly figures can be entered in Rows 6, 9 and 12.

The total weekly Priority Foods-Home (PF-Home) can now be calculated by completing rows 7, 10 and 13, first for each person and then add across to get the weekly total for the family.

Figure 55 – Household Priority Foods Requirements Worksheet

Row	Person =>	1	2	3	4	5	6	Total
1	Name	Mom	Dad	Sis	Bro			
2	Age/Gender	38/F	38/M	12/F	9/M			
3	Activity Level	Mod	Mod	Act	Mod			
4	Calories/Day (Fig 7 and Appendix II)	2,000	2,600	2,400	1,800			
	Veggies, c-eq							
5	Weekly Requirement (Figure 16)	17.5	24.5	21	17.5			80.5
6	Weekly Veggies Out (Figure 20 est.)	2	2.5	0	0			4.5
7	Weekly Veggies Home (Req't – Out)	15.5	22	21	17.5			76
	Fruit, c-eq							
8	Weekly Requirement (Figure 16)	14	14	14	10.5			52.5
9	Weekly Fruit Out (Figure 22 est.)	0	0	2.5	2.5			5
10	Weekly Fruit Home (Req't – Out)	14	14	11.5	8			47.5
	Protein, gm							
11	Weekly Requirement (Figure 16)	585	689	682	567			2,523
12	Weekly Protein Out (Figure 20 est.)	70	175	110	110			465
13	Weekly Protein Home (Req't – Out)	515	514	572	457			2,058

Step 2: Now we are going to take our Priority Foods Targets for Home and turn that into a shopping plan. Using the Baseline Priority Foods Plan Worksheet below (Figure 56), start by entering the household totals (from Figure 55) into Rows 2, 3 and 4.

Let's take a minute and review the totals with a critical eye, especially the produce. These targets represent 2 ½ - 3 ½ cups of vegetables and 1 ½ - 2 cups of fruit each day per person. Based on your family's history, are you thinking, "Sure – sounds fine." Or, "Holy Cow – are you kidding me?" We don't want to see any food wasted but we do want to push ourselves toward our nutritional objectives. This is where selecting foods with a forgiving food longevity can help. We can be aggressive in pursuing our targets but know that if we buy enough longer-longevity foods, we can let some roll over to next week.

Our fantasy family has a fairly stable schedule but still needs flexibility. We are going to start by applying a 33% : 33% : 33% longevity ratio to our Priority Foods. In the Baseline Priority Foods Plan Worksheet, record the chosen ratio on Row 1. Now distribute the Total-Home value for each of our Priority Foods types using the longevity ratio. For instance, the Total-Home Veggies for the week is 76 c-eq. Multiply 76 by 33% and record on Row 2 for each of the longevity categories. Do the same process for Fruit and for Protein.

Figure 56 – Baseline Priority Foods Plan Worksheet

					Longevity Distribution		
Row	Priority Foods	Total	Out	Total-Home	Fast-Fade	Fresh-Med	Long
1	Ratio =>				33%	33%	33%
2	Veggies, c-eq	80.5	4.5	76	25	25	25
3	Fruit, c-eq	52.5	5	47.5	16	16	16
4	Protein, g	2,523	468	2,058	679	679	679

Step 3: Let's get ready to go shopping! Take a blank Baseline Priority Foods Shopping Guide Worksheet and enter your targets on Rows 1, 14 and 27 as shown on Figure 57 below. Make a copy of the Vegetable and Fruit Buying Guides (Fig 31a and 31b), along with the Protein Buying Guide (Figure 32) for easy reference. At this point you could head out to the store and simply fill out the PF Shopping Guide as you go along. However, if you are new to this, I suggest you start filling in the table with items you normally buy. You will quickly see where your historical buying habits diverge from your goals. When you do go to the store, you can always substitute items based on what looks good and is a good value. This example includes meat as a primary protein source. However, this type of worksheet is equally valuable for vegetarians or any eating style. If you are getting significant protein from protein-fortified foods such as protein shakes and high-protein pasta, do include them in the protein section.

Figure 57 – Baseline Priority Foods Shopping Guide Worksheet

		Total	Fast-Fade	Fresh-Med	Long
1	**Veggie Target, c-eq =>**	76	25	25	25
2	Broccoli - 2 packages, Cauliflower - 2 heads	20		20	
4	Romaine - 2 heads	8	8		
5	Peas, frozen - 2 x 12 oz packages	8			8
6	Green beans, frozen - 24 oz package	5			5
7	Tomato - 2 large	4	4		
8	Cabbage - 1 head	8		8	
9	Potatoes - 3 lb	6.5		6.5	
10	Marinara sauce - 24 oz	4			4
11	Tomatoes - 28 oz can	4.25			4.25
12	Onions - 2	4		4	
13	Mushrooms - 16 oz	5	5		
14	Total	76.75	17	38.5	21.25
15	**Fruit Target, c-eq =>**	47.5	15.7	15.7	15.7
16	Bananas - 8	8	8		
17	Peaches - 4	5	5.3		
18	Apples - 6	9		9	
19	Applesauce - 48 oz	12			12
20	Berries - 16 oz, frozen	3.5			3.5
21	Orange juice - 52 oz	13		13	
22	Total	50.5	13.3	22	15.5
23	**Protein Target, g =>**	2,058	679	679	679
24	Milk - 1 gallon	128		128	
25	Eggs - 2 dozen	148		148	
26	Cheese - 32 oz	224			224
27	Ground beef - 3 lb, Ground turkey - 4 lb	700	700		
28	Chicken breast - 2 lb	200		200	
29	Peanut butter - 1 lb	110			110
30	Canned beans - 4 x 15oz	96			96
32	Pork tenderloin - 2 lb	200		200	
33	Canned chickpeas - 2 x 15 oz	48			48
34	Salmon fillets - 1.5 lb	150	150		
35	Greek yogurt - 32 oz	85		85	
36	Total	2,089	850	761	478

Looking at our example you will notice a few things. Firstly, things never add up perfectly but that's OK. This is just a guide to help us buy food according to our objectives. If you notice that the longevity ratios are too misaligned, you may change out a food item or make a mental note to prepare or freeze something right away. Secondly, the list makes it easy to check whether we are meeting our general guidelines about variety. For example, do we have enough different types of veggies? Do we have some fish? Legumes? Limited juice? Thirdly, this is a lot of food. Real food. Highly nutritious food. Your grocery cart is pretty full already and we have yet to buy everything else.

Step 4: Now let's buy carbs and fats. Carbs include all of the cereals, flours, rice, grains, pasta, and breads. Fats just really include butter, cooking and salad oils. The rest of the fat in your diet comes from either whole-food sources or processed food. As you are buying carbs and fats, the most important thing is to buy the least processed alternative. This means the least altered food with the least added sugar, industrial vegetable oils, and additives. Other than fresh breads, most of these items have a long shelf life so it is not critical to buy exactly the right amount for the week as these will keep for several weeks.

Lastly, buy the various staples that you need to stock your kitchen, as well as tea, coffee, and so on. If you normally buy snacks, chips, crackers, candy, ice cream, frozen pizza, sweetened drinks, etc. now is the time to consider if you need them at all, given all the food you already have in your cart.

When you get home, you still must figure out how and when you are going to prepare all this food. You may have favorite recipes for much of it but the "What to do with _____" charts in the next chapter can direct you to Agile Recipes™ specifically for the ingredients you have purchased.

Step 5: Next, we should distribute the Priority Foods we have bought by day for each person and then check that we are meeting our targets. This is a little tedious, but you really only have to do this once. Remember, we are only allocating the Priority Foods, not the bread, cereal, pasta, rice, snacks, etc. Figure 58 on the following page is an example of our hypothetical dad.

As you go through this process, you will start to get a better feeling for how portions relate to dietary guidelines. For example, on day 5 in Figure 58 on the following page, Dad is going to eat 3 c-eq of cauliflower at dinner. (Hope he likes cauliflower!) That is 3 cups raw but shrinks when cooked. If you bought a medium-sized head of cauliflower, this is half of the head. That's why we bought two heads. You may also notice that it can be challenging to get significant veggies at breakfast and lunch, especially if you are eating outside the home often.

Figure 58 – Daily Priority Foods Distribution Worksheet Example – Dad

	Priority Foods Distribution			Requirement Check		
Day	Breakfast	Lunch	Dinner	Veggie	Fruit	Protein
Daily Targets =>				3.5	2	98
1	8 oz milk (8 g) banana, 4 oz OJ	Lunch out: 35 g, 1/2 c-eq veggie	8 oz salmon (50 g), 2 C broccoli	2.5	2	93
2	2 eggs (12 g) canteloupe (2 c-eq)	Lunch out: 35 g, 1/2 c-eq veggie	Turkey chili (50 g + 1 c-eq veggie), salad (2 c-eq)	3.5	2	97
3	8 oz milk (8 g), banana, 4 oz OJ	Lunch out: 35 g, 1/2 c-eq veggie	8 oz pork (50 g), 2 C cabbage, 2 C peas	3.5	2	93
4	2 eggs (12 g) canteloupe (2 c-eq)	Lunch out: 35 g, 1/2 c-eq veggie	8 oz meatballs (50 g), sauce (1 C), mushrooms (1 C)	2.5	2	97
5	Gr yogurt (17 g) strawberries (1 C), 4 oz OJ	Lunch out: 35 g, 1/2 c-eq veggie	Chicken & chick-pea masala (45 g), cauliflower (3 C)	3.5	2	97
6	2 eggs (12 g) applesauce (1 C)	Pork & cheese flabread (33 g), cauliflower (1.5 C)	Chili tostadas w/ cheese (50 g + 1/2 V), 2 C green beans	3.5	2	95
7	Gr yogurt (17 g), 1 C OJ	2 oz peanut butter, 1 oz cheese, (214 g), 1 apple	6 oz chicken, 2 oz cheese (50 g), 2 C cabbage, 1.5 C potatoes	3.5	2.5	88

Step 6: Are we done now? Not quite. At the end of the week, we need to check on how we did; we need the feedback step. Did we eat all of the PFs that we bought? Did we throw anything away? Did the PFs run out before the end of the week? Consider what could be improved for next week. Do we need to change the PF targets? Change to a more forgiving longevity ratio? Find ways to make some of the PFs more appealing and/or quicker to prepare? This book has given you the strategies and techniques to achieve your goals. With each successive week, the process will become easier and soon feel automatic. With each successive week you will be making progress to put more Real Food on your table faster, easier, and cheaper.

Example – Key Points

Step 1 – Complete Fig. 55 - Priority Foods Req'ts Worksheet
  » Enter gender, age, activity levels in rows 1-3
  » Enter daily calories from Fig. 9 or Appendix B in row 4
  » Enter Priority Food targets per family member using Fig. 18 in rows 5, 8, 11
  » Calculate Priority Foods Out using Fig. 26 and enter in rows 6, 9, 12
  » Calculate Priority Foods Home and enter in rows 7, 10, 13
    » Priority Foods Home = Targets - Priority Foods Out

Step 2 – Create Figure 56 – Baseline Priority Foods Plan
  » Transfer data from Figure 55 to Figure 56 for rows 2, 3, 4
  » Determine food longevity ratio for your lifestyle and enter in row 1
  » Calculate what to buy and complete rows 2, 3, 4

Step 3 – Complete Figure 57 – Priority Foods Shopping Guide
  » Enter targets from Figure 56 in rows 1, 14, 27
  » Use Figures 31 and 32 to help complete Figure 57
  » First time: fill out trial form in preparation for shopping
  » Normally: use as guide and complete when shopping

Step 4 – In-store choices
  » Carbs and fats => minimally processed options
  » Staples to stock your kitchen
  » Last and least: ultra-processed snacks, drinks, etc.

Step 5 – Complete Figure 58 – Daily Priority Foods Distribution
  » Do this for each family member

Step 6 – Feedback Loop: Evaluate if you ate all the Priority Foods purchased. Adjust for the next week.

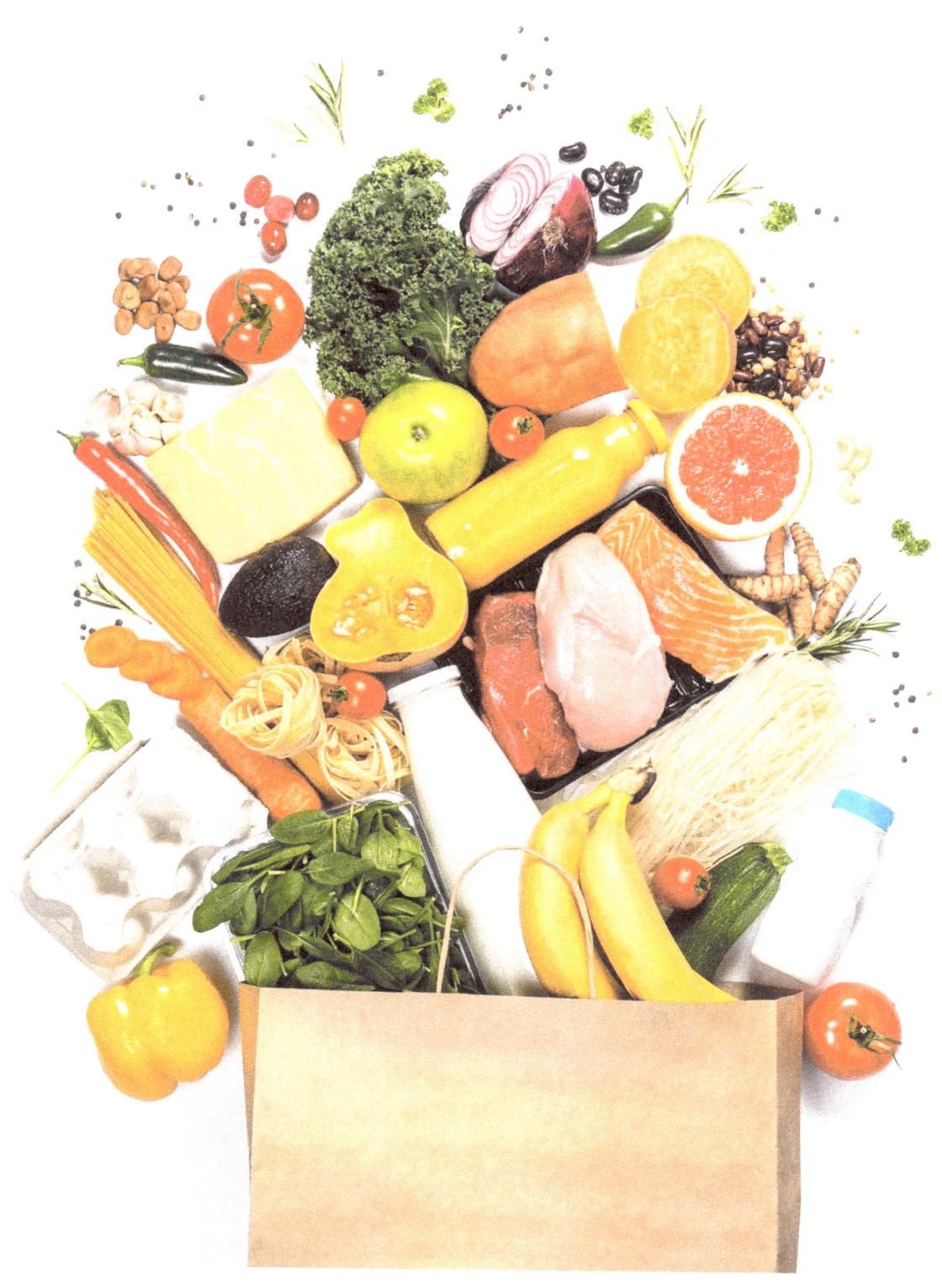

CHAPTER 18

WE HAVE GROCERIES – NOW WHAT?

Now that you have purchased your groceries for the week, you may be wondering what you are going to do with it all. Remember, you have purchased your target amount of Priority Foods based on quality and value, not ingredients for predetermined recipes. You may have a few ideas and favorite recipes for some of these foods (great!) but probably not for everything. Not to worry; we have a plan for that!

Included in this book are recipes that focus on simple ways to prepare many of the most common Priority Foods. But right now, we need a plan for the week. How do we decide what we are going to make and when? To make the process easy, we have "What to do with _____" tables. These tables allow you to look up recipe ideas by key ingredients. If you look up broccoli, you'll find four recipes to choose from. These tables also allow you to cross-reference the recipes to see potential variations in the key ingredient. For example, the recipe for Enchilada Surprise shows that it can be made with a variety of different proteins. This means that you can always purchase the priority foods that look best, confident that you have quick and easy preparation ideas handy.

Start by looking at the Priority Foods you just purchased. Plan for the Fast-Fade foods first knowing that you will need to prepare these in the next few days. Perhaps list out the key Priority Foods you plan to eat by day, keeping food longevity in mind as well as your personal schedule. Now jot down how you plan to prepare those foods. If you are stuck for ideas or just want some variation, look at the "What to do with _____" charts for possible options. The "What to do with _____" charts starting on the next page are organized around our Priority Foods. This is the start of your plan. Things may shift during the week and that is fine. However, if you have a plan for the week, it is much more likely that the food you purchased will be prepared and eaten.

In Chapters 19 and 20 we will introduce you to the new Agile Recipe™ format.

Page #	Figure 59 — What to do With Meat	Ground Beef	Steak	Skirt or Flank Steak	Canned Chicken	Ground Chicken	Chicken Breast Bnls	Chicken on Bone	Turkey (include ground)	Pork (include sausage)	Leftover/Cooked Meat	Shrimp	Canned Tuna	Fresh Fish
232	5-Minute Flatbread^V – 4 Ways						X			X	X			
233	Asian Glazed Anything^V		X				X			X	X	X		
234	Baked Rice Casserole^V				X	X	X	X	X	X	X			
235	Balsamic Glazed Chicken						X							
298	Beans and Rice^V									X				
236	Beef Stroganoff	X	X											
201	Breakfast Sausage					X			X	X				
238	Chicken Curry – 2 Ways				X		X	X	X		X			
239	Chicken Divan				X	X	X		X					
240	Chicken Mushroom Marsala						X				X			
241	Chicken Paillard						X							
242	Chicken Paprika						X	X						
243	Chicken Salad – 4 Ways						X	X						
244	Chili Express	X	X			X			X		X			
245	Citrus Grilled Shrimp											X		
247	Enchilada Surprise^V – 3 Ways	X			X	X	X	X	X	X	X			
248	Fajitas		X	X			X	X				X		
249	Fried Rice^V						X			X	X			
250	Glazed Salmon – 3 Ways													X
251	Hammered Chops									X				

Page #	Figure 59 What to do With Meat	Ground Beef	Steak	Skirt or Flank Steak	Canned Chicken	Ground Chicken	Chicken Breast Bnls	Chicken on Bone	Turkey (include ground)	Pork (include sausage)	Leftover/Cooked Meat	Shrimp	Canned Tuna	Fresh Fish
252	Italian Sausage – Scratch					X			X	X				
254	Lemon Butter Baked Fish													X
256	Marinated Flank Steak			X										
257	Meatballs – Italian	X				X			X	X				
258	Meatloaf – 5 Ways	X				X			X	X				
259	Oven-Fried Chicken – 4 Ways						X							
282	Pasta Salad^v – 4 Ways												X	
261	Picadillo	X								X				
262	Poached Chicken						X	X				X		X
263	Roasted Pork Tenderloin									X				
208	Sausage Brunch Bake								X	X				
264	Shrimp Scampi											X		
265	Sloppy Joes	X				X			X					
266	Spaghetti Sauce w/ Meat	X				X			X	X				
268	Tacos	X	X			X	X		X	X	X			
269	Teriyaki for All^v		X	X		X				X		X		
270	Tuna Cake												X	
284	Tuna Salad Niçoise												X	
271	Tuna Salad – 2 Ways												X	
272	Yogurt Marinated Chicken						X	X						

Page #	Figure 60 What to do With Legumes, Eggs, and Dairy	Chickpeas	Black Beans	Lentils	Red Beans	White Beans	Eggs	Cheese	Cottage Cheese/Ricotta	Milk/Cream	Tofu
296	$100 Macaroni & Cheese^V							X	X	X	
232	5-Minute Flatbread^V – 4 Ways							X			
233	Asian Glazed Aything^V										X
234	Baked Rice Casserole – 3 Ways						X	X		X	
191	Baked Salsa Dip^V							X			
276	Bean Salad^V – 4 Ways	X	X		X	X					
325	Bean Soup Express		X		X	X					
298	Beans and Rice^V – 3 Ways		X		X						
237	Black Bean & Sweet Potato Chili^V		X								
214	Bread Pudding^V – 5 Ways						X			X	
244	Chili Express		X		X	X					
302	Continental Beans^V		X		X	X					
192	Crispy Chickpea Snacks^V – 4 Ways	X									
202	Egg Cups^V – 5 Ways						X	X	X		
219	Egg Custard^V						X			X	
204	French Toast Casserole^V						X		X	X	

Page #	Figure 60 What to do With Legumes, Eggs, and Dairy	Chickpeas	Black Beans	Lentils	Red Beans	White Beans	Eggs	Cheese	Cottage Cheese/Ricotta	Milk/Cream	Tofu
249	Fried Rice^V						X				X
191	Hummus^V	X									
253	Lasagna Florentine^V						X	X	X		
255	Lentils del Sol^V			X							
328	Lentil Soup^V – 5 Ways			X							
224	Milk Pudding^V – 5 Ways						X			X	
206	Potato Frittata^V – 4 Ways						X	X			
316	Rice Pilaf^V – 4 Ways							X			
227	Rice Pudding^V – 2 Ways						X			X	
207	Ricotta Pancakes^V						X		X		
228	Ricotta Cheesecake^V						X		X		
208	Sausage Brunch Bake						X	X		X	
320	Savory White Beans^V					X					
209	Spinach Mushroom Bake^V						X	X	X		
267	Stuffed Shells^V						X	X	X		
210	Swedish Pancakes^V						X			X	

Page #	Figure 61 What to do With Fruit and Grain	Apple	Applesauce	Banana	Dried Fruit	Fresh Berries	Frozen Berries	Peach, Plum, Apricot	Pineapple	Bread, Tortillas	Oats	Rice, Quinoa	Flour, Wheat, Pasta, etc.
296	$100 Macaroni & Cheese[v]												X
232	5-Minute Flatbread[v] – 4 Ways									X			
211	Applesauce Oatmeal Crisp[v]		X		X						X		
234	Baked Rice Casserole[v]											X	
194	Banana Bread[v]			X									X
212	Bananas Foster[v]			X									
298	Beans and Rice[v] – 3 Ways											X	
195	Beer Bread[v]												X
196	Biscuits/Shortcake[v] – 5 Ways												X
213	Brandied Peaches[v]							X					
214	Bread Pudding[v] – 5 Ways				X					X			
216	Brownies[v]												X
217	Butter Berry Cobbler[v]					X	X	X					X
278	Carrot Salad w/ Fruit[v]	X			X				X				
218	Chocolate Applesauce Cake[v]		X		X								X
197	Corn Bread[v]												X
220	Essential Cake[v] – 6 Ways												X
223	Fast Fruit Filling[v]					X	X	X					

Page #	Figure 61 What to do With Fruit and Grain	Apple	Applesauce	Banana	Dried Fruit	Fresh Berries	Frozen Berries	Peach, Plum, Apricot	Pineapple	Bread, Tortillas	Oats	Rice, Quinoa	Flour, Wheat, Pasta, etc.
249	Fried Rice^V											X	
204	French Toast Casserole^V						X			X			
198	Irish Soda Bread^V												X
199	No Touch Bread^V												X
205	Oatmeal Pancakes^V										X		X
282	Pasta Salad^V – 4 Ways												X
225	Pantry Cake^V												X
226	Pumpkin Muffins^V												X
316	Rice Pilaf^V – 4 Ways											X	
227	Rice Pudding^V – 2 Ways				X							X	
283	Rice Salad^V – 3 Ways											X	
207	Ricotta Pancakes^V												X
229	Russian Tea Cakes^V												X
230	Spiced Poached Fruit^V	X					X	X					
210	Swedish Pancakes^V												X
268	Tacos, Tostadas, Enchiladas									X			
200	Yeast Rolls^V												X

Page #	Figure 62 What to do With Vegetables	Baby Bok Choy	Broccoli	Brussels Sprouts	Collard Greens	Kale	Salad Greens	Spinach	Cabbage
232	5-Min Flatbread^V							X	
297	Aloo Gobi^V								
276	Bean Salad^V – 4 Ways								
325	Bean Soup Express^V								
237	Black Bean and Sweet Potato Chili^V								
299	Braised Cabbage^V								X
277	Brussels Sprouts Salad^V			X					
278	Carrot Salad w/ Fruit^V								
300	Cauliflower Marinara^V								
301	Citrus Glazed Brussels Sprouts^V			X					
290	Classic Marinara Sauce^V								
326	Cream of Mushroom Soup^V								
303	Creamed Vegetables^V							X	X
279	Cucumber Salads^V								
292	Enchilada Sauce^V								
247	Enchilada Surprise^V								
327	French Onion Soup^V								
249	Fried Rice^V								
304	Frizled Cabbage^V – 3 Ways								X
305	Glazed Carrots^V – 4 Ways								
280	Green Bean Salad w/ Goat Cheese^V								
306	Green Beans^V – 4 Ways								

Cauliflower	Cucumber	Green Beans	Mushrooms	Onions	Summer Squash	Bell Peppers	Carrots	Spaghetti Squash	Sweet Potato	Winter Squash	Corn	Peas	Potato	Tomatoes
			X	X		X								X
X													X	
		X												
				X			X						X	
				X					X					X
				X			X							
							X							
X														X
				X										X
			X											
X		X	X								X	X	X	
	X													
				X										X
									X		X			
				X										
				X			X						X	
				X			X							
							X							
		X												
		X	X											

Page #	Figure 62 What to do With Vegetables	Baby Bok Choy	Broccoli	Brussels Sprouts	Collard Greens	Kale	Salad Greens	Spinach	Cabbage
307	Green Bean Sucotash^V								
308	Green Bean Un-Casserole^V								
309	Lemon Bacon Brussels Sprouts^V			X					
310	Lemon Garlic Kale^V					X			
311	Mediterranean Spaghetti Squash^V								
313	Moroccan Cauliflower^V								
294	Mushroom Parmesan Cream Sauce^V								
281	Napa Cabbage Salad^V								X
330	Potato Broccoli Soup^V		X						
206	Potato Frittata^V							X	
314	Quick Creamed Spinach^V							X	
315	Quick Spaghetti Squash^V								
316	Rice Pilaf^V - 4 Ways		X						
317	Roasted Vegetables^V – 5 Ways		X	X					
319	Sautéed Baby Bok Choy^V	X							
321	Simple Greens^V				X				
322	Spinach – Flash Sautéed^V							X	
209	Spinach Mushroom Bake^V							X	
323	Sweet Potato Casserole^V								
269	Teriyaki for All^V								
284	Tuna Salad Niçoise						X		
324	Vegetables au Gratin^V		X						
331	Vegetable Soup^V					X			X

Cauliflower	Cucumber	Green Beans	Mushrooms	Onions	Summer Squash	Bell Peppers	Carrots	Spaghetti Squash	Sweet Potato	Winter Squash	Corn	Peas	Potato	Tomatoes
		X									X			
		X												
				X	X	X		X						X
X														
			X											
													X	
													X	
				X										
				X				X						
			X	X			X						X	
X			X	X	X	X	X		X	X			X	
			X											
									X					
			X	X		X	X							
		X											X	X
X							X		X				X	
		X		X			X				X	X	X	X

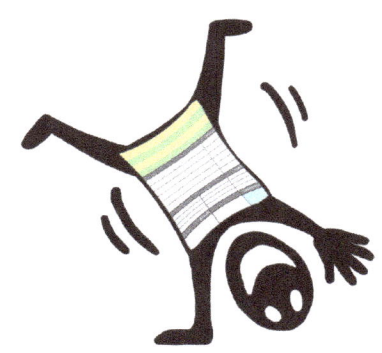

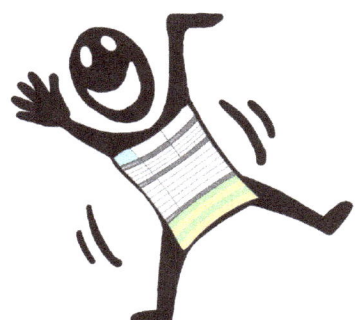

Celebrate – we've gone through the entire process.

Now its time to cook!

We Have Groceries – Now What? – Key Points

Lay out what to eat by day
  » Consider food longevity
  » Include preparation ideas

Use "What to do with _____" charts for ideas

"You don't have to cook fancy or complicated masterpieces – just good food from fresh ingredients."

– Julia Child

CHAPTER 19

INTRODUCING THE AGILE RECIPE™

So far, we have discussed improving our Food Cycle by determining our nutritional objectives and buying the right foods, including our important Priority Foods. We have an idea of what we are going to make with these foods by using a combination of our own favorite recipes and looking up recipes on the "What to do with _____" charts in the last chapter. The recipes in this book are focused on simple ways to prepare Priority Foods and homemade alternatives to ultra-processed foods. However, these recipes are not just "easy", they have been completely redesigned to be efficient and flexible. These recipes are a tool to help you implement the next step of the Re-Engineered Food Cycle by preparing Real Food more often.

The Best Recipe

How is it that, with the proliferation of recipes from cookbooks, online recipe collections, magazines, and television shows we still struggle to find the right recipe? I get food magazines and have a healthy collection of cookbooks, recipe cards, and stacks of loose paper recipes, complete with hand-scribbled notes and petrified food stains. I enjoy just reading recipes and I often learn some new technique or flavor combination. That doesn't mean I will ever make any of these recipes. Frequently, the recipe just doesn't fit my situation. It is too long and complicated. It has an ingredient that I am unlikely to buy, and I am unsure if the recipe will tolerate a substitution. I can't envision a scenario where I would purchase $25 worth of fresh herbs for a single dish. Or maybe something doesn't look "right" – so I waste time looking at other recipes for the same thing, trying to judge if the proportions are correct. Or worse, I go down the Internet rabbit hole of reading recipe reviews. Before I realize it, I have spent an improbable amount of time trying to find a recipe that works for the pork chops I need to cook right now.

I have many beloved recipes that are long and intricate; they require precise proportions and exact procedures. If I am going to make those dishes, I need to take the time to make them right. They may not happen often but, when they do, they play to rave reviews. Crème Brûlée is an example. It requires many steps, multiple pans, tempered eggs, pouring the liquid into ramekins that are bathed in hot water, gently baked, cooled, and, finally, glazed with that delightful, caramelized sugar. This is a celebratory treat that happens, at best, once per year. This may be a wonderful recipe, but you will not find it here in this book. It is too complicated, time-consuming, allows no substitutions, and is unforgiving.

How do you judge a recipe? It goes without saying that the result must be delicious. Other than that, the best recipe is the one that suits the situation at hand.

Updated Recipe Format

The format of recipes has changed very little in centuries. You can easily understand historical cookbooks, an attribute that makes them charming souvenirs. We may find the outdated terminology quaint (a thumb of butter, or glass of sugar), but the basic format is familiar to us: a list of ingredients then instructions. While this format has enjoyed centuries of acceptance and success, it does leave room for improvement. We have improved many of our processes at home, school, and work and, along with that, we have improved our communication and documentation of those processes. Think of all the instructions that have become visually accessible and intuitive: clothing and food labels, web navigation, electronic device operations, and DIY furniture assembly to name just a few.

Features to improve the old recipe format would include:

- Make it easy to understand the scope of the recipe at a glance.
- Clearly show the essential ingredients and possible substitutions.
- List options separate from the basic recipe.
- Ensure it is visually accessible – your eyes quickly find the information you seek.
- Keep it brief – eliminate unnecessary information.
- Be consistent with layout so the same information is always in the same place.

These format changes will improve the recipe by communicating more information and doing so more efficiently.

Streamlined Process

Whenever I cook, I am always looking for process-improvement opportunities. At each step, I am considering what value that action or ingredient adds. Can I consolidate steps? Is it really necessary to list oil as an ingredient when it is just a pan lubrication? Do you really need to mix the dry ingredients in a separate bowl? Can you make this without the special-purpose equipment? How can clean-up be minimized? How can we minimize wasted ingredients? (I hate it when a recipe calls for a partial container of something!) Which ingredients can be omitted or substituted?

All the recipes in this book are designed to taste great yet be simple, reliable, flexible, and forgiving. They have been re-engineered to achieve our many objectives, including reducing waste.

Process improvement changes have been made to:

- Minimize steps and effort.
- Use commonly available ingredients and list substitutions.
- Include information to meet some dietary requirements.
- Proportion recipe to fit common package sizes.
- Reduce the required equipment to the minimum, include low-tech options.
- Minimize the amount of kitchen clean-up required

Why streamline a recipe at all?

For example, most traditional biscuit recipes require many steps using a pastry cutter, multiple bowls and measuring cups, a pastry board and rolling pin, etc. – resulting in a second "project" to clean-up afterward! The streamlined recipe for biscuits used here only requires a single glass bowl, knife, fork, measuring spoon and a scoop as shown in the photo: low impact, minimal clean-up.

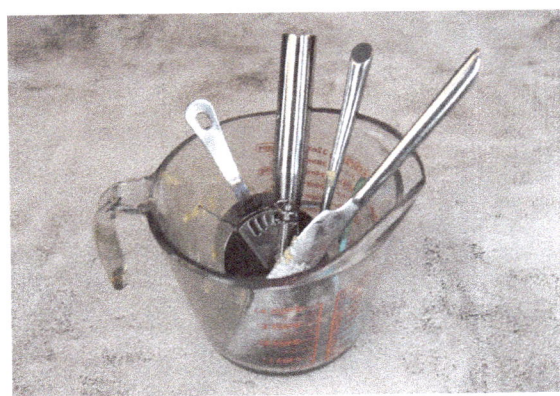

After re-designing the format and re-engineering the processes, the result is so different from a conventional recipe that it deserves a new name: the Agile Recipe™!

Guide to Agile Recipes™

Every Agile Recipe™ follows the same, intuitive layout so that information is accessible at a glance. The graphic features make it easier to find the information as you look back and forth between your cooking and the Agile Recipe™. The one-page layout will display concisely on paper or the screen of your device (download PDFs of Agile Recipes™ at www.ReEngineeringtheKitchen.com). A sample recipe is shown on the following page.

Figure 63 – Sample Agile Recipe™

New Graphic Layout
Visually Accessible at a Glance
Intuitive and Consistent

Key Ingredient Type

Substitutions

Type of Dish

Essential
Ingredients

Streamlined
Steps

Variations

GRAIN	Biscuit/Shortcake^V Makes 6 Biscuits		BREAD
INGREDIENTS		**SUBSTITUTE**	
3 Tbsp	Butter	Crisco or margarine	
1½ C	Flour (180 g)	1 C rice flour + ½ C tapioca flour (GF) or substitute up to 50% whole grain flour	
½ Tbsp	Baking powder		
½ Tbsp	Sugar	Brown sugar or dry sugar substitute	
½ tsp	Salt		
½ C	Milk	Half & Half or buttermilk or half cream/half water	
STEPS			
1	Preheat oven to 400°F. Grease pan or line with parchment.		
2	In a heat-proof glass bowl or 4 C glass measuring cup, warm butter to room temp in micro.		
3	Add flour to bowl with butter. If you have a scale, weigh flour directly into your bowl.		
4	Add baking powder, salt and sugar to flour. Stir to distribute dry ingredients.		
5	With a fork, work the flour mixture and butter together until it becomes coarse and grainy.		
6	Add milk and stir just enough to fully incorporate.		
7	Use scoop or spoon to make 6 rounded biscuits. Each should be about 1½ inches high.		
8	Bake for 12-18 minutes, until golden brown at edges.		
9	Store covered. May reheat for 5 minutes in 350° F oven or 15 seconds in micro.		
OPTIONS			
A	**Rolled Biscuits:** Roll dough on floured surface to about ¾ inch thickness. Cut with cookie cutter or with a glass or jar of desired diameter.		
B	**Cheese Biscuits:** Stir in ½ C any shredded cheese into dough. Can add ½ tsp garlic powder to dry ingredients for more savory flavor.		
C	**Cinnamon Bun Biscuits:** Place biscuits close together in 9" pan, flatten each slightly by hand. Mix 2 Tbsp soft butter with 1 tsp cinnamon and 2 Tbsp sugar. Spread paste over biscuits prior to baking.		
D	**Shortcake:** Add another ½ Tbsp of sugar to the dough. For decoration, brush with butter and sprinkle with sugar prior to baking.		

The Agile Recipes™ will give the basic recipe and then several variations or options, so you can make it work for you. The variations might suggest additional ingredients, variable flavor combinations, options using store-bought vs. homemade components, sweet and savory renditions or a list of compatible ingredients.

Referring to the sample Biscuit/Shortcake Agile Recipe™ on the previous page, here are some of the features that make it an Agile Recipe™ compared to a typical recipe:

Revised Process:

- Use only one prep bowl:
    - Use tempered glass so cold or frozen butter can be microwaved.
    - Measure dry ingredients directly into the bowl with butter. Incorporate baking powder and salt by stirring into flour while on top of the butter.
- Use scale to measure flour – increases accuracy, less measuring overspill, and no measuring cup to wash.
- Use a fork to cut in flour and butter (eliminates hard-to-clean pastry cutter).
- Use a scoop or rounded spoon to get rounded biscuits – eliminates messy rolling but looks better than "drop biscuits".

Substitutions:

- » Substitutions for different fats.
- » Proportions for common gluten-free flours.
- » Substitutions for milk.

Options:

- Option to make a sweeter shortcake.
- Can be rolled and cut for a fancier presentation.
- Savory cheese biscuits.
- Cinnamon bun biscuits.

Would I use this recipe when hosting a fancy brunch? Absolutely. Perhaps I would "flex" it toward the higher-end result by using buttermilk and rolling/cutting the biscuits for a prettier presentation. On the other hand, I am willing to make the basic version of these biscuits at the drop of a hat because they can be so easy and low impact. I have never had anyone turn down a fresh biscuit, hot out of the oven. The "best" recipe is the one that meets your needs at the moment.

Why is this collection of Agile Recipes™ unique?

What is the difference between this collection of recipes and other cookbooks, websites, and cooking shows? The Agile Recipes™ here are included for one reason and one reason only: to help you put Real Food on your table faster, easier, and cheaper. This means having easy preparation methods for your Priority Foods and homemade options for often ultra-processed foods. There is no discussion of the recipe's origin or history. There is no charming story about Aunt Bertie making this dish for every holiday. There is no lengthy description of technique or pictures of the steps. I admit that I do enjoy reading such things elsewhere, but not when I need to get a meal prepared right now. The two approaches to presenting recipes represent two entirely different objectives.

This makes sense when you consider that we are now living in the "Attention Economy", a term coined by political scientist Herbert A. Simon. Our most valuable companies are those that command your attention the most effectively. Everyone who develops and delivers content is trying to make money from ads. Most food-related content is developed primarily as entertainment, with a modicum of information for value. They make money by maintaining your attention. This applies to everyone from the busy-mom-with-a-cooking-website to the multi-channel behemoths with a print, web, and television presence. With this perspective in mind, you can see that brevity is not aligned with the objective of maintaining attention for the longest time. It is not to say that one approach is inherently better or worse – it just means that they are different.

Another way that this collection of Agile Recipes™ is different than the norm is how the recipes are structured. Agile Recipes™ have a "Theme and Variation" structure. Historically, each normal recipe leads to one outcome. For instance, making tacos with ground chicken, turkey, or beef would involve at least three distinct recipes (or more if you can find ways to vary the recipe and photos with different accents). The Agile Recipe™ for Tacos is one "theme" recipe, with several "variations" outlined. It is a waste of the readers' time to repeat the same core information multiple times – and make them hunt and peck to find what they need. But remember, commandeering your time is their primary objective! How many ads did you view while you were sifting through six recipes?

The unique Theme and Variation structure of Agile Recipes™ requires a new way of organizing the recipes to support our Re-Engineered Food Cycle. First, we organize the recipes around the primary ingredients: Vegetables, Protein (meat), Protein (other), Fruits, and Grains. Protein (meat) includes beef, pork, poultry, and fish. Protein (other) includes dairy products, eggs, and legumes. You may notice that many recipes have ingredients from multiple categories, but we choose the primary to be the most prevalent ingredients and/or one of our Priority Foods. For each category of ingredient, there is a "What to do with _____" matrix as discussed in the prior chapter. This allows us to efficiently find preparation alternatives for our Priority Foods and homemade options for commonly processed foods. Next, the recipes are categorized by the type of dish, e.g. Main, Side, Dessert.

Also included are recipes for Salad Dressings, Brines & Marinades, and Sauces. There are Agile Recipes™ for several key "from scratch" sauces. However, the rest of the recipes for each category are so super-simple and quick to assemble that they are in charts. There is a chart each for Salad Dressings, Sauces, and Brines & Marinades so that it is efficient to review and then quickly prepare one. The charts list the ingredients and instructions as needed.

Biases

You will notice that the recipes included here start with very basic ingredients and are average American in their taste. While this may reflect my own taste and relative expertise, it is also very intentional. I reasoned that, if you have purchased an expensive cut of meat or seafood, you probably either already know how to prepare it or it is a special occasion that warrants figuring out how to do so properly. Similarly, I avoided getting too deeply into specific international cuisines (e.g., Asian, Indian). I tried to include only recipes that could be made without visiting a specialty grocer in person or online. If you have an interest in, say, Thai cooking then you either already know more than I do and/or are going to look elsewhere to learn. I do include a few international recipes that use prepared sauces and/or spice blends that are widely available.

Using salt

You may also notice (and any professional chefs will be aghast) that I frequently include only a small amount of salt or note salt as optional. Our family intentionally tries to moderate our sodium intake. Any packaged food and restaurant foods are likely to be heavily salted, so we compensate with lower-sodium home-prepared foods. However, this is a personal choice, and you may find the recipes taste bland if you are used to more salt. (I will say that your taste will shift if you let it: restaurant foods often taste "too salty" to me now.) If you are considering increasing the salt in a recipe, don't forget that all canned and jarred ingredients already have salt, as well as any condiments and spice blends. However, here are some common rules of thumb for how much salt is typically recommended in cooking:

- Meat: 1-2 tsp per pound of raw meat
- Flour: ¼- ½ tsp per cup of flour
- Grains/Cereals: ½ - 1 tsp per cup of water
- Pasta: 1 tsp per quart of water
- Soup: 1 tsp per quart

Using sugar

Like salt, we are also trying to minimize the amount of sugar we consume. The obvious solution would be to simply skip all desserts, baked goods, pancakes, and other sweets. However, since these are some of the foods that are most likely to be ultra-processed, it makes sense to give you homemade options. These are often quite simple to make at home where you can control the ingredient quality and reduce the sugar content. Accordingly, many of the recipes that have significant sugar show a range of how much sugar to add. I personally always use the lowest end of the range and have never had anyone turn up their nose. The upper range is consistent with a more standard recipe. Like salt, your sweetness threshold will change over time if you let it. For example, I love cake but no longer enjoy it in a restaurant as commercially prepared cakes taste too sweet; too much like candy and not enough like cake.

You will notice that many of the savory recipes include small amounts of sugar or honey. When a recipe calls for just one to two teaspoons sugar, the sweetener is just to smooth out the flavor profile. Feel free to omit it if you prefer.

Real Food – Real Photos

Artistically stylized photos of food are lovely to look at, but you won't find them in this book. The photos accompanying the recipes here are pictures of Real Food, prepared according to the recipe in a normal home kitchen. No tricks, no special equipment, no exaggerated proportions: just the food as you can expect it to look when you prepare it at home. For example:

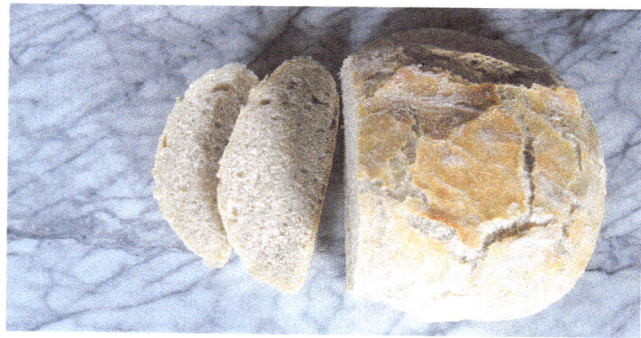 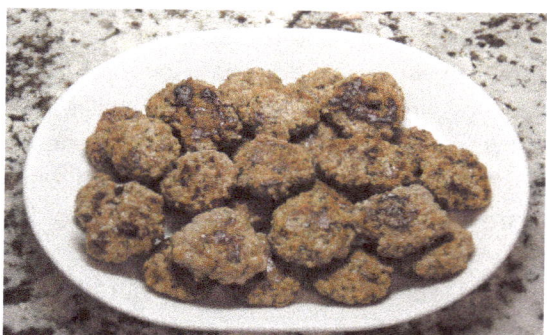

Vegetarian Dishes

You may notice that there are a lot of Agile Recipes™ in the "Veggie" category. Remember that this means that the recipe's major component(s) falls in the Priority Foods category of "Veggie." This is just one more tool to help you manage your Priority Foods; it does not mean that the dish is vegetarian.

Any recipe that is (or could be) vegetarian will have a superscript V at the end of the title. For example, the recipe for Cauliflower Marinara^V is both in the "Veggie" category and is a vegetarian dish. In this book, the vegetarian notation means that the recipe can be made without meat but there could be dairy products or eggs.

Agile Recipes™

The more than 120 Agile Recipes™ that follow in Chapter 20 are organized by meal type to enable you to find the information you need as quickly and efficiently as possible. In the following chapters we will move on to Phase IV – Efficient Kitchen Management.

The Agile Recipe™ – Key Points

The best recipe is the one that fits the situation
- » **Updated recipe format**
- » **Streamlined processes**

Agile Recipes™
- » **Visually accessible graphic layout**
- » **Simplified steps**
- » **Substitutions listed**
- » **Theme and variation – options included**

Why is this recipe collection unique?
- » **Organized around Priority Foods**
- » **One recipe for multiple results**
- » **Basic ingredients, simple preparation**
- » **Charts for Salad Dressings, Sauces, and Brines & Marinades**

You can download PDFs of Agile Recipes™ for your use at www.ReEngineeringtheKitchen.com

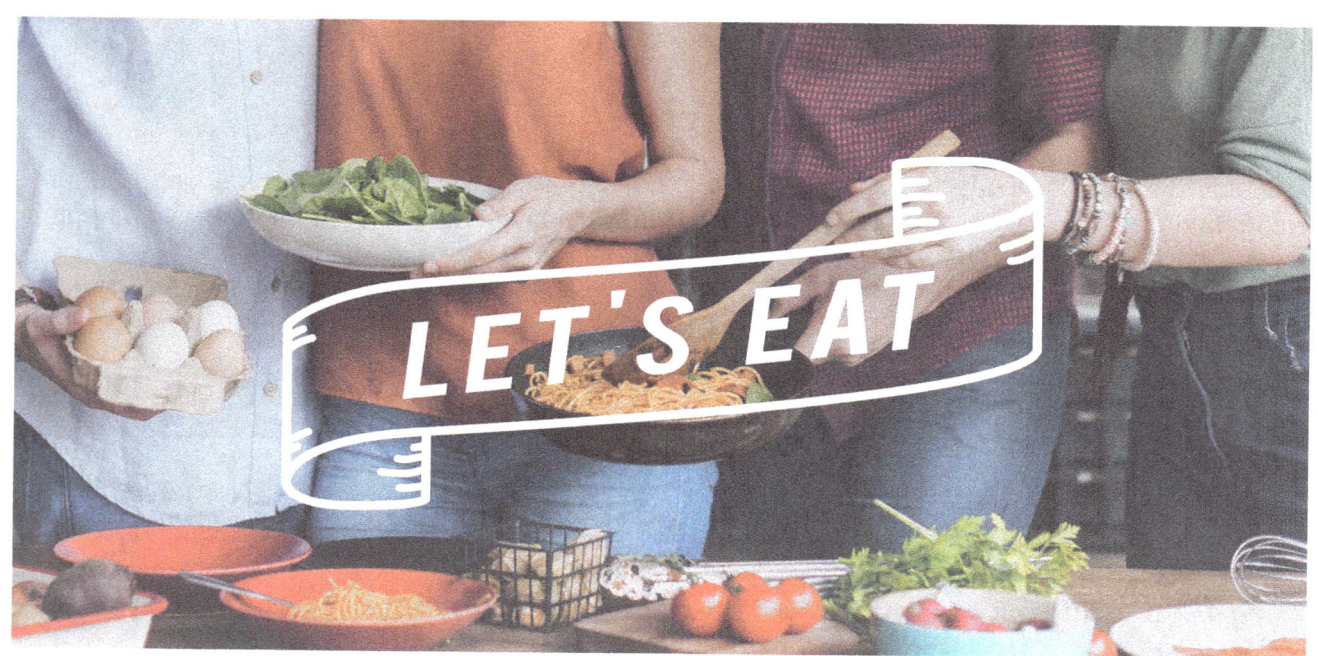

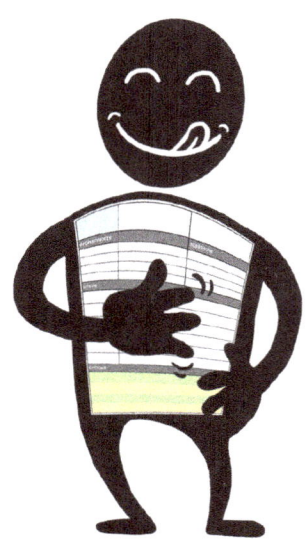

CHAPTER 20

AGILE RECIPES™

AGILE RECIPES

Any recipe that is or could be vegetarian has a superscript V at the end of the title.

AGILE RECIPES

BREAKFAST (CONT.)

208	SAUSAGE BRUNCH BAKE
209	SPINACH MUSHROOM BAKE^V
210	SWEDISH PANCAKES^V

DESSERT

211	APPLESAUCE OATMEAL CRISP^V
212	BANANAS FOSTER^V
213	BRANDIED PEACHES^V
214	BREAD PUDDING^V

- VANILLA
- PRALINE
- RAISIN CINNAMON
- CHOCOLATE
- AUTUMN HARVEST

216	BROWNIES^V
217	BUTTER BERRY COBBLER^V
218	CHOCOLATE APPLESAUCE CAKE^V
219	EGG CUSTARD^V
220	ESSENTIAL CAKE^V

- VANILLA
- CONFETTI CAKE
- CHOCOLATE CHIP
- MAPLE PECAN
- BERRY
- CINNAMON COFFEE CAKE

221	FAST FLEX FROSTING^V

- VANILLA
- LEMON
- CHOCOLATE
- ALMOND

DESSERT (CONT.)

223	FAST FRUIT FILLING^V
224	MILK PUDDING^V

- VANILLA
- CHOCOLATE
- BANANA
- MAPLE BROWN SUGAR
- FRUITY PARFAIT

225	PANTRY CAKE^V
226	PUMPKIN MUFFINS^V
227	RICE PUDDING^V

- VANILLA
- CHOCOLATE

228	RICOTTA CHEESECAKE^V
229	RUSSIAN TEA CAKES^V
230	SPICED POACHED FRUIT^V

MAIN

232	5-MINUTE FLATBREAD^V

- MARINARA PEPPERONI
- BBQ
- VEGETABLE
- CAPRESE

233	ASIAN GLAZED ANYTHING^V
234	BAKED RICE CASSEROLE^V

- CHICKEN BROCCOLI
- CHICKEN POT PIE
- SAVORY MUSHROOM

235	BALSAMIC GLAZED CHICKEN
236	BEEF STROGANOFF

AGILE RECIPES

AGILE RECIPES

AGILE RECIPES

AGILE RECIPES

PROTEIN OTHER	Baked Salsa Dip^V Makes about 1 cup		Appetizer
INGREDIENTS		**SUBSTITUTE**	
1	Jar of salsa, 16 oz		
8 oz	Goat cheese log		
STEPS			
1	Preheat oven to 350°F.		
2	Cut goat cheese log into disks about 1 inch thick. Arrange in the bottom of a shallow baking dish or pan (at least 1 quart).		
3	Pour salsa over the cheese.		
4	Bake until golden on top and bubbly, about 35-45 minutes.		
5	Serve with bread, chips, or crackers.		

PROTEIN OTHER	Hummus^V Makes about 1 cup		Appetizer
INGREDIENTS		**SUBSTITUTE**	
1	15.5 oz can chickpeas (~2 C), drained	Any canned or cooked white beans	
3 Tbsp	Extra Virgin Olive Oil		
2 Tbsp	Lemon juice - fresh	Any lemon juice	
2 cloves	Garlic	Jarred minced garlic or garlic powder	
½ tsp	Salt		
¼ tsp	Ground cumin		
0-3 Tbsp	Tahini (optional)		
2-4 Tbsp	Water - just enough so that mixture will blend		
STEPS			
1	Combine all ingredients including 2 Tbsp of water in blender, food processor or immersion blender cup.		
2	Blend until the mixture is a smooth texture. Add water in 1 tsp increments if necessary.		
3	Serve with a spinkle of paprika on top. Great with any flat bread, crackers, or raw veggies.		

AGILE RECIPES

PROTEIN OTHER	Crispy Chickpea Snacks[V] Makes 3 cups		Appetizer
INGREDIENTS		**SUBSTITUTE**	
2	15.5 oz cans chickpeas, drained		
1 Tbsp	Extra Virgin Olive Oil	Any olive oil, avocado oil or any other neutral cooking oil	
1 tsp	Salt		
½ tsp	Cracked black pepper	Other spices - see options below	
STEPS			
1	Preheat oven to 375°F.		
2	Rinse chickpeas and dry well by rubbing between paper towels. Remove any skins that have come loose in the drying.		
3	Spread dry chickpeas on a rimmed baking sheet lined with parchment paper.		
4	Bake for 35 minutes until chickpeas are crispy but still a bit soft in the middle. Shake the pan a few times during cooking.		
5	Remove from oven, put chickpeas into a bowl and toss with oil, salt and spices. Return to sheet pan and roast for another 10 minutes until crispy but not burnt.		
6	Remove from oven and allow to cool. Store loosely covered.		
OPTIONS			
A	**Spicy**: Replace black pepper with 1 tsp each of chili powder, cumin and paprika. Add ¼ tsp cayenne for an extra kick.		
B	**Herb-y**: In addition to black pepper, toss with ¼ tsp garlic powder and 2 tsp thyme, Italian seasoning or oregano.		
C	**Sweet**: Cut salt in half and replace black pepper with 1 Tbsp brown sugar and 2 tsp cinnamon or pumpkin pie spice.		
D	**Spice Blend**: Replace pepper with 2-3 tsp of your favorite prepared spice blend, e.g. Chili-Lime, Seasoning Salt, Adobe, Cajun, etc. Omit salt if your blend contains salt.		

AGILE RECIPES

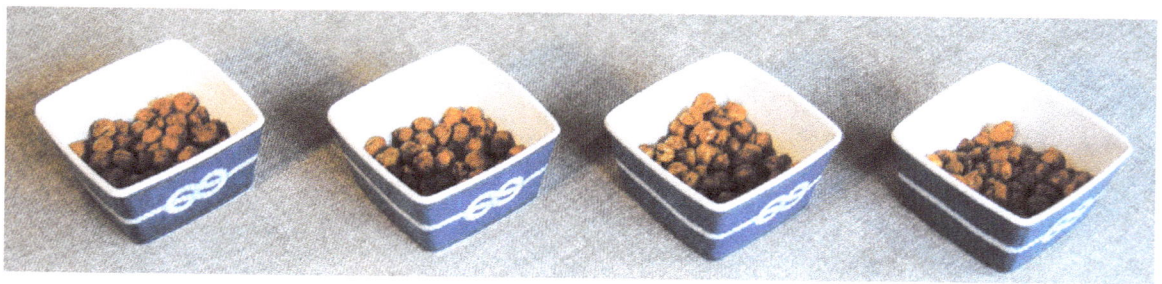

MEASUREMENTS CONVERSIONS
· COOKING - BAKING ·

CUP	ONCES	MILLILITERS	TBSP.
1/16	1/2 oz	15 ml	1
1/8	1 oz	30 ml	3
1/4	2 oz	59 ml	4
1/3	2.5 oz	79 ml	5.5
3/8	3 oz	90 ml	6
1/2	4 oz	118 ml	8
2/3	5 oz	158 ml	11
3/4	6 oz	177 ml	12
1	8 oz	240 ml	16

GRAIN	Banana Bread^v Makes 2 loaves		Bread
INGREDIENTS		**SUBSTITUTE**	
8 Tbsp	Butter, melted	Margarine	
¾ C	Sugar	Brown sugar or dry artificial sweetener	
3	Eggs, large or XL		
½ C	Milk	Cream or Half & Half or half cream/half water	
4-5	Bananas, ripe and smashed		
2 C	Flour (240 g)	Substitute up to half whole wheat flour	
1 Tbsp	Baking soda		
1 tsp	Baking powder		
¼ tsp	Salt (optional)		

STEPS	
1	Preheat oven to 350°F or 325°F if using glass loaf pans.
2	In a large mixing bowl, mix bananas, eggs, milk, and sugar together well.
3	Add dry ingredients to banana mixture and mix well.
4	Stir in melted butter.
5	Pour batter into two 8 inch greased loaf pans.
6	Bake for 40-60 minutes. Center will become firm. Test for doneness by inserting knife near the center; knife will not be clean, but should not be gooey.
7	Store covered or wrapped in foil. Freezes well.

OPTIONS	
A	Stir ½ C chopped nuts or ½ C chocolate into batter.
B	If using a muffin pan or larger loaf pans, start checking for doneness after 30 minutes.

Photo on page 203

GRAIN	Beer Bread^V Makes 1 loaf		Bread
INGREDIENTS		**SUBSTITUTE**	
3 C	Flour (360 g), up to 1/3 whole wheat	Self rising flour - omit baking powder and salt	
1½ Tbsp	Baking powder		
1½ tsp	Salt		
2 Tbsp	Sugar or honey	Up to ¼ C	
¼ C	Butter, melted	2 Tbsp more for top crust, optional	
12 oz	Beer, any type		
STEPS			
1	Preheat oven to 350°F. Coat inside of 8" x 4" loaf pan with oil.		
2	Mix dry ingredients together in large bowl.		
3	Stir beer and melted butter into dry ingredients. Mix only enough to combine.		
4	Pour into loaf pan. Pour additional 2 Tbsp melted butter on top if desired.		
5	Bake for about one hour. Start checking for doneness after 45 minutes; center will spring back when pressed and toothpick or knife will come out clean.		
6	Serve with butter, cheese, soup, or stew. Great option to stretch a meal on short notice. Warm bread is a welcome addition to any appetizer tray.		

AGILE RECIPES

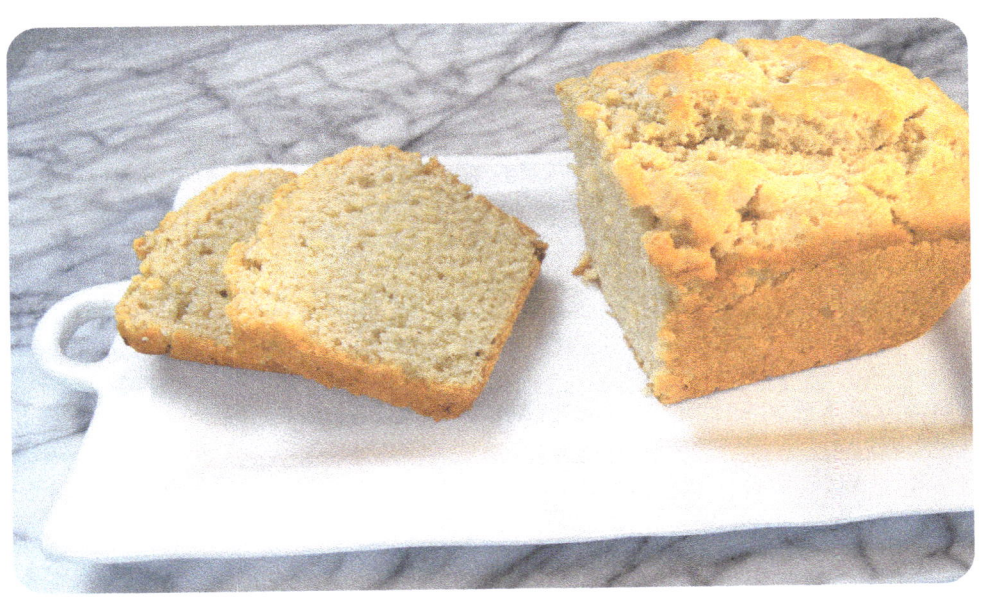

AGILE RECIPES

GRAIN	Biscuit/Shortcake^V Makes 6 biscuits		Bread
INGREDIENTS		**SUBSTITUTE**	
3 Tbsp	Butter	Crisco or margarine	
1½ C	Flour (180 g)	1 C rice flour + ½ C tapioca flour (GF) or substitute up to 50% whole grain flour	
½ Tbsp	Baking powder		
½ Tbsp	Sugar	Brown sugar or dry sugar substitute	
½ tsp	Salt		
½ C	Milk	Half & Half or buttermilk or half cream/half water	
STEPS			
1	Preheat oven to 400°F. Grease pan or line with parchment paper.		
2	In a heat-proof glass bowl or 4 C glass measuring cup, warm butter to room temp in micro.		
3	Add flour to bowl with butter. If you have a scale, weigh flour directly into your bowl.		
4	Add baking powder, salt, and sugar to flour. Stir to distribute dry ingredients.		
5	With a fork, work the flour mixture and butter together until it becomes coarse and dry.		
6	Add milk and stir just enough to fully incorporate.		
7	Use scoop or spoon to make six rounded biscuits. Each should be about 1½ inches high.		
8	Bake for 12-18 minutes, until golden brown at edges.		
9	Store covered. May reheat for 5 minutes in 350°F oven or 15 seconds in micro.		
OPTIONS			
A	**Rolled Biscuits:** Roll dough on floured surface to about ¾ inch thickness. Cut with cookie cutter or with a glass or jar of desired diameter.		
B	**Cheese Biscuits:** Stir in ½ C any shredded cheese into dough. Can add ½ tsp garlic powder to dry ingredients for more savory flavor.		
C	**Cinnamon Bun Biscuits:** Place biscuits close together in 9 inch pan, flatten each slightly by hand. Mix 2 Tbsp soft butter with 1 tsp cinnamon and 2 Tbsp sugar. Spread paste over biscuits prior to baking.		
D	**Shortcake:** Add another ½ Tbsp of sugar to the dough. For decoration, brush with butter and sprinkle with sugar prior to baking.		

GRAIN	Corn Bread^V Makes one 9 inch pan		Bread
INGREDIENTS		**SUBSTITUTE**	
1¼ C	All purpose flour (150 g)		
¾ C	Corn meal		
1 Tbsp	Baking powder		
½ tsp	Salt		
4 Tbsp	Sugar, white		
1	Egg, large or XL, beaten		
3 Tbsp	Butter, melted		
1 C	Milk		
1 C	Corn, cooked and well drained (optional)	Fresh, canned or frozen	
STEPS			
1	Preheat oven to 400°F.		
2	Prepare baking pan. Can use well oiled cast iron skillet, cake pan or pie pan.		
3	In a large bowl mix together flour, corn meal, baking powder, salt and sugar.		
4	Add milk, egg, and melted butter to bowl and mix. Fold in corn if using.		
5	Pour batter into pan and bake for 30-40 minutes, until golden. A toothpick inserted in the center should come out clean.		

AGILE RECIPES

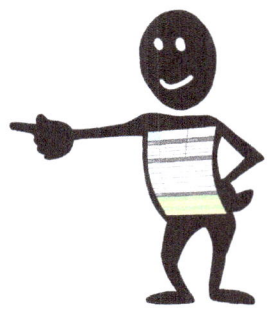

Scoop Biscuits

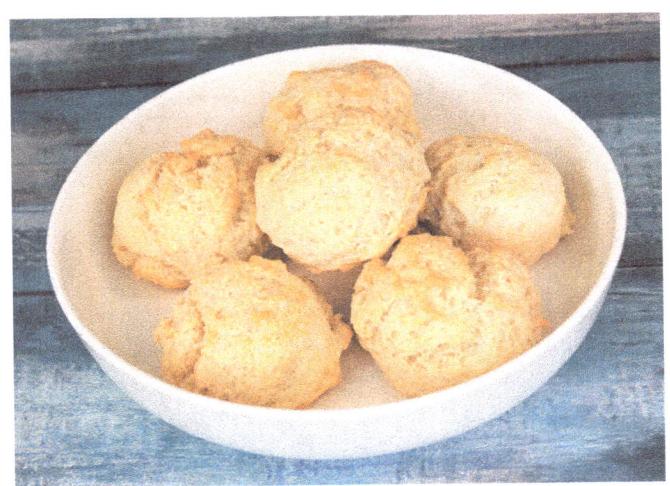

GRAIN	Irish Soda Bread^V Makes 1 loaf		Bread
INGREDIENTS		**SUBSTITUTE**	
4 C	All purpose flour (480 g)	Up to ⅓ whole wheat	
1 tsp	Baking powder		
1 tsp	Baking soda		
½ tsp	Salt		
2 Tbsp	Sugar, white or brown	Up to ¼ C	
1	Egg, large or XL		
4 Tbsp	Butter, room temperature		
1½ C	Buttermilk	1½ Tbsp vinegar + 11 oz Milk	
1 C	Raisins (optional)		
STEPS			
1	Preheat oven to 375°F.		
2	Prepare baking pan. Can use seasoned cast iron skillet or dutch oven. A baking sheet or cake pan can be oiled or lined with parchment paper.		
3	In a large bowl mix together flour, baking powder, baking soda, salt and sugar.		
4	Work butter into the flour mixture with pastry cutter, fork or fingers until crumbly.		
5	Beat buttermilk and egg together then pour into flour mixture. Add raisins if using.		
6	Stir until no dry flour remains. If dough is too sticky, add a little bit of flour. Knead dough about eight times.		
7	Form a round loaf with the dough and place on the prepared pan. Cut a shallow X across the top surface of the dough to ensure the loaf bakes evenly.		
8	Bake for 40-50 minutes.		

GRAIN	No Touch Bread^V Makes one 1½ lb loaf		Bread

INGREDIENTS		SUBSTITUTE
4 C	Flour, all purpose (480 g)	Bread flour
2¼ tsp	Instant yeast (1 packet)	Active dry yeast
1 tsp	Kosher salt	
1⅔ C	Warm water (105-115°F)	

STEPS	
1	In a large bowl, mix the flour, salt and yeast. Add the warm water and mix. The temperature of the water should feel slightly hot, but not scalding.
2	Mix until all of the flour is incorporated with spatula or spoon - silicone is best as the dough will not stick to it. Dough should be soft and sticky.
3	Cover the bowl and allow dough to rise in a warm, but not hot, place. Dough should double in bulk in 1-2 hours.
4	OPTIONAL STEP: When the dough has risen, you can refrigerate the dough for up to 2 days to allow the flavor to develop further. Allow the dough to warm up prior to next step.
5	Preheat the oven to 450°F. Put your covered baking pan (Dutch oven or roasting pan with lid) in to preheat with the oven.
6	Scrape from sides and fold the dough a few times forming a round loaf in the bowl. A silicone spatula is best, but you can use floured hands.
7	Turn loaf onto a large sheet of parchment paper dusted with flour. Cover dough with the overturned bowl and allow to rise for 30 minutes.
8	Using the parchment paper, lift loaf into the pre-heated covered pan and replace lid.
9	Bake for 30 minutes with lid on. Remove lid and continue baking for an addition 10-15 minutes or until bread is done (internal temperature of about 200°F).
10	Lift loaf out of pan with paper and allow to cool before slicing.

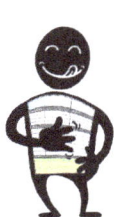

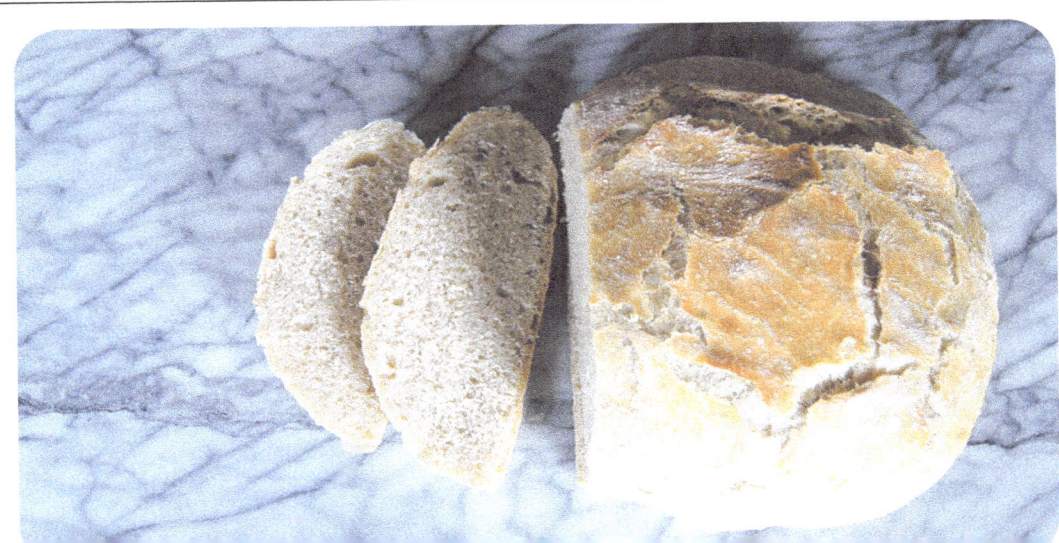

GRAIN	Yeast Rolls^V Makes 24 dinner rolls		Bread
INGREDIENTS		**SUBSTITUTE**	
1 C	Milk		
½ C	Butter	Margarine	
4 Tbsp	Sugar		
1 tsp	Salt		
1	Package active dry yeast (2¼ tsp)	Rapid rise yeast	
2	Eggs, large or XL		
4 C	Flour, all purpose (480 g)		
STEPS			
1	Preheat oven to 375°F. Prepare a 9"x13" pan by coating with cooking spray. Can use two 8"x8" baking pans.		
2	Scald milk in a large pan. Add butter, sugar and salt and allow to cool to lukewarm (110-115°F).		
3	Mix in yeast and eggs with mixer or whisk.		
4	Mix half the flour into the liquid with a whisk or mixer. Mix in the remaining flour with a spoon or spatula (silicone works well as the dough sticks less).		
5	Turn dough onto floured surface and knead only until dough becomes smooth and elastic. Avoid adding more flour than necessary for handling.		
6	Cover the dough and put in a warm place. Allow to rise until doubled in bulk, about 1 hour.		
7	Punch down the dough to release the gas. Dough may be refrigerated at this point for up to 24 hours.		
8	Divide the dough into 24 pieces, shaping each into a ball. Arrange dough balls in the pan(s).		
9	Cover the dough with a clean towel and allow to rise in a warm place for about 1 hour. Dough should double in size.		
10	Bake for 20-25 minutes or until golden brown. Rolls may be brushed with melted butter.		

AGILE RECIPES

PROTEIN MEAT	Breakfast Sausage Makes 8 patties		Breakfast
INGREDIENTS		**SUBSTITUTE**	
1 lb	Ground pork	Ground turkey or chicken	
2 tsp	Sage, ground		
2 tsp	Thyme		
1 tsp	Fennel seed, ground		
1 tsp	Salt		
¾ tsp	Black pepper, ground		
½ tsp	Red pepper flakes (optional)		
⅛ tsp	Nutmeg, ground		
STEPS			
1	Mix meat with all spices until thoroughly incorporated. May use immediately, but better if allowed to rest for 4-24 hours in refrigerator.		
2	Shape into patties, if desired.		
3	Fry with a little oil if needed. Sausage made with turkey will be drier and need oil to brown nicely.		

AGILE RECIPES

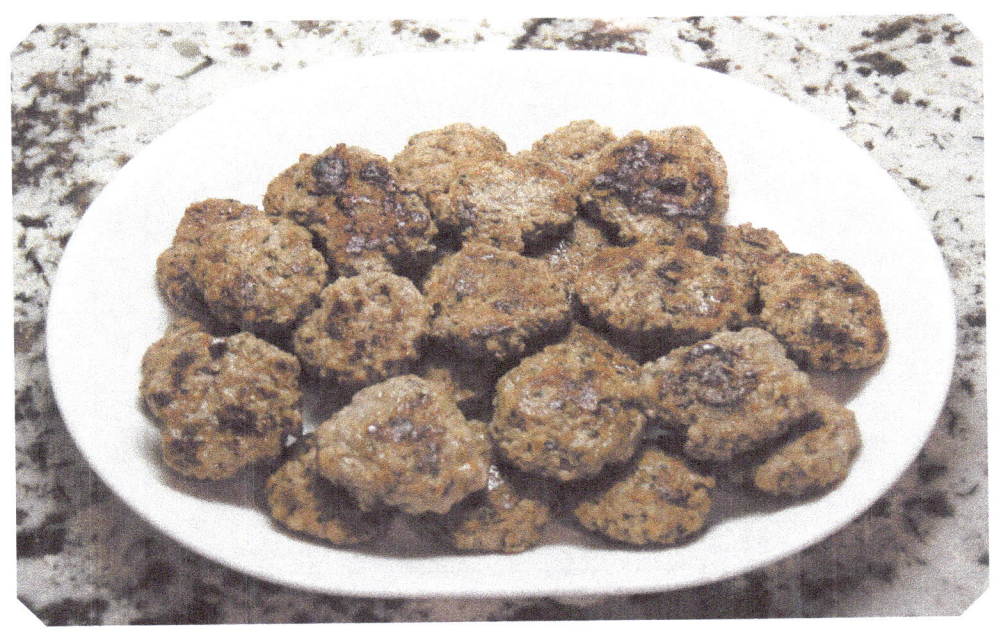

PROTEIN OTHER	Egg Cups^V Makes 12 cups		Breakfast
INGREDIENTS		**SUBSTITUTE**	
8	Eggs, large or XL		
1 C	Cottage cheese		
1½ tsp	Corn starch		
¼ C	Bacon, cooked and diced (optional)	Sausage, pancetta, diced onion or pepper	
6 oz	Shredded cheese		
½ tsp	Black pepper		
½ tsp	Salt		
½ tsp	Onion flakes or red pepper flakes (optional)		

STEPS

1	Preheat oven to 325°F. On lower oven rack, place a pan with 1 inch of hot water in it. This step is not essential, but the humidity keeps the eggs from drying out.
2	Spray muffin tin with cooking spray.
3	Brown and dice the bacon or other meat if using.
4	Combine the eggs, cottage cheese, corn starch and spices together, mixing well. Best done in a blender or mixer, but can use a bowl, and whisk vigorously.
5	In each muffin tin, put 1 tsp of bacon, ½ oz shredded cheese.
6	Pour egg mixture into tins and fill almost to the top, about ¼ C each. If there is a little extra egg mixture, it can be baked in either silicone cups or custard cups.
7	Bake for 25 minutes or until eggs are cooked. A knife inserted should come out clean.
8	Serve warm. Extras freeze well.

OPTIONS

A	**Ham & Swiss**: Use finely diced ham instead of bacon and shredded Swiss or Gruyere cheese.
B	**Veggie**: Replace bacon with finely diced onion and red pepper. Start with ½ C veggies and put 2 tsp in each cup.
C	**Sausage & Cheddar**: Replace bacon with cooked sausage crumbles and use a sharp shredded cheddar cheese.
D	**Greek**: Replace bacon with ½ C cooked and well drained spinach. Use 2 tsp spinach per tin. Replace shredded cheese with crumbled feta.

Photo on page 203

AGILE RECIPES

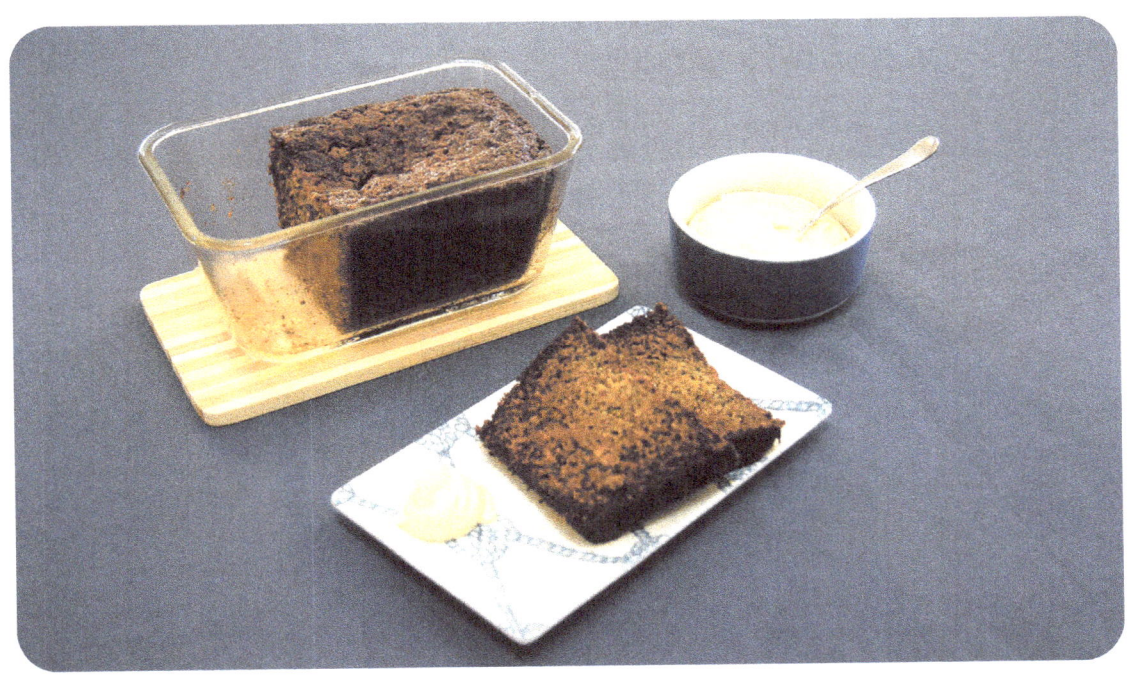

Banana Bread - Recipe on page 194

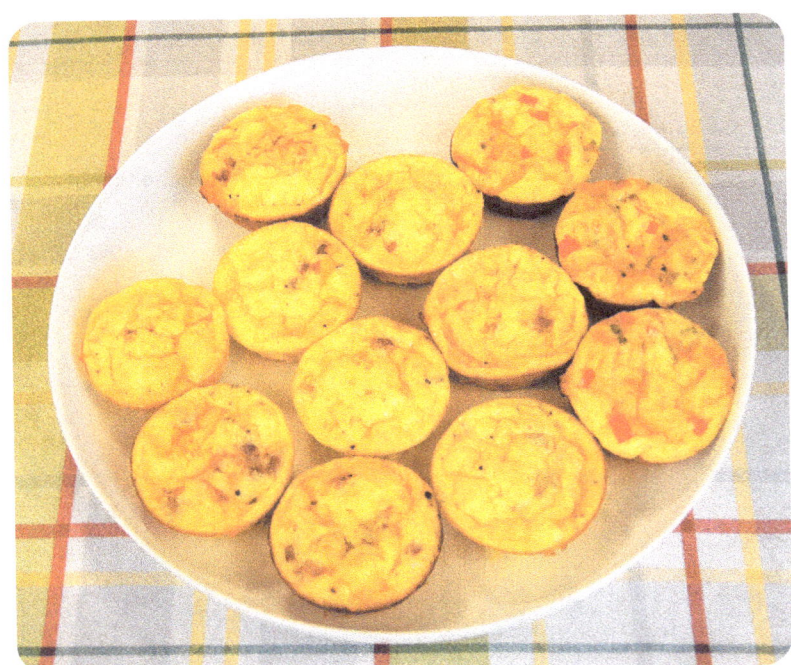

Egg Cups

Recipe on previous page

PROTEIN OTHER	French Toast Casserole[V] Makes 6-10 servings		Breakfast
INGREDIENTS		**SUBSTITUTE**	
12 oz	Bread, cubed or torn into chunks	Buns, rolls, or bagels	
¾ C	Milk		
1 C	Cottage cheese	Ricotta cheese	
3	Eggs, large or XL		
¼ C	Sugar, white	Brown sugar, honey, or sugar substitute	
1 tsp	Vanilla extract	Lemon extract	
2 C	Berries, fresh	Frozen berries, thawed and drained	
STEPS			
1	Preheat oven to 350°F. Generously grease a 9 x 13 inch pan or 2½ quart casserole dish.		
2	Put bread in a large bowl and pour milk over it. If your bread is dry, add another ¼ C of milk. Stir and allow all milk to soak in.		
3	In a separate small bowl, add cottage cheese, eggs, sugar, and vanilla. Beat well - an immersion blender is ideal, but can be whisked vigorously by hand.		
4	Pour cottage cheese and egg mixture over bread and stir to incorporate.		
5	Gently fold berries into bread/cheese/egg mixture and pour into baking pan.		
6	Bake for 35-45 minutes, until top is golden and center is firm.		
7	Serve with syrup, powdered sugar, or whipped cream.		

AGILE RECIPES

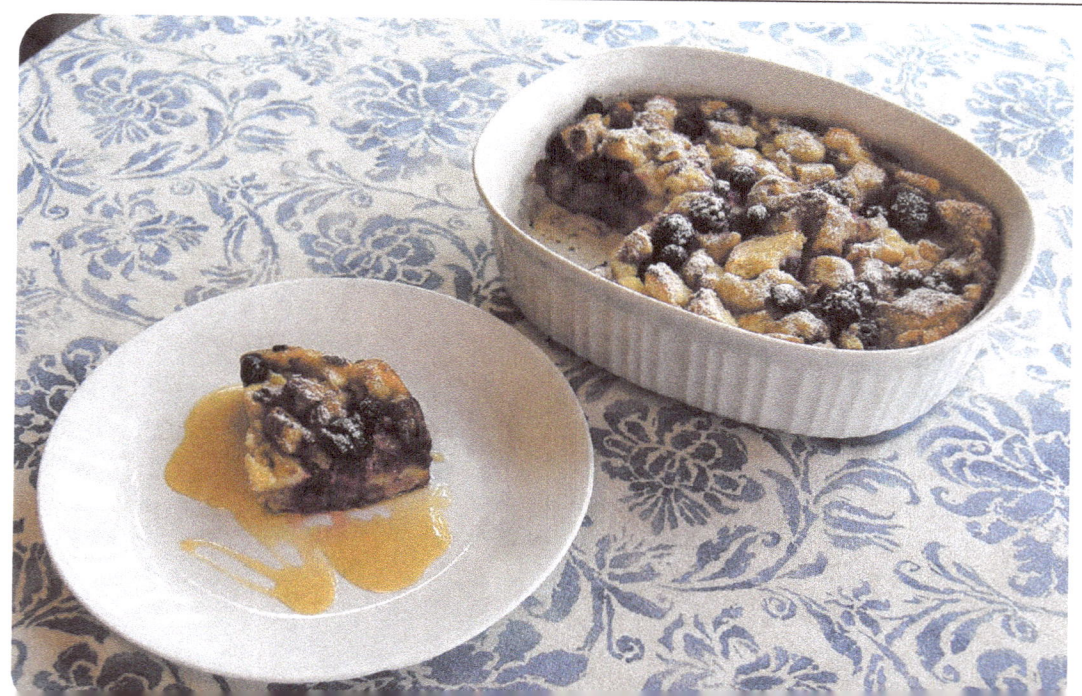

GRAIN	Oatmeal Pancakes^v Serves 2-3		Breakfast
INGREDIENTS		**SUBSTITUTE**	
1 C	Flour (120 g)	Up to ⅓ whole wheat	
¾ C	Oats, Old Fashioned	Quick oats	
1 tsp	Baking powder		
¼ C	Brown sugar	White sugar	
¼ tsp	Salt		
1 C	Milk	½ C cream + ½ C water	
1	Egg, large or XL		
1 Tbsp	Oil	Melted butter	
STEPS			
1	In a large bowl, mix all dry ingredients.		
2	Beat milk, egg and oil together then add to dry ingredients. Mix well.		
3	Allow to stand 5-10 minutes.		
4	Cook batter ¼ to ½ cup at a time in a medium hot pan or griddle that has been lightly oiled.		
5	Makes 2 cups batter, approximately 8 four inch diameter pancakes.		
Copyright © 2024 Alin E. Steele May be copied for personal use only. www.ReEngineeringtheKitchen.com			

AGILE RECIPES

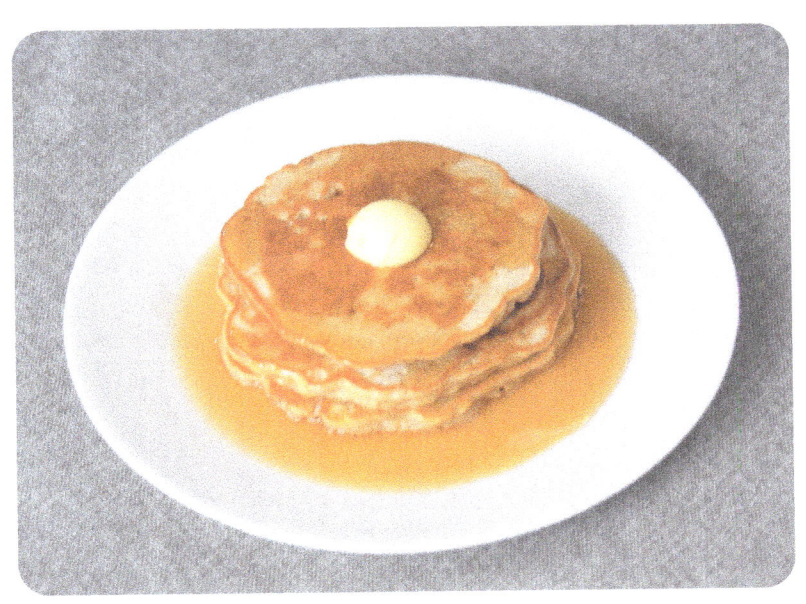

PROTEIN OTHER	Potato Frittata^V Serves 6		Breakfast

AGILE RECIPES

INGREDIENTS		SUBSTITUTE
8	Eggs, large or XL	
2	Potatoes, medium (approx. 1 lb)	Leftover potatoes
1	Medium onion, sliced thinly	
2 Tbsp	Extra Virgin Olive Oil	
¼ C	Milk	Cream
½ tsp	Salt	
¼ tsp	Cracked black pepper	

STEPS	
1	Preheat oven to 350°F.
2	Cook potatoes to tender by either boiling in water or microwaving. Can use leftover potatoes. Cut potatoes into slices or cubes no thicker than ¼ inch.
3	In a large (12 inch) oven-proof skillet, sauté onion until soft. Add potatoes and brown slightly. Distribute onions and potatoes evenly in pan.
4	In a bowl, whip eggs, milk, salt and pepper together.
5	Pour egg mixture over onions and potatoes, spreading evenly.
6	Bake in oven for 20-25 minutes, until eggs are set.
7	Serve warm or room temperature.

OPTIONS	
A	**Bacon & Cheddar**: Fry 3 strips of diced bacon in pan. Omit olive oil. Use the residual bacon fat to saute onions and potatoes. Add ½ C shredded cheddar cheese into egg mixture.
B	**Veggie**: Increase the vegetable content by adding up to ½ C chopped bell peppers, spinach, or asparagas. If you add more than ½ C, decrease onion or potato proportionately.
C	**Pasta**: Replace potatoes with 2 C cooked pasta. Stir ½ C Parmesan cheese into egg mixture.

Photo on page 215

PROTEIN OTHER	Ricotta Pancakes^V Makes ~ twelve 5" pancakes		Breakfast
INGREDIENTS		**SUBSTITUTE**	
4	Eggs, large or XL		
1 tsp	Vanilla extract		
¼ C	Sugar		
1 C	Milk		
1 C	Ricotta cheese	Cottage cheese	
1½ C	Flour (180 g)		
3 Tbsp	Butter, melted		
STEPS			
1	Whisk egg, vanilla and sugar together.		
2	Add milk and ricotta cheese, mixing well. If using cottage cheese, use an immersion blender to fully mix.		
3	Add flour and baking powder and whisk until smooth.		
4	Pour in melted butter slowly while continuing to stir.		
5	Preheat sauté pan lightly coated with oil over medium heat. The pan is hot enough when a drop of water will "dance" but oil is not smoking.		
6	Pour about ⅓ C batter into hot pan, spreading batter if necessary so that it is not too thick.		
7	Cook until the pancake is set, then flip to cook an additional couple minutes.		
8	Serve with your favorite topping: fruit and whipped cream, syrup, jam, chocolate-hazelnut spread, powdered sugar.		

AGILE RECIPES

PROTEIN MEAT	Sausage Brunch Bake Makes 8-10 servings	Breakfast
INGREDIENTS		**SUBSTITUTE**
1 lb	Pork breakfast sausage	Turkey breakfast sausage
9	Eggs, large or XL	
1 C	Milk	
12 oz	Co-Jack cheese, shredded	Any mild cheese or cheese blend
8 oz	Bread, in 1 inch cubes or chunks	Any type of yeast bread or roll
½ tsp	Salt and pepper, each	
STEPS		
1	Preheat oven to 350°F and prepare 9 x 9 inch (or 2½ quart) baking dish by coating interior of pan with oil.	
2	Brown sausage and then drain well.	
3	In a bowl, whisk eggs, salt, pepper, and milk together.	
4	Put bread, sausage crumbles and half of the cheese in the pan.	
5	Pour egg and milk mixture over the bread in the pan. Turn gently to distribute and ensure everything is coated with the liquid.	
6	Sprinkle the remaining cheese on top.	
7	Bake until eggs are set, about 45 minutes. A knife inserted in the middle should come out clean at an internal temperature of 165°F	
8	For a double recipe, use a 9 x 13 in pan. Leftovers freeze and reheat well.	

AGILE RECIPES

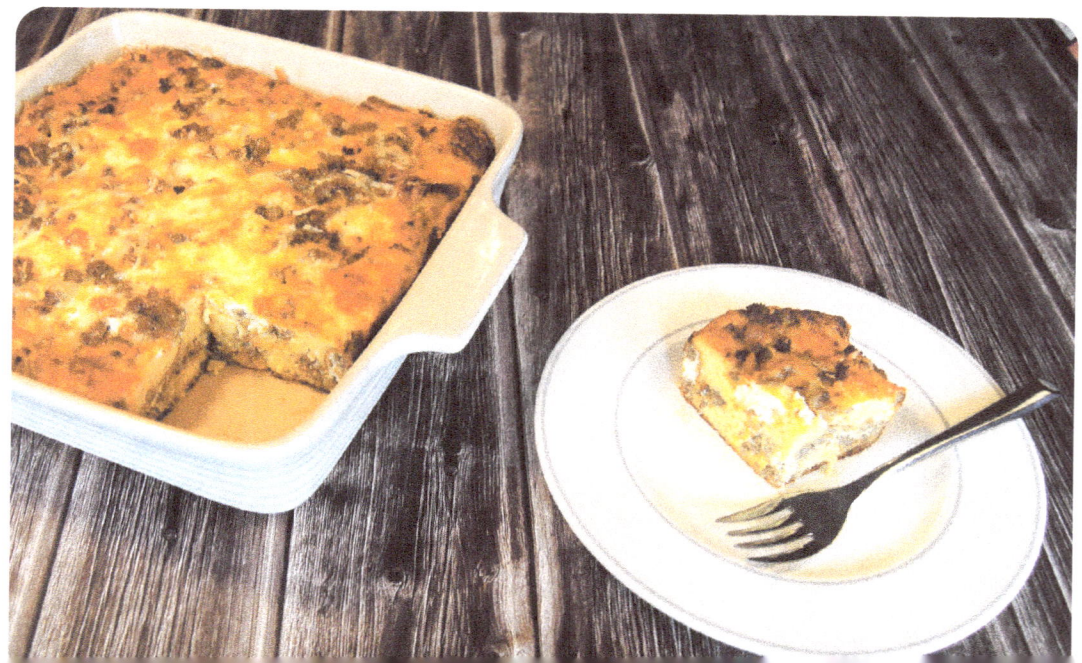

PROTEIN OTHER	Spinach Mushroom Bake^v Makes 12 servings		Breakfast

INGREDIENTS		SUBSTITUTE
12	Eggs, large or XL	
16 oz	Cottage cheese	Ricotta cheese
16 oz	Shredded cheese, cheddar or blend	
8 Tbsp	Butter	
½ C	Corn starch	Tapioca flour or rice flour
10 oz	Chopped spinach, cooked and drained	
8 oz	Mushrooms, sliced	Fresh, frozen or canned
1	Onion, medium, diced	
1¼ tsp	Baking powder	
½ tsp	Salt	
½ tsp	Black pepper	

STEPS	
1	Preheat oven to 350°F. Prepare 9 x 13 inch pan by coating interior with oil.
2	Sauté onion and mushrooms in butter until onion is soft. Add spinach and set aside to cool slightly.
3	In a large bowl, whisk eggs then add cottage cheese, ¾ of the grated cheese, corn starch, baking powder, salt and pepper. Mix well.
4	Stir spinach, onion and mushrooms into the egg mixture.
5	Pour into prepared baking pan. Pan will be full.
6	Spread remaining grated cheese on top.
7	Bake until eggs are set and knife inserted into the center comes out clean, 45-60 minutes.
8	Popular vegetarian and gluten free option for brunch. Leftovers freeze and reheat well.

AGILE RECIPES

GRAIN	Swedish Pancakes[v] Makes ~ twelve 6" pancakes		Breakfast
INGREDIENTS		**SUBSTITUTE**	
4	Eggs, large or XL		
1 tsp	Vanilla extract		
¼ C	Sugar		
2 C	Milk		
1½ C	Flour (180 g)		
3 Tbsp	Butter, melted		
STEPS			
1	Whisk eggs, vanilla and sugar together.		
2	Add milk and mix well.		
3	Add flour and whisk until smooth.		
4	Pour in melted butter slowly while continuing to stir. Batter will be thin. At this point, the batter may be stored in the refrigerator overnight.		
5	Preheat sauté pan lightly coated with oil over medium heat. The pan is hot enough when a drop of water will "dance".		
6	Pour about ⅓ C batter into hot pan, turning the pan so that the batter covers the entire bottom surface.		
7	Cook until the pancake is set, then flip to cook an additional couple minutes.		
8	Serve with your favorite topping: fruit and whipped cream, syrup, lingonberries, orange butter, chocolate-hazelnut spread, or powdered sugar.		

AGILE RECIPES

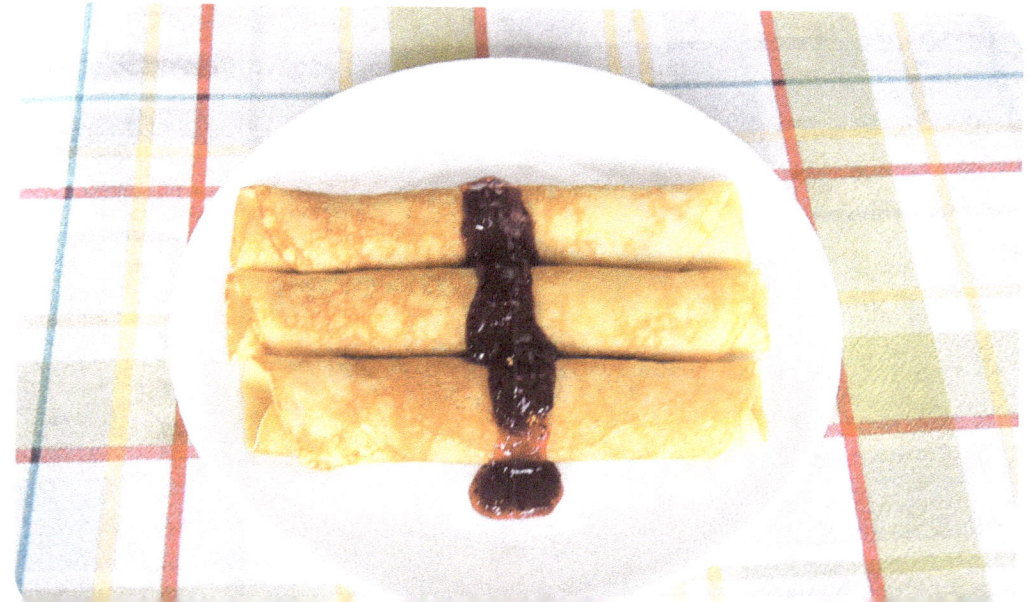

FRUIT	Applesauce Oatmeal Crisp^V Makes one 9" x 9" pan		Dessert
INGREDIENTS		**SUBSTITUTE**	
2½ C	Rolled oats (Old Fashioned or Quick)		
1 C	Brown sugar	White sugar	
½ C	Butter, room temperature	Margarine (regular, not reduced fat)	
24 oz	Applesauce, unsweetened (one jar)	Sweetened applesauce (reduce sugar by ⅓)	
1 tsp	Cinnamon	Pumpkin pie spice	
STEPS			
1	Preheat oven to 350°F.		
2	Mix oats, brown sugar and cinnamon together. Put ⅓ of the dry mixture in a 9" x 9" baking pan or 2½ quart baking dish.		
3	Pour applesauce over the dry oat mixture in the pan and mix.		
4	Add softened butter to the remaining dry oatmeal mixture and mix well. There should be no lumps of butter and the oats covered with butter. Spread over top of applesauce mixture.		
5	Bake for 45-60 minutes until top is crunchy and golden.		
6	Serve warm or cold, plain or garnished with whipped cream, ice cream or caramel sauce.		
OPTIONS			
A	**Additions**: Stir ⅓ C raisins, dried cranberries or cherries or chopped walnuts or pecans to the appleasauce mixture.		
B	**Extra Fruit**: Use a 46 oz jar of applesauce to increase the applesauce to topping ratio.		
C	**Any Fruit**: Replace the applesauce with Fast Fruit Filling (see recipe on page 223).		

The text "AGILE RECIPES" appears on the vertical tab at the right edge.

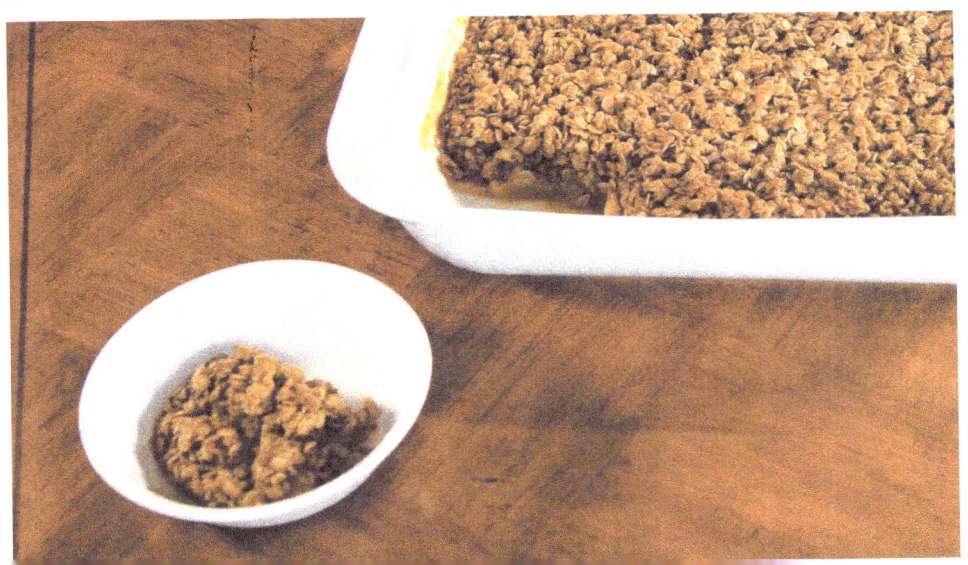

FRUIT	Bananas Foster[V] Serves 4		Dessert
INGREDIENTS		**SUBSTITUTE**	
4	Bananas, peeled and sliced in half		
4 Tbsp	Butter		
½ C	Brown sugar, packed		
½ tsp	Cinnamon		
¼ C	Dark rum (optional)	Light rum or brandy	
STEPS			
1	In a large skillet or sauté pan, melt butter and mix brown sugar and cinnamon in well.		
2	Over medium heat, add the banana slices to the bubbly butter/sugar mixture. Heat on each side for about 2 minutes. Bananas should start to caramelize.		
3	Pour rum over bananas and gently shake pan to mix.		
4	Optional Step: Flambe the rum upon addition by igniting it carefully with a long lighter. Flame should go out in just a few seconds.		
5	Serve warm over vanilla ice cream, pancakes, waffles, pound cake, or bread pudding.		
Copyright © 2024 Alin E. Steele May be copied for personal use only. www.ReEngineeringtheKitchen.com			

AGILE RECIPES

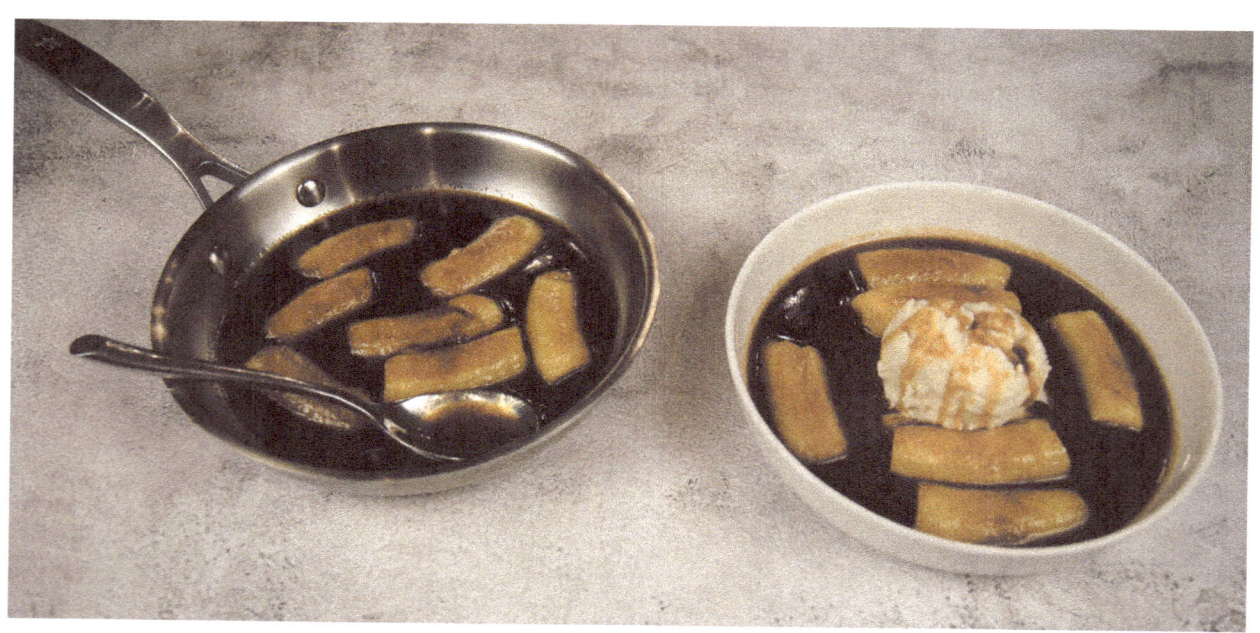

FRUIT	**Brandied Peaches**^V **Makes about 5 cups**		**Dessert**
INGREDIENTS		**SUBSTITUTE**	
4	Ripe peaches, medium to large		
1¾ C	White granulated sugar		
1½ C	Water		
2 tsp	Ground cloves		
½ C	Brandy		
STEPS			
1	Have clean glass jars with lids ready – mason jars or any heavy glass jars are fine.		
2	Clean the peaches well and cut into cubes or slices. They do not need to be peeled. Put peach pieces into glass jar(s), filling only ½ to ¾ full.		
3	In a sauce pan, heat water and sugar to boiling. It should thicken slightly, making a syrup that will coat the back of a spoon.		
4	Remove syrup from heat and stir in the ground cloves. Next stir in the brandy and mix well.		
5	When syrup is still warm, pour over the peaches. Cool before sealing the jars.		
6	Allow to set for at least 12 hours before serving. Store in the refrigerator for up to a week.		
7	Serve over vanilla ice cream, pancakes or french toast.		

AGILE RECIPES

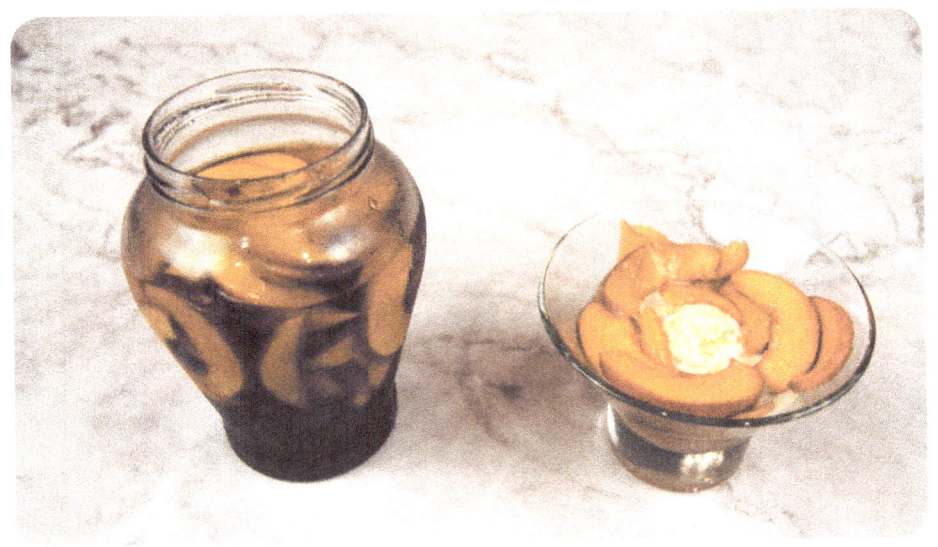

GRAIN	Bread Pudding^V Makes 8-12 servings		Dessert
INGREDIENTS		**SUBSTITUTE**	
12 oz	French bread, cut into 1 inch cubes	Any bread but stale and crusty is better	
3 C	Milk	Half cream + half water	
3	Eggs, large or XL		
½ - 1 C	Sugar	Brown sugar (affects appearance)	
2 tsp	Vanilla extract		
½ tsp	Cinnamon		
¼ tsp	Nutmeg		
1-2 Tbsp	Butter, melted		
STEPS			
1	Preheat oven to 350°F.		
2	In a large bowl, mix bread cubes and milk and allow to stand until milk is mostly absorbed.		
3	In a second bowl, beat eggs, sugar and spices together.		
4	Pour egg mixture over the bread and milk, then gently fold together. Ensure that the bread is well coated.		
5	Prepare a 9 x 13 baking pan, casserole dish or individual baking dishes by coating interior with oil. Scoop mixture into pan. Drizzle with melted butter.		
6	Bake for about 60 minutes or until center is set. Individual baking dishes will take closer to 50 minutes.		
OPTIONS			
A	**Praline**: Fold in ½ -1 C of chopped pecans before baking then top with a caramel sauce.		
B	**Raisin Cinnamon**: Fold in ½ -1 C of raisins and sprinkle top with cinnamon sugar before baking. Serve with whipped cream or vanilla ice cream.		
C	**Chocolate**: Fold in ½ -1 C of chocolate chips or chocolate chunks (semi-sweet or dark chocolate) before baking. Serve with a drizzle of chocolate sauce and whipped cream.		
D	**Autumn Harvest**: Fold in ½ -1 C of chopped dried apricots or cherries before baking then serve with a drizzle of maple syrup.		

AGILE RECIPES

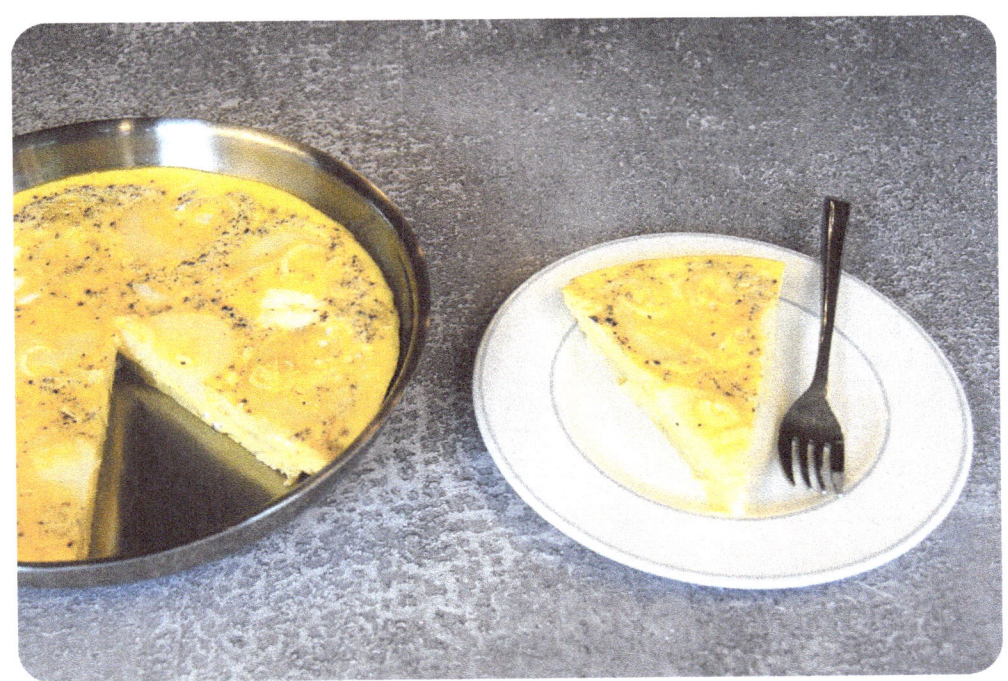

Potato Frittata

Recipe on page 206

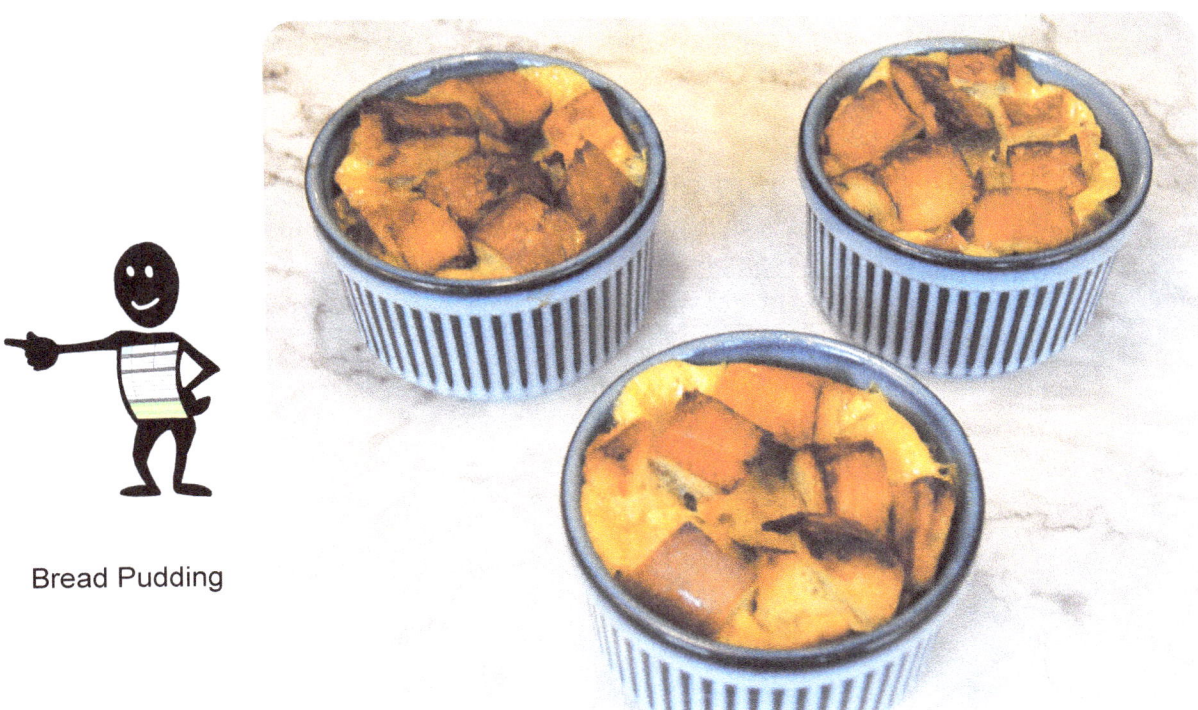

Bread Pudding

GRAIN	Brownies[V] Makes one 8" x 8" pan		Dessert
INGREDIENTS		**SUBSTITUTE**	
½ C	Butter, room temperature	Margarine or coconut oil	
1 C	Sugar	½ C white sugar + ½ C brown sugar	
2	Eggs, large or XL		
1 tsp	Vanilla extract		
½ C	Baking cocoa, unsweetened	Dark chocolate baking cocoa	
½ C	Flour, all purpose (60 g)	Self rising flour (omit baking powder and salt)	
1 tsp	Baking powder		
½ tsp	Salt		
½ C	Chocolate chips (optional)	Any flavor baking chips, M&Ms, crushed candy canes	
½ C	Chopped nuts (optional)		
STEPS			
1	Preheat oven to 350°F. Prepare a 8" x 8" pan by coating with cooking spray. Use a 9' x 13" pan for a double recipe.		
2	In a bowl, beat the sugar and butter together then add eggs and vanilla. Beat with a whisk or mixer until fully incorporated.		
3	Stir cocoa, flour, baking powder and salt together in a small bowl then pour into the egg mixture and mix until smooth.		
4	Fold optional chocolate chips and/or nuts into batter, if using.		
5	Spread batter in pan and bake for 20-25 minutes. Brownies are done when a toothpick inserted in the middle comes out clean. Cool before cutting.		

GRAIN	Butter Berry Cobbler^v Makes 8 - 12 servings	Dessert
INGREDIENTS		**SUBSTITUTE**
8 Tbsp	Butter	Margarine
2 C	Flour, all purpose (240 g)	Up to ⅓ whole wheat
1 Tbsp	Baking powder	
2 C	Sugar (white or brown)	Reduce by ½ C for a less sweet result
2 C	Milk	
¼ tsp	Salt	
16 oz	Any Berries, fresh or frozen (3-4 C)	Canned or frozen peaches
STEPS		
1	Preheat oven to 350°F.	
2	Thaw fruit if using frozen.	
3	Put butter in 9 x 13 inch pan then place in oven to melt butter and heat pan.	
4	In a bowl, mix the flour, salt, baking powder and sugar.	
5	Stir in the milk and mix. It is OK to leave slightly lumpy.	
6	Remove hot pan from oven with melted butter. Pour the batter mixture into pan – do not stir.	
7	Drop fruit into batter, evenly distributing over the entire surface. Any residual fruit juice may be drizzled in, avoiding the center.	
8	Bake for 50-60 minutes until golden brown and center is firm.	
9	Serve warm or cool. Great with vanilla ice cream.	
	Copyright © 2024 Alin E. Steele May be copied for personal use only. www.ReEngineeringtheKitchen.com	

AGILE RECIPES

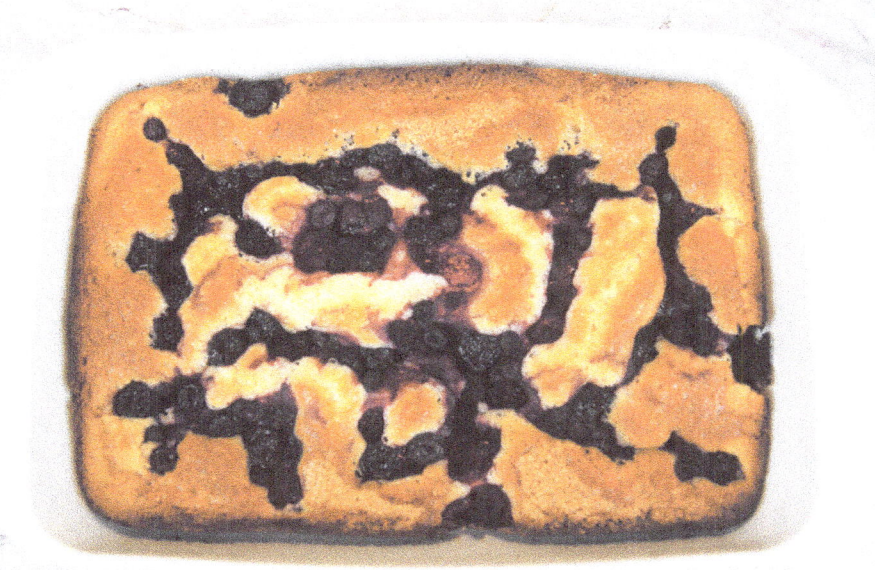

GRAIN	Chocolate Applesauce Cake Makes one 9" x 9" cake		Dessert

INGREDIENTS		SUBSTITUTE
2 C	All purpose flour (240 g)	Substitute up to one half whole wheat flour.
1-1½ C	Sugar	
3 Tbsp	Cocoa powder	
1 Tbsp	Baking soda	
1 tsp	Cinnamon	
½ tsp	Nutmeg	
½ tsp	Cloves	
¼ tsp	Salt	
1 Tbsp	Corn starch	
½ C	Vegetable oil	Melted butter
2 C	Applesauce, unsweetened	Sweetened applesauce (use ½ C less sugar)

STEPS	
1	Preheat oven to 325°F.
2	Prepare pan (either bundt pan or 9 x 9 baking pan) by coating with oil then dusting with flour.
3	Place all dry ingredients in bowl and mix well.
4	Warm applesauce and oil together in oven or microwave to about 110°F.
5	Add applesauce and oil to the dry ingredients and mix thoroughly.
6	Pour batter into prepared baking pan.
7	Bake for one hour. Check for doneness after 45 minutes. A knife or toothpick inserted in the middle should come out clean when cake is done.

OPTIONS	
A	**Additions**: Add ½ C of chopped nuts or raisins or dried cranberries.
B	**Toppings**: Whipped cream or fresh berries or lemon curd or Fast Flex Frosting shown on page 221.

Photo on page 222

PROTEIN OTHER	Egg Custard^v Makes 6-8 cups		Dessert
INGREDIENTS		**SUBSTITUTE**	
3 C	Milk	Commercially prepared eggnog (omit sugar)	
½ C	Sugar		
4	Eggs, large or XL		
1	Egg white		
1 tsp	Vanilla extract		
STEPS			
1	Preheat oven to 325°F.		
2	Mix all ingredients and beat well. May be done with a blender, mixer or whisk.		
3	Place 6-8 custard cups into a shallow baking pan. Fill each cup with 4-5½ oz of the mixture.		
4	Pour about 1 inch of hot water into the baking pan so that the cups are surrounded by water.		
5	Carefully set pan with the water and cups into the oven. Bake for 45-60 minutes, until the custard has just set. A knife inserted into the custard will come out clean.		
6	Remove from oven and allow to cool. Cover and chill before serving.		
7	Serve plain or with a sprinkle of nutmeg, cinnamon sugar, caramel sauce, fruit preserves or fresh berries.		

AGILE RECIPES

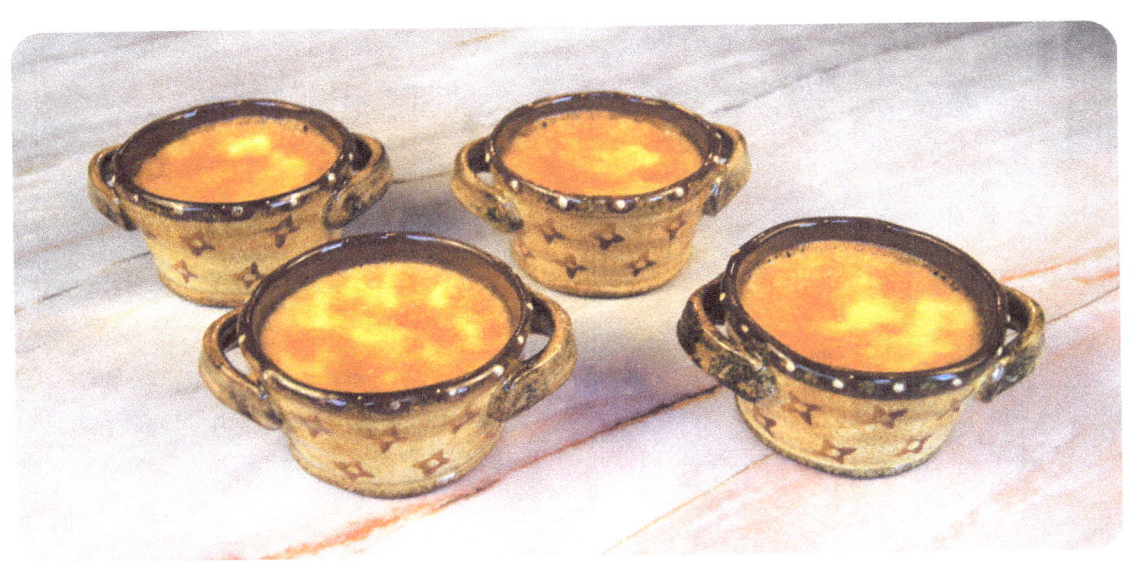

GRAIN	Essential Cake^V **Makes one 8" - 9" cake**		Dessert
INGREDIENTS		**SUBSTITUTE**	
8 Tbsp	Butter, softened	Margarine	
¾ C	White sugar	Brown sugar	
2	Large or XL eggs, room temperature		
1½ tsp	Vanilla extract	Almond or other flavor extract	
1½ C	All Purpose Flour or Cake Flour (180 g)	1 C rice flour + ½ C tapicoa flour (GF)	
1½ tsp	Baking powder		
½ tsp	Salt		
¾ C	Milk	Buttermilk	

STEPS	
1	Preheat oven to 350°F.
2	Prepare pan by coating with oil (or cooking spray) and then dusting with flour. May use 8-9 inch square or round pan, loaf pan or 12 cupcake pan.
3	In a large bowl, beat butter and sugar until it is well combined, light and fluffy.
4	Add eggs to the bowl and beat well. Add vanilla extract and beat.
5	Measure flour (weighing is best), baking powder and salt into a bowl and stir to mix.
6	Add half of the flour and half of the milk to the butter/egg bowl then beat to incorporate. Add remaining flour and milk and beat until batter is smooth, about two minutes.
7	Pour into prepared pan and bake for about 20 minutes for cupcakes or 30-35 minutes for a pan. Cake is done when a toothpick inserted in the middle comes out clean.
8	Allow to cool. May be topped with frosting, ice cream, whipped cream, fruit compote, caramel or chocolate sauce.

OPTIONS	
A	**Confetti Cake**: Stir ¼ C colorful sprinkles into batter right before baking. Frost with vanilla frosting and decorate with more sprinkles.
B	**Chocolate Chip**: Stir ½ C mini chocolate chips into batter right before baking.
C	**Maple Pecan**: Use maple extract instead of vanilla and then stir in ½ C finely chopped pecans into batter right before baking.
D	**Berry**: Wash & dry one cup of blueberries or raspberries & fold into the batter prior to baking.
E	**Cinnamon Coffee Cake**: Mix ½ C brown sugar, 2 tsp cinnamon, 2 Tbsp flour and 3 Tbsp melted butter together, then sprinkle over batter prior to baking.

Fast Flex Frosting^V Makes ~ 3 cups		Dessert
INGREDIENTS		**SUBSTITUTE**
2-3	Sticks butter - softened (unsalted preferred)	Margarine, Crisco
0-1	Package (8 oz) cream cheese - softened	
4 C	Powdered sugar	Use 1¼ C brown or white granulated sugar (affects texture)
1½ tsp	Vanilla extract	Other extract - lemon, almond
STEPS		
1	Use 3 sticks of butter or 2 sticks of butter plus one package cream cheese.	
2	Beat butter and cream cheese (if using) in bowl with mixer until fluffy.	
3	Add vanilla extract.	
4	Add powdered sugar in four increments, beating well between additions. Frosting should be firm yet spreadable.	
5	Adjust consistency: Add sugar in 1 Tbsp increments to thicken or milk by 1 tsp increments to thin.	
6	Yields about 3 cups of frosting. Enough for 24 cupcakes (2 Tbsp each) or one 9" x 13" sheet cake.	
OPTIONS		
A	**Spread**: Can be made with white granulated sugar or brown sugar (reduce volume). However, the texture will be softer, and a bit grainy. Tastes ok in a pinch but not workable for decorating.	
B	**Lemon**: Use 2 tsp lemon extract instead of vanilla, and for extra flavor, add 1 Tbsp lemon zest.	
C	**Chocolate**: Add ½ C melted chocolate chips to the butter/cream cheese mixture in step 3. Add vanilla and sugar as usual.	
D	**Almond**: Use 2 tsp almond extract in place of vanilla. Use almond slices as decoration.	

AGILE RECIPES

Photos of Essential Cake and Fast Flex Frosting on page 222

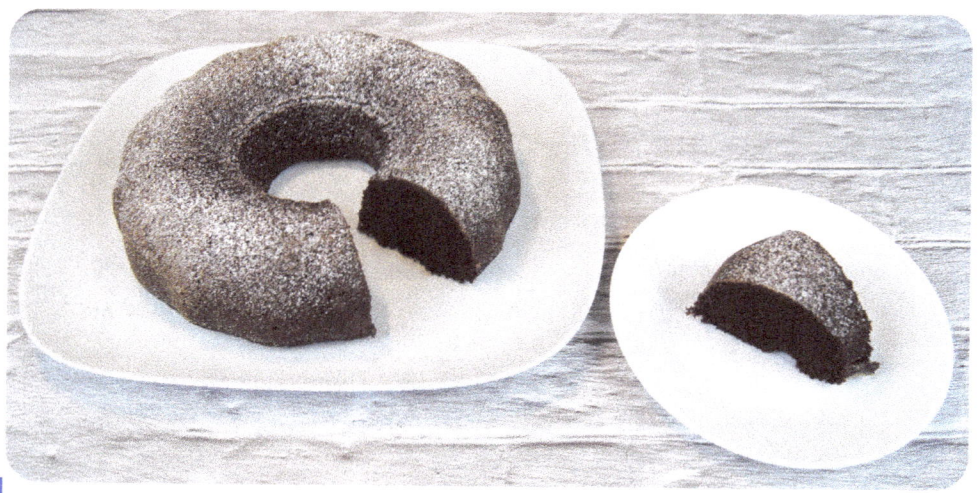

Chocolate Applesauce
Cake

Recipe on page 218

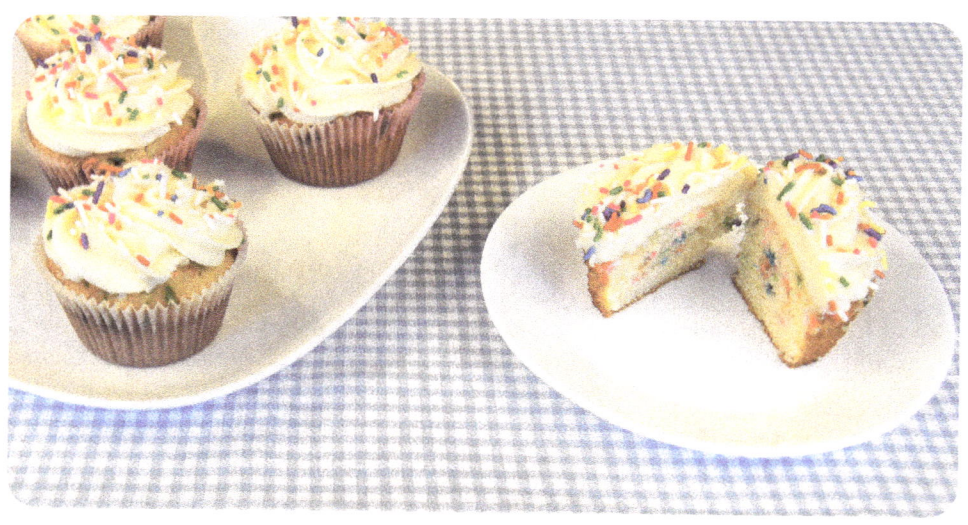

Essential Cake & Fast Flex Frosting - Recipes on pages 220 & 221

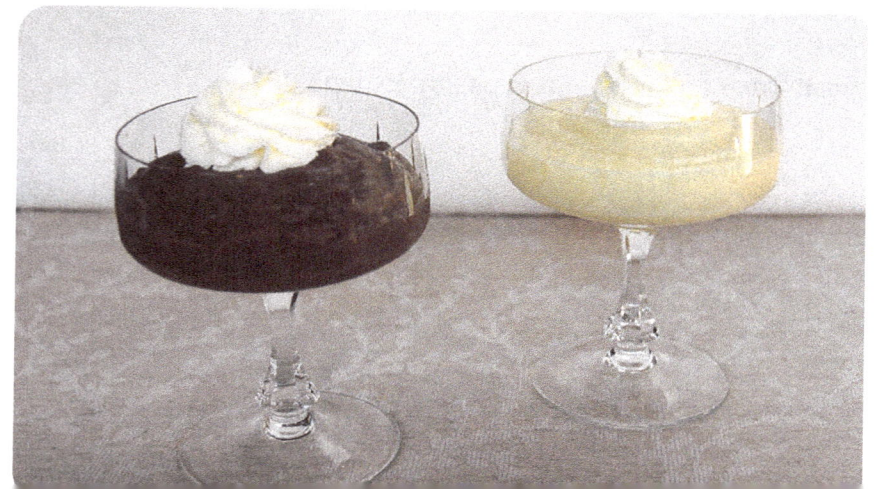

Milk Pudding

Vanilla & Chocolate

Recipe on page 224

FRUIT	Fast Fruit Filling^V Makes 1¾ cups		Dessert
INGREDIENTS		**SUBSTITUTE**	
1	Bag (16 oz) frozen berries	Any non-citrus frozen, fresh (A) or canned fruit (B)	
½ C	Sugar	Any natural or artificial sweetener. If using liquid, add 1 tsp corn starch per ½ C liquid.	
2 Tbsp	Corn starch	Rice flour	
1 tsp	Lemon juice	Any juice or OJ concentrate	
STEPS			
1	In a heat-proof glass bowl or measuring cup, microwave fruit for 3 minutes on high until thawed but still cold.		
2	Stir sugar, lemon juice and corn starch into fruit and mix well.		
3	Microwave on high for four minutes then stir.		
4	Microwave on high for another four minutes. Should be steamy and look glossy.		
5	If it is not yet steamy and glossy, continue heating in microwave in one minute increments until it is.		
6	Serve hot or cold. Makes about 1¾ Cups.		
7	Use as a topping for ice cream, pancakes, french toast, or cheesecake. Layer in a parfait or to fill a pie shell or tart shell. Use as a fruity complement to roast poultry or pork.		
OPTIONS			
A	**Fresh Fruit**: Skip the initial thawing step and add 2-5 minutes to the microwave time until fruit is cooked and thickened.		
B	**Canned Fruit**: Skip the initial thawing step, reduce sugar if fruit is sweetened, and add 1 Tbsp more cornstarch.		
C	**Spices**: Add 1 tsp cinnamon, nutmeg, ginger or other spices to complement fruit.		
D	**Liquor**: For a sophistiacted flavor, add 2 Tbsp liquor and an additional 1 tsp cornstarch in step 2. Grand Marnier, brandy, Amaretto and Chambord are suggestions.		

AGILE RECIPES

Photo on page 228

PROTEIN OTHER	Milk Pudding^V Makes about 2½ cups		Dessert
INGREDIENTS		**SUBSTITUTE**	
2 C	Milk	1 C cream + 1 C water, almond or oat milk	
½ C	Sugar		
2 Tbsp	Corn starch		
2	Eggs, large or XL		
1 tsp	Vanilla extract		
STEPS			
1	In a medium sauce pan, mix cold milk, corn starch and sugar well. Bring mixture to almost a boil over medium heat stirring constantly. It will start to thicken. Remove from heat.		
2	In a small bowl, beat eggs.		
3	Temper the eggs by slowly adding a cup of hot milk mixture to the eggs, 1-2 tablespoons at a time while stirring briskly.		
4	Pour tempered egg mixture back into the warm milk mixture in the pan stirring constantly.		
5	Cook over low heat stirring continuously until pudding almost boils and it thickens. Pudding will thicken more as it cools.		
6	Remove from heat and stir in the vanilla extract. Cover when cool. Serve warm or cold.		
OPTIONS			
A	**Vanilla Pudding**: Recipe above. Serve plain or with whipped cream, berries, or in a parfait.		
B	**Chocolate Pudding**: Stir ⅔ C chocolate chips or small pieces of chocolate bar into hot pudding. Stir to mix melted chocolate into pudding.		
C	**Banana Pudding**: Layer pudding with vanilla wafer cookies and bananas.		
D	**Maple Brown Sugar Pudding**: Use brown sugar instead of white sugar and stir in 1 tsp of maple extract along with the vanilla extract.		
E	**Fruity Parfait**: Layer pudding with fresh fruit, canned fruit, or jam, and granola or crushed cookies.		

Why make pudding from scratch?
  » It is super easy and you already have all the ingredients.
  » This recipe has about 8 g of protein per serving.
  » It costs about half vs making pudding from a mix.
  » There are no artificial ingredients.

Photo on page 222

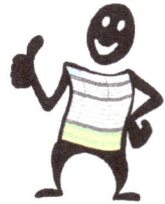

GRAIN	Pantry Cake^V Makes one 8" x 8" cake		Dessert
INGREDIENTS		**SUBSTITUTE**	
1½ C	Flour, all purpose (180 g)		
5 Tbsp	Cocoa powder		
¾ C	White sugar		
1 tsp	Baking powder		
½ tsp	Salt		
1 C	Coffee, cold	Water	
1 tsp	Vanilla extract		
2 tsp	Vinegar, white	Apple cider vinegar	
⅓ C	Canola oil	Coconut oil, melted butter	
STEPS			
1	Preheat oven to 350°F. Prepare a 8" x 8" pan by coating with cooking spray.		
2	Whisk dry ingredients in a bowl to combine well.		
3	Add liquid ingredients to dry and mix well with a whisk or large fork until there are no lumps.		
4	Pour into prepared pan.		
5	Bake for 25-30 minutes or until a toothpick comes out clean. Allow to cool before frosting or cutting.		
6	Serve topped with a sprinkle of powdered sugar, whipped cream or any frosting.		

AGILE RECIPES

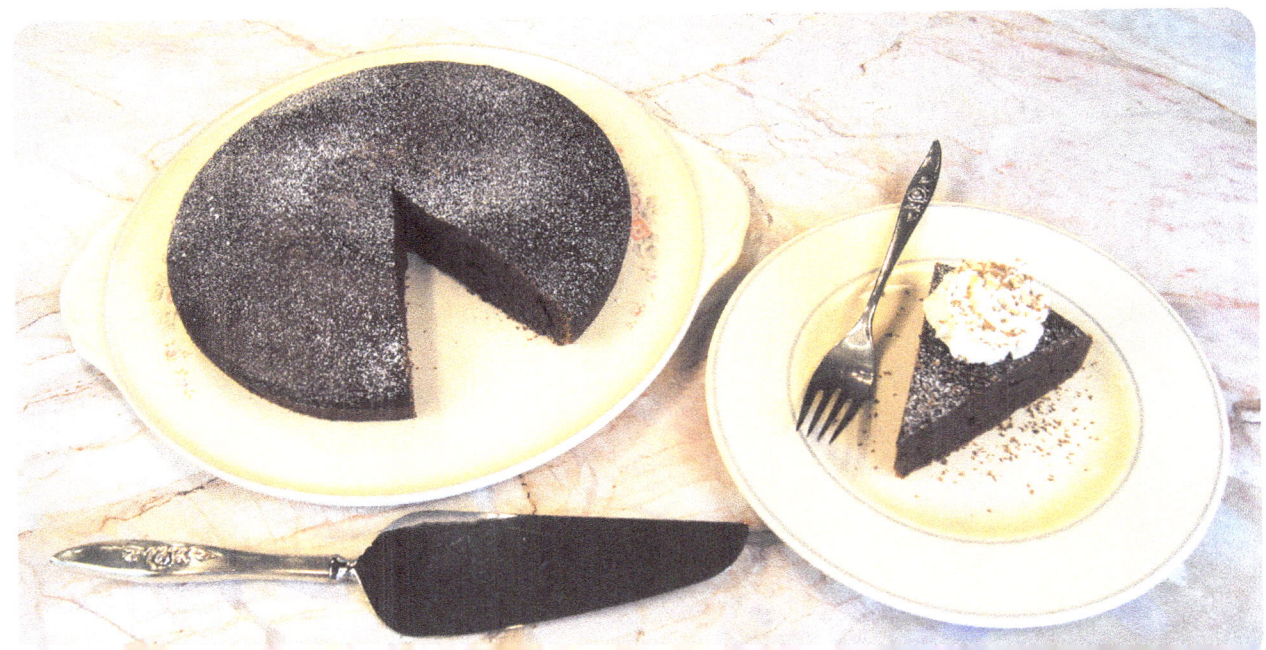

GRAIN	Pumpkin Muffins[V] Makes 24 muffins		Dessert
INGREDIENTS		**SUBSTITUTE**	
2 C + 1½ Tbsp	Flour, all purpose (251 g)	1½ C rice flour + ⅔ C tapioca flour or corn starch	
1½ tsp	Baking powder		
½ tsp	Baking soda		
1 tsp	Salt		
1½ tsp	Ginger		
1 tsp	Cinnamon		
½ tsp	Cloves, ground		
½ tsp	Nutmeg		
¾ C	Sugar, white		
¾ C	Sugar, brown		
1 C	Butter, melted	Light vegetable oil	
4	Eggs, large or XL		
1	Pumpkin puree, 15 oz can		
STEPS			
1	Preheat oven to 350°F. Prepare muffin pans by coating with cooking spray or using paper liners.		
2	In a large bowl, mix the flour, baking powder, baking soda and spices together.		
3	In a second bowl, mix the sugars, butter, eggs and pumpkin puree together.		
4	Pour the wet mixture into the dry and stir until fully incorporated and smooth.		
5	Pour batter info the muffin pans.		
6	Bake for 20-25 minutes, or until done and a toothpick inserted in the middle comes out clean.		
7	Serve plain or add frosting to serve as cupcakes (vanilla or cream cheese frosting are good choices).		

GRAIN	Rice Pudding^V Makes ~ 5 cups		Dessert

INGREDIENTS / SUBSTITUTE

INGREDIENTS		SUBSTITUTE
3 C	Cooked rice (white or brown)	Quinoa or wild rice
2 C	Milk	Almond or oat milk or half cream and half water.
½-1 C	Sugar	
2	Eggs, large or XL	
1 tsp	Vanilla extract	

STEPS

STEPS	
1	In a medium suace pan, bring rice, milk and sugar almost to a boil, stirring constantly.
2	Reduce heat and simmer for 15 minutes, stirring often.
3	In a small bowl, beat eggs.
4	Temper the eggs by adding a cup of hot milk/rice mixture to the eggs, 1-2 tablespoons at a time while stirring well.
5	Pour tempered egg mixture back into warm pan and mix well.
6	Cook over low heat for about 5 minutes stirring continuously.
7	Remove from heat and stir in the vanilla extract. Allow to cool then cover. Serve warm or cold, sprinkled with nutmeg or cinnamon sugar.

OPTIONS

OPTIONS	
A	**Chocloate Rice Pudding**: Stir ½ C chocolate chips or pieces of chocolate bar into hot pudding.
B	**Additions**: Stir in ⅓ C raisins or other dried fruit.

AGILE RECIPES

PROTEIN OTHER	Ricotta Cheesecake^V Makes one 9" cake		Dessert
INGREDIENTS		**SUBSTITUTE**	
32 oz	Ricotta cheese, well drained		
1½ C	Powdered sugar	½ C sugar	
4	Eggs, large or XL		
2 Tbsp	Corn starch		
1 tsp	Almond extract	1 Tbsp lemon or orange zest, 1 Tbsp Amaretto or Grand Mariner	
STEPS			
1	Preheat oven to 350°F.		
2	Prepare 9 inch springform pan by either coating it with butter and then flour, or lining it with parchment paper.		
3	In a bowl, beat the ricotta cheese and sugar until smooth.		
4	Add the eggs, corn starch and extract and beat gently until fully combined.		
5	Pour batter into the prepared pan.		
6	Bake about 60 minutes or until the center of the cake is just set. Cool fully before cutting. Serve plain or with a dusting of powdered sugar, whipped cream and berries.		

AGILE RECIPES

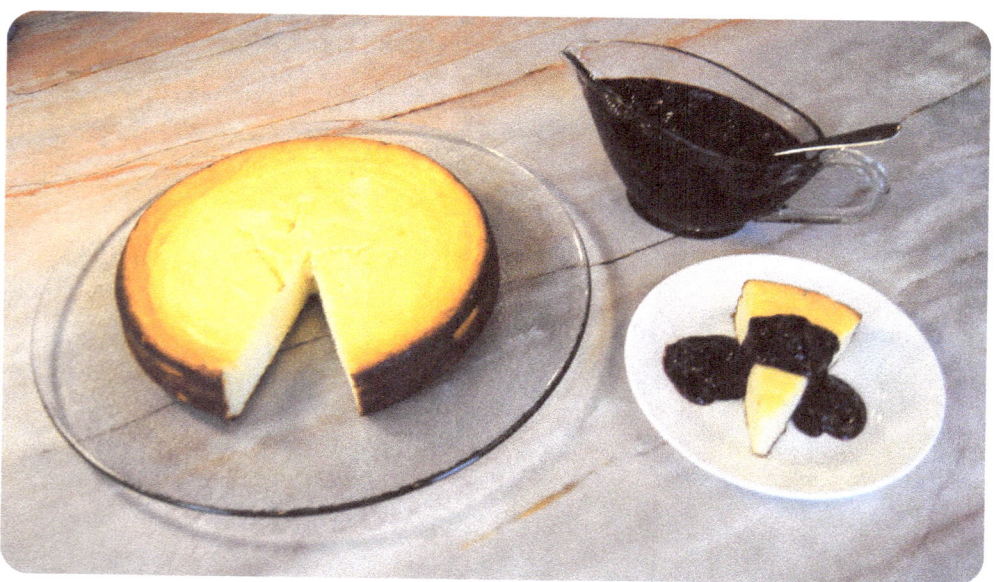

Shown with

Fast Fruit Filling

Recipe on page 223

GRAIN	Russian Tea Cakes^V Makes ~ 24		Dessert
INGREDIENTS		**SUBSTITUTE**	
1 C	Butter, room temperature		
½ C	Confectioners sugar (plus more for coating)		
1 tsp	Vanilla extract		
2½ C	All purpose flour (300 g)	2¾ C cake flour or substitute up to one fourth whole wheat flour	
¼ tsp	Salt		
¾ C	Finely chopped walnuts or pecans	Almond meal (nuts are not optional)	
STEPS			
1	Preheat oven to 400°F. Line cookie sheet with parchment paper if desired.		
2	In a large mixing bowl, cream butter, sugar and vanilla with mixer until smooth. A hand whisk may be used with good vigor.		
3	Add salt and flour. If you have a scale, you can weigh the flour directly into the bowl. Mix well.		
4	Add nuts and mix well. Dough should come together but be crumbly.		
5	Scoop rounded tablespoons of dough and roll into ~1" balls. Place on ungreased cookie sheet.		
6	Bake for 10-16 minutes, until set but not brown.		
7	Roll in confectioners sugar while warm and then again when cool. Store tightly covered.		

AGILE RECIPES

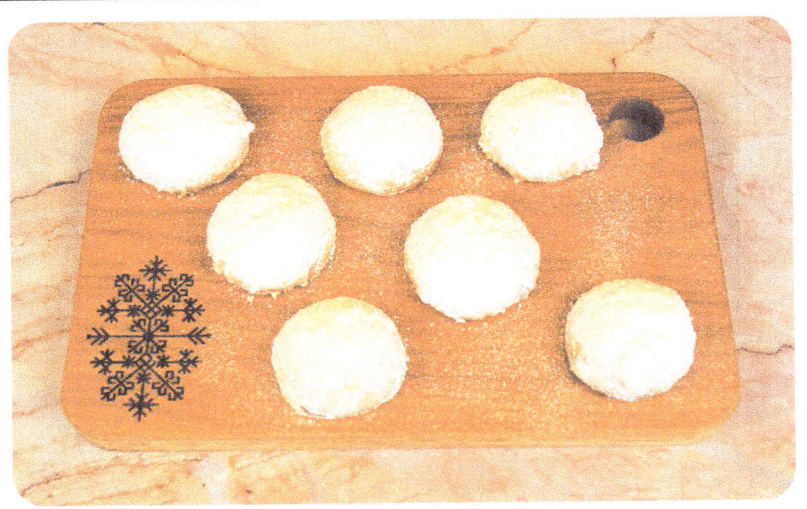

FRUIT	Spiced Poached Fruit^V Makes 4-6 servings		Dessert
INGREDIENTS		**SUBSTITUTE**	
1½ C	White wine		
½ C	Water		
¾ C	White sugar	Brown sugar	
1 Tbsp	Ginger paste or minced candied ginger	Cinnamon	
3 C	Fresh fruit - apple, peach, or pineapple		
STEPS			
1	In a sauce pan boil wine, water and sugar until it reduces slightly and starts to thicken, about 15 minutes.		
2	Remove from heat and stir in the ginger or other spice.		
3	Cut the fruit into slices or chunks and place in a heat resistant covered dish.		
4	Pour hot liquid over fruit, cover and allow to cool to room temperature. Refrigerate for an additional 1-24 hours.		
5	Served chilled fruit and syrup over ice cream or sorbet.		

AGILE RECIPES

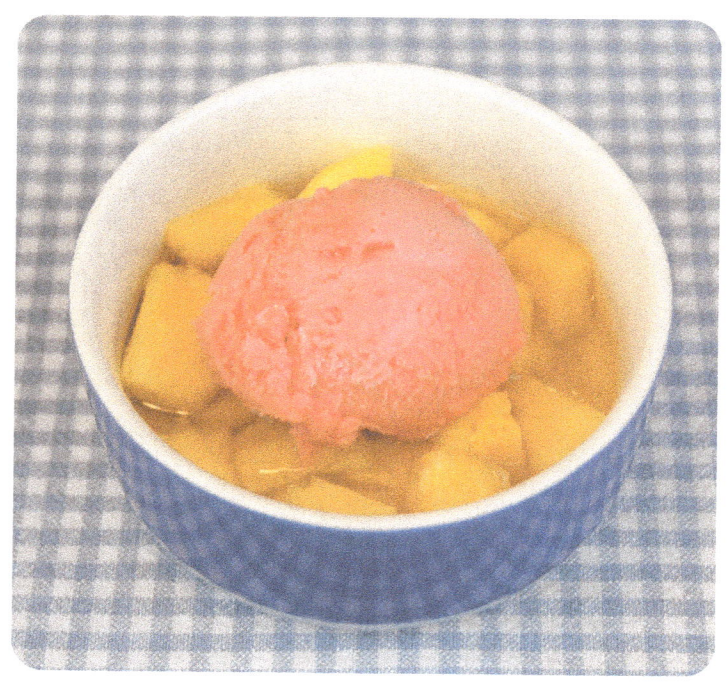

"Anything worth cooking generally starts with sautéed onion and garlic."

- Bette C. Martinoff

GRAIN	5-Minute Flatbread^V Serves 2		Main
INGREDIENTS		**SUBSTITUTE**	
2	Naan, fresh or frozen	Any flat bread, wrap or wheat tortilla	
½ C	Marinara sauce or pizza sauce	See Instant Marinara Sauce recipe page 289	
2 oz	Pepperoni	Hard salami	
6 oz	Mozzarella, grated		
STEPS			
1	Preheat oven to 400°F and line a baking sheet with parchment paper.		
2	Spread sauce over the top of the bread then add the toppings and cheese.		
3	Bake for 5-8 minutes, or until cheese is melted and bubbly.		
OPTIONS			
A	**BBQ**: Replace marinara suace with BBQ sauce, use cooked diced chicken or pork instead of pepperoni, and cheddar cheese instead of mozzarella. Sliced red onion is nice.		
B	**Veggie**: Replace pepperoni with thinly sliced veggies such as mushrooms, onion, peppers, spinach		
C	**Caprese**: Replace marinara with pesto and top with slices of fresh tomato and fresh mozzarella.		

AGILE RECIPES

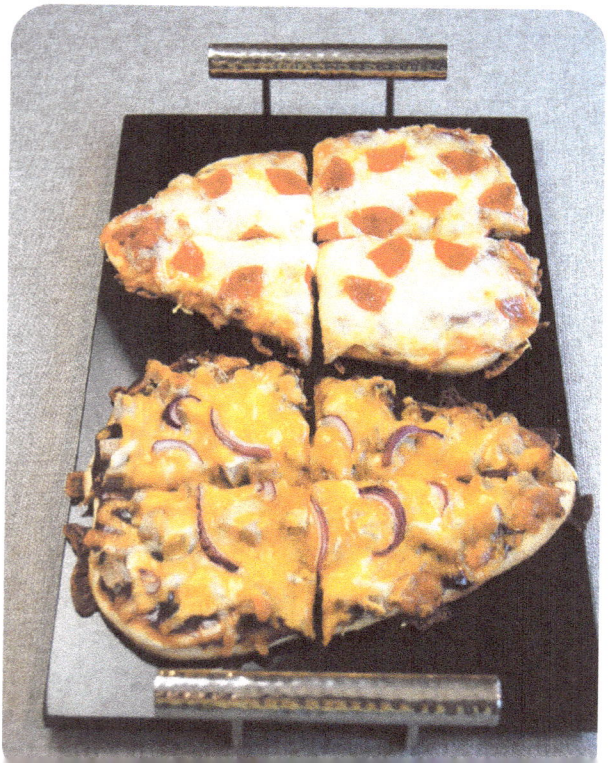

Marinara Pepperoni

Option A - BBQ

PROTEIN MEAT	Asian Glazed Anything^V Serves 3-4		Main

INGREDIENTS		SUBSTITUTE
1 lb	Chicken breast	Firm tofu, steak, pork, shrimp
1 Tbsp	Canola oil	Peanut oil
4 Tbsp	Soy sauce	
3 Tbsp	Water	
2 Tbsp	Brown sugar	
2	Cloves garlic, minced	1 tsp jarred minced garlic
1 tsp	Sesame oil	
1 tsp	Chili sauce	½ tsp red pepper flakes
1 Tbsp	Corn starch	
¼ C	Green onions, sliced	

STEPS	
1	Cut the meat or tofu into 1/2 inch thick slices. Leave shrimp whole.
2	In a large skillet, heat the oil to shimmering. Add meat and cook over medium high heat for three minutes per side. Should be nicely browned and almost completely cooked.
3	Whisk together remaining ingredients except green onions in a small bowl. Corn starch should form a smooth slurry.
4	Add sauce to the pan and continue to cook for about three minutes, stirring. Sauce should thicken.
5	Serve with white rice and garnished with green onions.

AGILE RECIPES

GRAIN	Baked Rice Casserole^V Serves 6-8	Main

INGREDIENTS		SUBSTITUTE
4 C	Cooked rice, white or brown	Packaged cooked rice, microwaved
1 lb	Cooked chicken, diced or shredded	Two 12.5 oz cans of chicken meat, cooked turkey or roast pork
½	Onion, finely diced	2 Tbsp dehydrated onion
4 C	Broccoli or broccolini, cut into bite size pieces	12 oz bag of frozen broccoli florets
4 C	Milk	
4 Tbsp	Flour	
2 C	Cheddar cheese, grated (8 oz)	Co-Jack cheese
1 Tbsp	Mushroom seasoning	Complete seasoning or other seasoning blend.
2 tsp	Salt (omit if your seasoning has salt in it)	
1 C	Panko bread crumbs (optional)	Any bread or cracker crumbs

STEPS	
1	Preheat oven to 350°F. Prepare a 9" x 13" pan or 2-3 qt baking dish by coating with cooking spray.
2	In a cup or bowl, mix the flour and milk together until a smooth, lump free slurry is achieved.
3	In a large stock pot, pour the milk and flour slurry together with the remaining milk and cook over medium heat until the mixture starts to thicken. Stir in the seasoning and salt.
4	Add the rice, chicken, onion, broccoli and half of the cheese to the milk mixture and stir to mix.
5	Pour rice mixture into the baking dish and top with remaining cheese and bread crumbs (if using)
6	Bake for 45 minutes or until bubbly and golden on top.

OPTIONS	
A	**Chicken Pot Pie Rice**: Replace broccoli with peas and carrots (thawed, if frozen) and replace mushroom seasoning with chicken bullion powder.
B	**Savory Mushroom**: Double the amount of onion and sauté the onion with 8-16 ounces of fresh, sliced mushrooms. Delete the broccoli. Replace mushroom seasoning with 2 tsp thyme or Herbs de Provence.

PROTEIN MEAT	Balsamic Glazed Chicken Serves 3-4		Main
INGREDIENTS		**SUBSTITUTE**	
1-1½ lb	Boneless chicken breast		
1 Tbsp	Extra Virgin Olive Oil	Any olive or cooking cil	
1 tsp	Minced garlic	½ tsp garlic powder	
1 tsp	Salt (optional)		
2 tsp	Herbs de Provence	Oregano or any mix of oregano, basil, rosemary and thyme	
¼ C	Balsamic vinegar	¼ C vinegar + 2 tsp any sugar or honey	
4 oz	Goat cheese, crumbled		
STEPS			
1	Slice chicken breast into pieces ¼ - ½ inches thick.		
2	Toss sliced chicken with oil, garlic, herbs, and salt (if using).		
3	Sauté chicken over medium high heat until nicely browned and nearly cooked through.		
4	Reduce heat to medium low and add balsamic vinegar. Cook for a few minutes, turning chicken to coat. Vinegar should thicken and become syrupy.		
5	Serve chicken drizzled with the balsamic reduction from pan and top with crumbled goat cheese.		

AGILE RECIPES

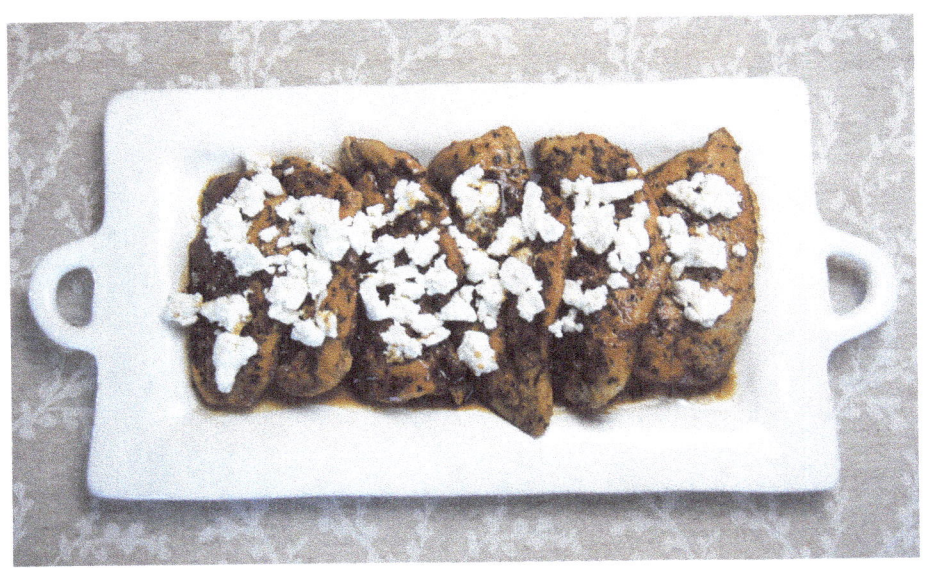

PROTEIN MEAT	Beef Stroganoff Serves 4-6		Main
INGREDIENTS		**SUBSTITUTE**	
1-1½ lb	Beef steak, finely sliced	Lean ground beef	
1	Onion, medium, finely sliced		
1 lb	Mushrooms, sliced (white or cremini)		
2 Tbsp	Extra Virgin Olive Oil	Any olive or light cooking oil	
1 C	Sour cream		
1 tsp	Thyme		
1 tsp	Salt		
STEPS			
1	Sauté the onion and mushrooms in the olive oil over medium-high heat until the liquid has nearly completely evaporated.		
2	Stir in the sliced meat and continue to cook until the meat is just cooked through. Stir often so all sides of the meat are cooked. This should go quickly – maybe 2-3 minutes		
3	Remove from the heat and stir in the sour cream, thyme and salt.		
4	Serve with noodles, rice or potatoes.		

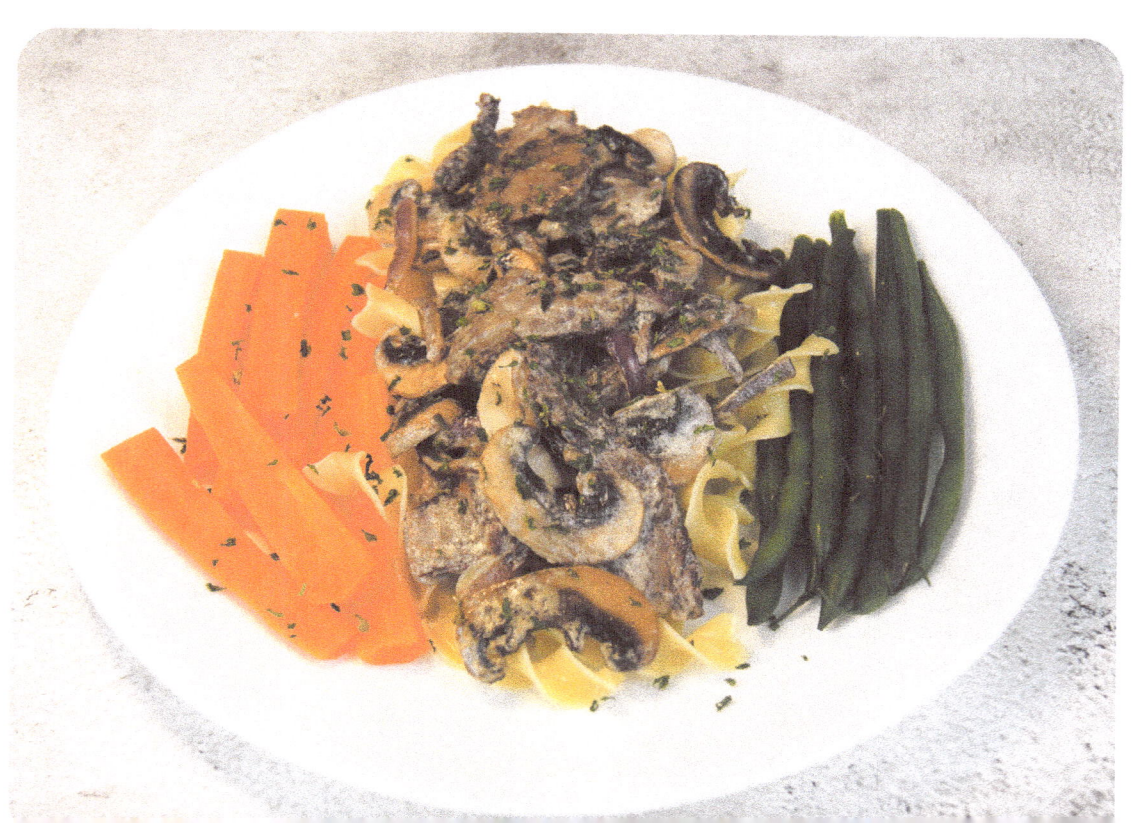

PROTEIN OTHER	Black Bean & Sweet Potato Chili^V Serves 6		Main

INGREDIENTS		SUBSTITUTE
2 Tbsp	Extra Virgin Olive Oil	Any olive, coconut or other light cooking oil
1	Onion	
4	Cloves garlic	2 tsp minced jarred garlic
1½ Tbsp	Chili powder	
1 Tbsp	Cumin	
½ tsp	Paprika	
½ tsp	Oregano	
1	28 oz can diced tomatoes	Fire roasted or with green chilies
2	15 oz cans of black beans, drained	
1 lb	Sweet potatoes, diced (3-4 small)	Butternut squash
2 Tbsp	Lime juice	Lemon or orange juice
2 C	Vegetable or chicken stock	Water

STEPS	
1	In a large stock pot, sauté onion in the oil until soft. Add the garlic and cook for another 2 minutes.
2	Add all other ingredients, stirring to mix well.
3	Bring to a boil and then reduce heat and simmer for 20-30 minutes or until sweet potatoes are tender.
4	Smash some of the sweet potatoes if you prefer a thicker consistency.
5	Serve plain or garnished with diced red or green onions, cheese, sour cream, avocado, or cilantro. Great with steamed corn tortillas or corn bread.

AGILE RECIPES

PROTEIN MEAT	Chicken Curry^V Serves 3-5		Main

INGREDIENTS		SUBSTITUTE
2 Tbsp	Extra Virgin Olive Oil	Any olive oil, butter, Ghee or light oil
½	Onion, medium, diced	1½ Tbsp dehydrated onions
2	Garlic cloves, minced	1 tsp garlic powder or granules
2 -3 Tbsp	Curry paste	Any preferred curry spice paste
1-1½ lb	Chicken breast, cubed	Diced turkey, canned chicken
8 oz	Tomato sauce (1 can)	Diced tomatoes (blended, optional)
8 oz	Water	Broth or coconut milk
8 oz	Chopped spinach, frozen or fresh	Sweet potatoes (diced), peas or chickpeas
½ C	Cream	Yogurt or aerosol whipped cream

STEPS	
1	In a heavy bottomed sauce pan, sauté onion over medium heat until soft.
2	Add garlic and curry paste to pan and cook another two minutes.
3	Add tomato sauce and water to pan, stir and bring to a boil.
4	Reduce heat, add chicken and any desired veggies. Simmer for 15 minutes or until chicken is cooked and veggies are tender.
5	Remove from heat and stir in the cream.
6	Serve with rice, naan, paratha or cooked cauliflower.

OPTIONS	
A	**Vegetarian:** Replace chicken with two 15 oz cans of chickpeas (drained). Include one diced sweet potato and spinach if desired.
B	**Thickened:** For a thicker sauce, use a flour/butter paste. Mix 1 Tbsp each of flour & butter, then stir the paste ½ tsp at a time into the simmering sauce to reach desired consistency.

AGILE RECIPES

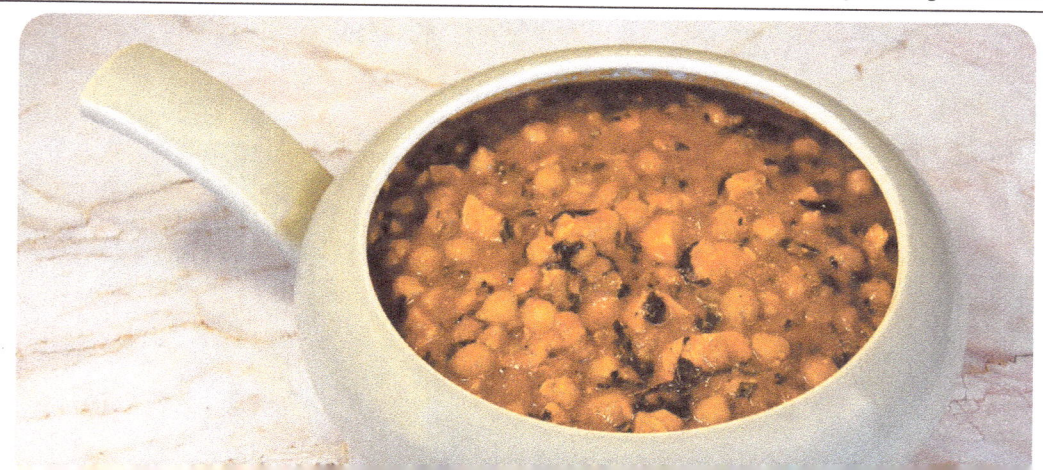

PROTEIN MEAT	Chicken Divan Serves 2		Main

INGREDIENTS		SUBSTITUTE
1 - 2	Cans chicken (6-12 oz total)	Any cooked and diced chicken or turkey
2 C	Chicken stock or broth	Bouillon cubes or stock paste + water
1 tsp	Dehydrated onions	2 Tbsp finely minced onions
⅓ C	Sherry	Any wine or 1 Tbsp of vinegar + 2 Tbsp water
2 Tbsp	Corn starch	
1 Tbsp	Mayonnaise	
1 Pkg	Broccoli spears, cooked and drained	Fresh or frozen
1 C	Shredded cheese (optional)	
½ C	Bread crumbs (optional)	Crushed crackers or unsweetened corn flakes

STEPS	
1	Warm chicken stock to almost boiling and add onions. Remove from heat.
2	Stir corn starch into cold wine, mixing well.
3	Stir wine and corn starch slurry into warm stock and return to heat. Warm over medium heat until thickened.
4	Add chicken to thickened sauce and heat thoroughly over medium heat.
5	Remove from heat and stir in mayonnaise.
6	Can serve chicken and sauce over a bed of cooked broccoli.
7	For a casserole, place brocolli and chicken in an oven proof casserole dish, top with cheese and/or bread crumbs. Bake for 10 minutes at 350°F for a crispy/melty top.

OPTIONS	
A	**Nutritious Pantry Meal**: Serve alone for a quick and easy low-carb meal.
B	**Extend the Meal**: Serve with rice, noodles, or grain to serve more people.
C	**Complete Casserole**: Layer 2 C cooked rice or noodles wth brocolli and chicken mixture. Top with cheese and bread crumbs and bake for 20 minutes at 350°F.

AGILE RECIPES

PROTEIN MEAT	Chicken Mushroom Marsala Serves 3-6		Main
INGREDIENTS		**SUBSTITUTE**	
8-16 oz	Mushrooms, sliced	Frozen or canned mushrooms	
1 tsp	Garlic, minced	½ tsp garlic granules	
3 Tbsp	Olive oil	Any light oil	
1-1½ lb	Chicken breast, sliced into thin cutlets	Veal or pork loin	
½ C	Flour		
¾ C	Masala or Sherry (sweet wine)	Any red wine + 3 tsp sugar	
½ Tbsp	Corn starch		
½ tsp	Salt and pepper, each		
STEPS			
1	Sauté mushrooms and garlic in 1 Tbsp of olive oil until mushrooms are cooked and most of the liquid is gone.		
2	Mix the corn starch into the cool wine then add to the mushroom pan. Stir over medium heat until the sauce thickens. Set aside and keep warm.		
3	Add salt and pepper to the flour in a shallow bowl.		
4	In a large skillet or sauté pan, heat the remaining 2 Tbsp of oil on medium heat until shimmering but not smoking.		
5	Dredge the chicken cutlets in the flour and place in the hot pan.		
6	Cook chicken until cooked through and lightly brown. Remove to platter.		
7	Serve chicken cutlets with mushroom and sweet wine sauce.		

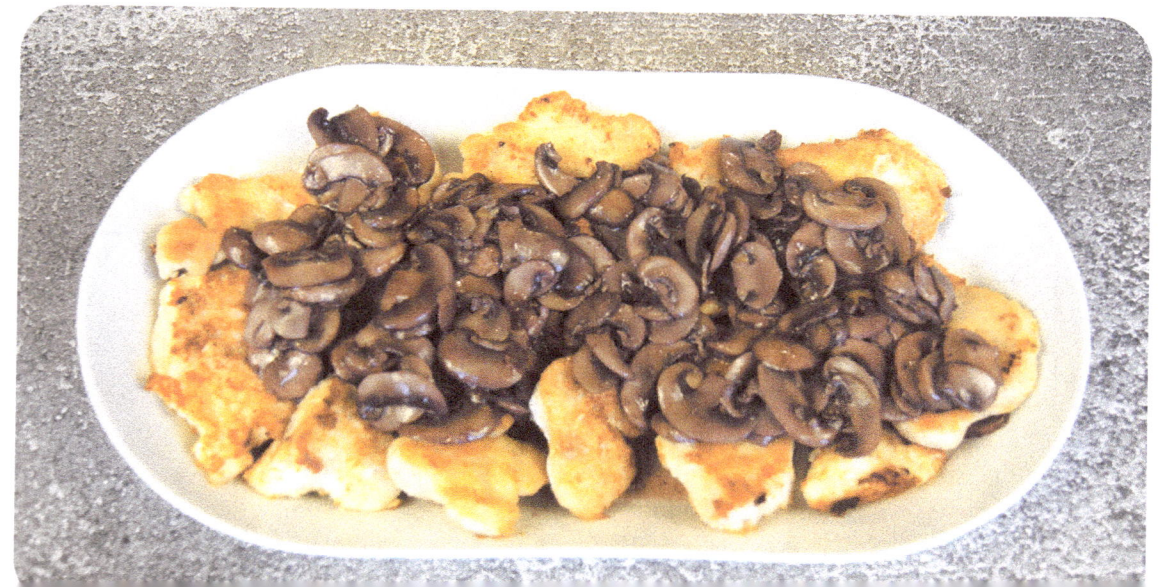

PROTEIN MEAT	Chicken Paillard Serves 4-6		Main
INGREDIENTS		**SUBSTITUTE**	
1-1½ lbs	Boneless chicken breast	Chicken tenders or medallions	
2 Tbsp	Extra Virgin Olive Oil		
1 tsp	Garlic, minced	Shallot or chives	
2 Tbsp	Fresh thyme (2 tsp if dried)	Basil	
2 Tbsp	Lemon juice (fresh is best) + lemon zest	White wine	
¾ C	Chicken stock (used in optional sauce)	¾ C water + ¾ tsp bullion powder	
	Salt and pepper to taste		
STEPS			
1	Slice each chicken breast into two or three cutlets, each ½ to ¾ inch thick.		
2	Place cutlets one or two at a time, between sheets of plastic cling wrap. Use a meat mallet or rolling pin to pound the cutlets to half thickness.		
3	Put pounded cutlets in a shallow dish and add the oil, lemon juice, and spices. Turn to coat and allow to rest for 15 minutes up to over night.		
4	Reserve the residual marinade if you are making the optional sauce.		
5	In a large sauté pan or skillet, pan fry the cutlets until golden on both sides. Use two pans or work in shifts so that the cutlets are not crowded in the pan.		
6	Chicken cutlets may be served without optional sauce, for example on a green salad.		
7	**Optional Sauce**: Add any remaining marinade and the chicken stock to the pan. Deglaze the pan over medium heat, stirring to fully incorporate. Cook a few minutes to allow sauce to thicken slightly. Drizzle over cutlets and serve.		

AGILE RECIPES

PROTEIN MEAT	Chicken Paprika Serves 2-4		Main
INGREDIENTS		**SUBSTITUTE**	
1½ -2 lb	Boneless chicken, thighs or breast	Bone-in chicken	
1	Onion, large, diced		
1 Tbsp	Paprika		
1 tsp	Garlic, minced	½ tsp garlic powder or granules	
8 oz	Tomato sauce	Diced tomatoes, canned or fresh	
½ C	Sour cream	Yogurt	
1 Tbsp	Flour		
	More paprika, salt and pepper to taste		
STEPS			
1	In a larger, heavy bottomed pot, sauté the onions with a little oil until soft. Add the garlic and paprika then cook an additional 2-3 minutes.		
2	Add the chicken, tomato sauce and water to the pot.		
3	Reduce heat, cover and simmer for at least 30 minutes. Chicken should be tender and cooked through.		
4	Stir the flour into the sour cream, mixing well. Add this to the warm sauce and stir continuosly over low heat while the sauce thickens.		
5	Serve with noodles, rice, potatoes or bread.		
OPTIONS			
A	**Bone-in**: If you use pieces with skin and bones, then allow the chicken to simmer for 45 minutes to ensure it is thoroughly cooked.		

AGILE RECIPES

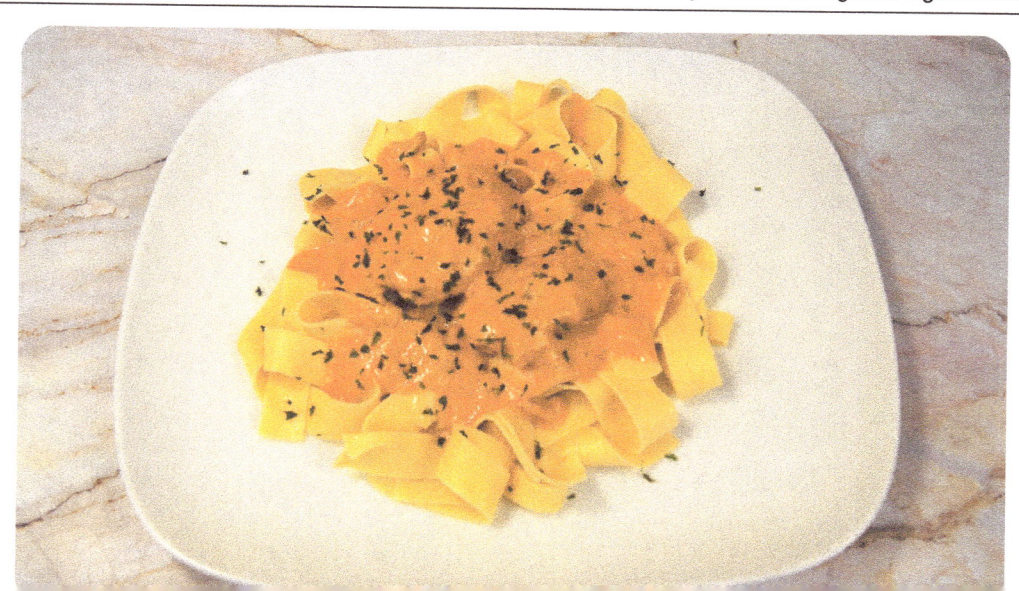

PROTEIN MEAT	Chicken Salad Serves 4		Main

INGREDIENTS		SUBSTITUTE
1 lb	Chicken breast, poached (see Poached Chicken recipe on page 262), diced	Any cooked chicken, cut up or shredded
¾ C	Mayonnaise	
¼ C	Sour cream	Yogurt
2	Green onions, finely sliced	2 Tbsp onion, finely minced
1-2	Celery stalks, finely diced	
1 tsp	Dijon mustard	
2 Tbsp	Fresh dill or tarragon	2 tsp dried dill or tarragon
2 Tbsp	Fresh parsley	2 tsp dried parsley
½ C	Seedless grapes, halved (optional)	Diced apples or dried cherries
¼ C	Slivered almonds (optional)	Chopped walnuts

STEPS	
1	In a large bowl, mix the mayonnaise, sour cream and Dijon mustard together.
2	Add all remaining ingredients and stir to mix.
3	Serve on bread, crackers or on a bed of greens.

OPTIONS	
A	**Classic:** Recipe above.
B	**Napa:** Include grapes and slivered almonds.
C	**Cherry Chicken:** Include dried cherries and chopped walnuts.
D	**Waldorf Chicken** Include grapes, apples and walnuts. Increase mayonnaise by ¼ C and add 1 Tbsp of honey.

PROTEIN MEAT	Chili Express Makes ~ 5 cups		Main
INGREDIENTS		**SUBSTITUTE**	
1 Tbsp	Extra Virgin Olive Oil	Any olive or light oil	
1	Onion, medium, diced	3 Tbsp dry onion or 1 Tbsp onion powder	
2	Cloves garlic, minced	1 tsp garlic powder or granules	
1 lb	Ground turkey	Ground chicken or beef	
1	Can (14.5 oz) cannellini beans, drained	Any canned beans	
1	Can (14.5 oz) diced tomatoes (with chilis, optional)	Any canned tomatoes or sauce	
1½ C	Chicken broth	1½ C water + 1/2 tsp bouillon or 1½ C water	
2 Tbsp	Chili powder		
1 Tbsp	Cumin		
STEPS			
1	In a large heavy bottomed stock pot, sauté onion in oil until soft. Add garlic & cook for 1 min.		
2	Add turkey, chili powder and cumin. Cook over medium high heat, stirring to crumble turkey, until meat is cooked.		
3	Add tomatoes, beans and broth. For a less chunky result, the tomatoes may be blended first.		
4	Bring to a boil then reduce heat and simmer for at least 20 minutes.		
5	Serve alone or with with diced green onion, warm tortillas, corn bread, sour cream or melted cheese. Freezes well.		

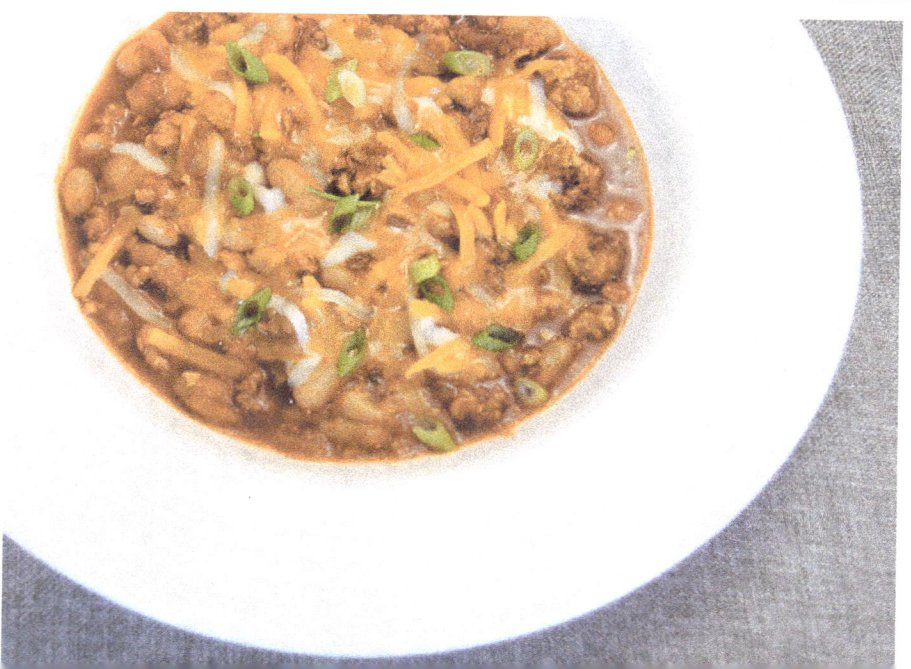

PROTEIN MEAT	Citrus Grilled Shrimp Serves 2 - 4		Main
INGREDIENTS		**SUBSTITUTE**	
1 lb	Large shrimp or prawns		
1 tsp	Garlic powder		
1 tsp	Onion powder		
1 Tbsp	Chili powder		
1 Tbsp	Canola oil	Coconut oil or sesame oil	
2 Tbsp	Orange juice concentrate	Orange juice	
2 Tbsp	Grand Marnier	Any orange liquor or brandy	
STEPS			
1	Rinse and devein shrimp. Remove tails if desired. Pat dry with a paper towel.		
2	Arrange shrimp in one layer on a plate. Apply half of the dry spices to one side, then flip and apply the rest to the other side.		
3	Heat oil in a large sauté pan – should be large enough that shrimp will fit in one layer.		
4	Over medium high heat, add the shrimp and cook for two minutes on one side. Flip and cook other side until shrimp is cooked: i.e. pink and not grey.		
5	Add orange juice and liquor to the pan, turning shrimp to coat and thicken sauce.		
6	Serve shrimp with rice, asian noodles, quinoa, or over salad greens.		

AGILE RECIPES

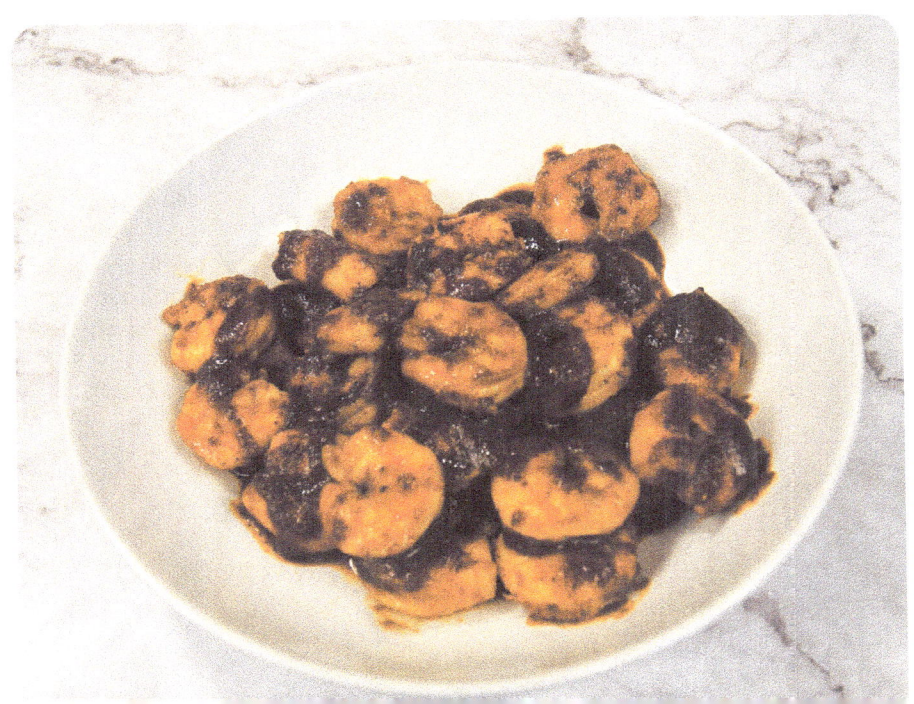

Safe Minimum Internal Temperature Chart for Cooking

Food	Type	Internal Temperature
Beef & Red Meats	Steaks, roasts, chops	145°F (63°C)
	Ground meat & sausage	160°F (71°C)
Poultry	Whole bird, breasts, legs, thighs, wings, ground, and sausage.	165°F (74°C)
Eggs	Raw eggs	Cook until yolk & white are firm
	Egg dishes (such as frittata or quiche)	160°F (71°C)
Ham	Raw ham	145°F (63°C) Rest time: 3 minutes
	Pre-cooked ham (reheat)	165°F (74°C)
Leftovers	Any type	165°F (74°C)
Pork	Steak, roasts, chops	145°F (63°C) Rest time: 3 minutes
	Ground meat & sausage	160°F (71°C)
Seafood	Fish such as salmon, tuna, cod, snapper, and sole	145°F (63°C) or cook until flesh is no longer translucent and separates easily with a fork
	Shrimp, lobster, crab, and scallops	Cook until flesh is pearly or white, and opaque

Source: Cook to a Safe Minimum Internal Temperature | FoodSafety.gov
March 14, 2024

PROTEIN MEAT	Enchilada Surprise^V Serves 4-6		Main

INGREDIENTS / SUBSTITUTE

INGREDIENTS		SUBSTITUTE
1	Medium onion, diced	
16	Corn tortillas	
16 oz	Grated cheese, Mexican blend	Co-Jack or mild cheddar or Queso Blanco
1	Can enchilada sauce (19 oz)	2-2½ C homemade Enchilada Sauce (see recipe on page 292)
½ -1 lb	Chicken, ground or diced	Beef, pork or turkey; precooked is OK.
1-2	15 oz cans black beans, drained	Other whole beans or refried beans
1	15 oz can corn, drained	½ bag of frozen corn, cooked and drained
1-2	Sweet potato, cooked and either mashed or diced	Canned sweet potato

STEPS

STEPS	
1	Preheat oven to 350°F.
2	If using uncooked meat, sauté onion and meat until meat is cooked through. For precooked meat, just add onion to the meat; it is fine to leave the diced onion uncooked.
3	In a 9" x 9" pan (or 2½ quart casserole dish) just cover the bottom with sauce: about ⅓ cup. Place four tortillas on top of the sauce, spread out to cover the bottom.
4	Spread one third of the meat, beans, corn and sweet potatoes over the tortillas, one-quarter of the cheese and then drizzle with one-third cup of sauce.
5	Make the second layer with 4 tortillas then repeat step 4. Repeat to make the third layer.
6	Use last four tortillas for the top layer, then cover with remaining sauce and then cheese.
7	Bake for 30-45 minutes, until hot and bubbly. Serve with sour cream, green onion, avocado or salsa as desired.

OPTIONS

OPTIONS	
A	**Vegetarian**: Omit the meat and use black beans, corn and sweet potato for a delicious combination.
B	**Tex-Mex**: Omit the sweet potatoes then use ground beef, corn, and red kidney beans or refried beans for a classic flavor.
C	**Leftover Meat**: Use any precooked, diced meat including roast beef, chicken, pork or turkey.
D	**Double Up**: Make a double recipe in a 9" x 13" pan.

Photo on page 260

PROTEIN MEAT	Fajitas Serves 4-6		Main
INGREDIENTS		**SUBSTITUTE**	
1½ - 2 lb	Steak - flank, skirt or other	Chicken breast, sliced horizontally, shrimp	
¾ C	Fajita Marinade (recipe on page 275)		
2 Tbsp	Canola oil		
1	Onion, large, cut into slices		
2-3	Bell peppers, sliced (red, yellow and green)		
12	Tortillas, corn or flour	Naan, pita bread	
STEPS			
1	Place the meat in a Ziploc bag or covered bowl with the Fajita Marinade and refrigerate for 2-24 hours. For shrimp, marinate for two hours.		
2	Ideally, grill the meat over a medium high fire to get nice caramelization on the outside. Steak takes about five minutes per side for medium rare. Chicken will take longer, shrimp less.		
3	Alternatively, use a large heavy skillet to cook the meat. Heat 1 Tbsp of the oil to shimmering and add the meat in one layer. Cook to desired doneness.		
4	Remove meat from the heat and allow to rest while cooking the vegetables.		
5	Add 1 Tbsp of oil to the heavy skillet, then cook the onions and peppers quickly over a medium high heat.		
6	Slice the meat into strips and serve with the vegetables and tortillas. Grated cheese, sour cream, salsa and guacamole compliment nicely.		

AGILE RECIPES

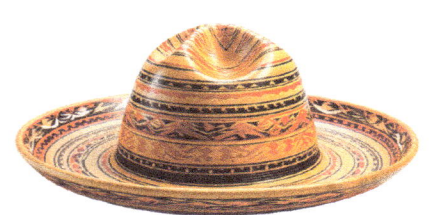
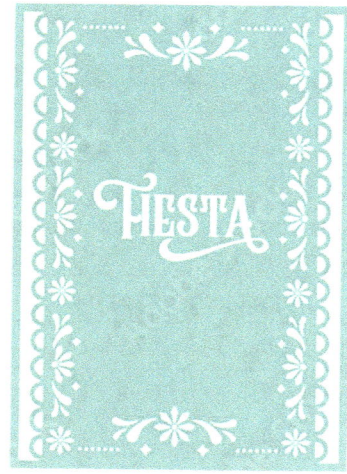
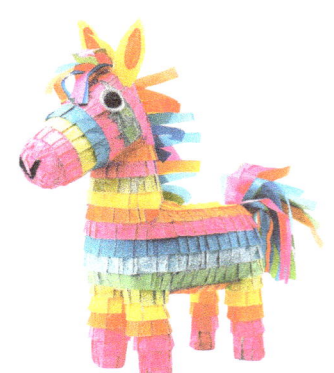

GRAIN	Fried Rice^V Serves 2		Main

INGREDIENTS		SUBSTITUTE
2 C	Cooked rice, refrigerated day old preferred	
2 Tbsp	Canola oil	
3	Eggs, large or XL, beaten	
3	Green onions, sliced	
2	Carrots, diced, cooked	
1 Tbsp	Soy sauce	
1 tsp	Sesame oil	
1½ C	Peas, cooked	
4 oz	Cooked chicken or pork, diced (optional)	Firm tofu, diced, for vegetarian dish

STEPS	
1	Heat 1 Tbsp oil in a large skillet or wok. Pour in the eggs and stir to scramble.
2	Once the eggs are set, add the rice and continue to cook over medium high heat, stirring to break up the rice and thoroughly mix.
3	Push the eggs and rice to the side, add the remaining 1 Tbsp of oil and green onions to the middle. Cook for a minute then stir into the rice mixture.
4	Add the cooked peas and meat (if using), along with the soy sauce and sesame oil to the pan. Continue to cook long enough to heat and mix.

AGILE RECIPES

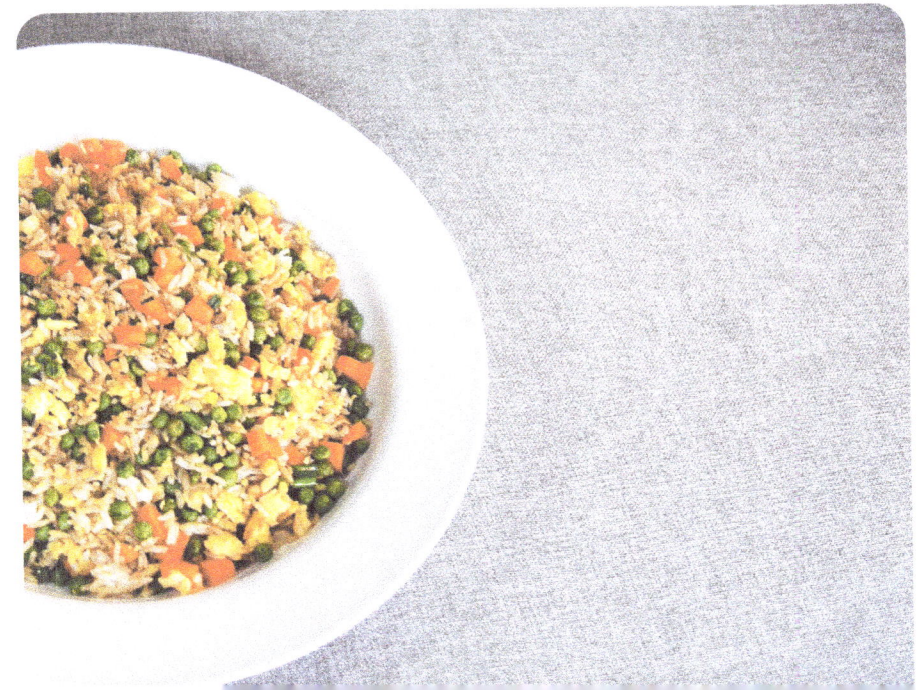

PROTEIN MEAT	Glazed Salmon Serves 4		Main
INGREDIENTS		**SUBSTITUTE**	
4	Salmon fillets, 6-8 oz each	Skin on or skinless, fresh or previously frozen	
4 Tbsp	Brown sugar		
1 tsp	Ginger paste	1 tsp dried ginger	
2 Tbsp	Dijon mustard		
2 Tbsp	Soy sauce		
STEPS			
1	Preheat oven to 400°F. Prepare baking pan or sheet pan by coating with oil.		
2	Prepare the salmon by removing any bones, rinsing and then patting dry.		
3	Mix the remaining ingredients together which will form both the glaze and a dipping sauce.		
4	Place the fillets in the pan and brush half of the mixture on top of the fillets.		
5	Bake for about 10-15 minutes until desired doneness. An internal temperature of 135°F for medium and 145°F for well done.		
6	If you would like a crispy upper crust, you can turn on the broiler for 3-5 minutes.		
7	Once cooked, the flesh may be easily separated from the skin by slipping a very thin metal spatula between them.		
OPTIONS			
A	**Sweet Mustard Glaze:** Recipe above. Serve with the remaining sauce on the side.		
B	**Citrus Glazed**: Replace the soy sauce, Dijon, and ginger with 2 Tbsp orange juice concentrate and ½ tsp each salt and paprika. Use all glaze.		
C	**Blackened**: Replace the soy sauce, ginger, Dijon, and brown sugar with 2 Tbsp Cajun seasoning mix. Use all to glaze. For a sweeter result, include 2 Tbsp of the brown sugar.		

Photo on page 260

PROTEIN MEAT	Hammered Chops Serves 2-4		Main
INGREDIENTS		**SUBSTITUTE**	
2 lbs	Pork chops, boneless		
½ C	Flour		
2 tsp	Garlic salt	Any savory spice blend	
1 tsp	Black pepper		
¼ C	Oil – for pan frying		
STEPS			
1	Start with chops between ½ - ¾ inch thick. If your chops are thicker than this, slice them to get the right thickness.		
2	Place the chops one or two at a time between sheets of plastic wrap, on top of a cutting board.		
3	Using a meat mallet, pound the chops until they are about half the thickness.		
4	Mix the flour and spices in a shallow dish or container. Dredge each chop and set aside until ready to fry.		
5	In a large fry pan, heat the oil until shimmering but not smoking. Cook the chops in one layer until golden and cooked through, about 3 minutes per side.		
6	Cooked chops may be kept warm by placing them in one layer on a sheet pan in a 350°F oven until ready to serve.		

AGILE RECIPES

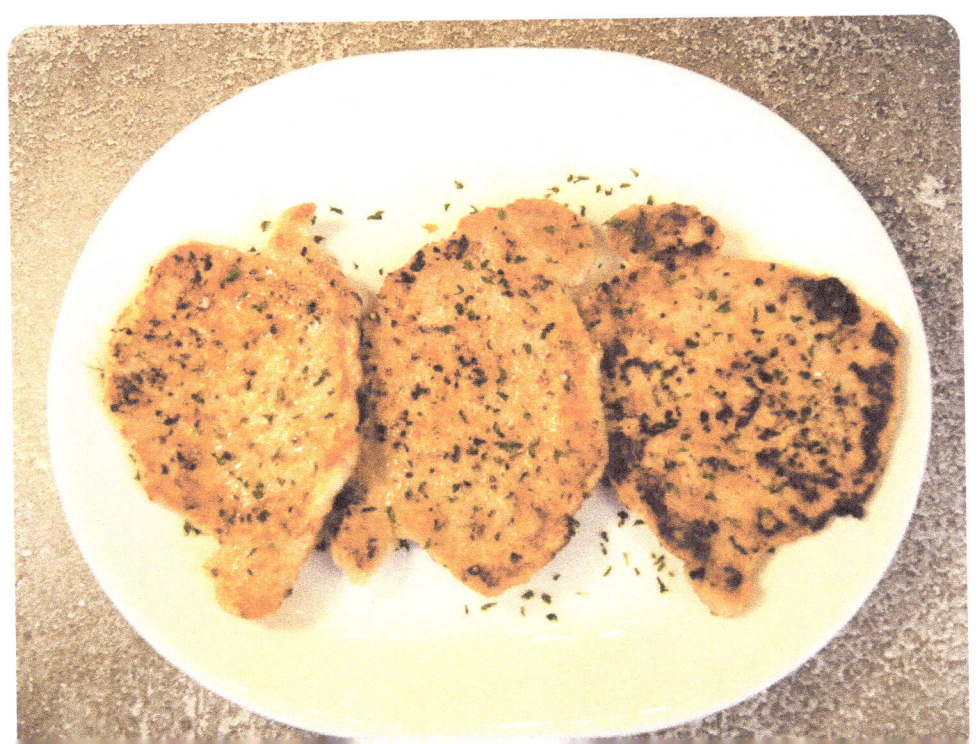

Dish in photo was made with 12 oz of pork, not the full recipe

PROTEIN MEAT	Italian Sausage – Scratch Makes 1 lb		Main
INGREDIENTS		**SUBSTITUTE**	
1 lb	Ground pork	Ground turkey or chicken	
1 Tbsp	Apple cider vinegar	Any vinegar or lemon juice	
¾ tsp	Salt		
¾ tsp	Black pepper		
1½ tsp	Dried parsley		
2 tsp	Onion powder		
2 tsp	Garlic powder		
2 tsp	Oregano		
1 tsp	Paprika		
1 tsp	Fennel seeds, ground		
½ tsp	Thyme		
½ tsp	Basil		
½ tsp	Brown sugar	Any sugar or sweetener	
¾ tsp	Red pepper flakes	For mild, use less or no red pepper flakes	
STEPS			
1	In a bowl, mix ground meat with vinegar.		
2	Spread all dry spices over meat and mix until evenly distributed.		
3	For sausage logs, divide sausage into thirds and then form 1 inch diameter cylinders. Wrap cylinders in plastic wrap. (Skip this step if you want sausage crumbles.)		
4	Refrigerate 12-24 hours prior to cooking.		
5	Use as you would any uncooked italian sausage; e.g., spaghetti, lasagna, pizza.		

PROTEIN OTHER	Lasagna Florentine^V Makes two 9" x 13" pans	Main
INGREDIENTS		**SUBSTITUTE**
6	Cloves garlic, minced	3 tsp jarred minced garlic
1 Tbsp	Extra Virgin Olive Oil	Butter
12 oz	Spinach, fresh, baby (8-16 oz)	Frozen spinach, thawed and drained
32 oz	Ricotta cheese	Cottage cheese, small curd
2	Eggs, large or XL	
48 oz	Marinara sauce	Store bought or use the Classic Marinara recipe on page 290
4 C	Mozzarella cheese, shredded (16 oz)	
2 ib	Lasagna noodles	Can use "oven ready" noodles

STEPS	
1	Sauté garlic in olive oil then add spinach and stir until just wilted.
2	Mix ricotta cheese with eggs, then stir in spinach.
3	Cook lasagna noodles until al dente, then drain and rinse. If using oven ready noodles, dip in sauce before putting them in the pan.
4	In two 9"x13" greased pans, make four layers. The first three layers are sauce, noodles, ricotta, and mozzarella. The top layer is noodles, sauce and mozzarella.
5	Cover pans tighly with greased foil. At this point, may be refrigerated for one day or frozen.
6	Bake at 350°F covered for 45 minutes then for 15 minutes uncovered. (From frozen: 75 minutes covered then 10 minutes uncovered)
7	Let stand for 10-15 minutes before slicing.

AGILE RECIPES

PROTEIN MEAT	Lemon Butter Baked Fish Serves 4		Main
INGREDIENTS		**SUBSTITUTE**	
4	Mild fish fillets, about 6 oz each, skinless	Cod, haddock, snapper, sole	
6 Tbsp	Butter		
2 Tbsp	Lemon juice		
¾ C	Panko bread crumbs	Any bread crumbs, crushed crackers	
1 Tbsp	Lemon pepper seasoning		
1 Tbsp	Dried parsley		
STEPS			
1	Preheat oven to 400°F.		
2	Melt 3 Tbsp of the butter in a shallow baking dish or pan, just big enough for your fillets. Add the lemon juice and stir.		
3	Melt the remaining 3 Tbsp of butter in a small bowl and mix in the seasoning, parsley and bread crumbs.		
4	Take each fillet and dip the top in the lemon butter then turn them over and place them in the pan.		
5	Top the fillets with the buttery crumb mixture.		
6	Cook for 20-25 minutes or until the fish has reached an internal temperature of 145°F.		

AGILE RECIPES

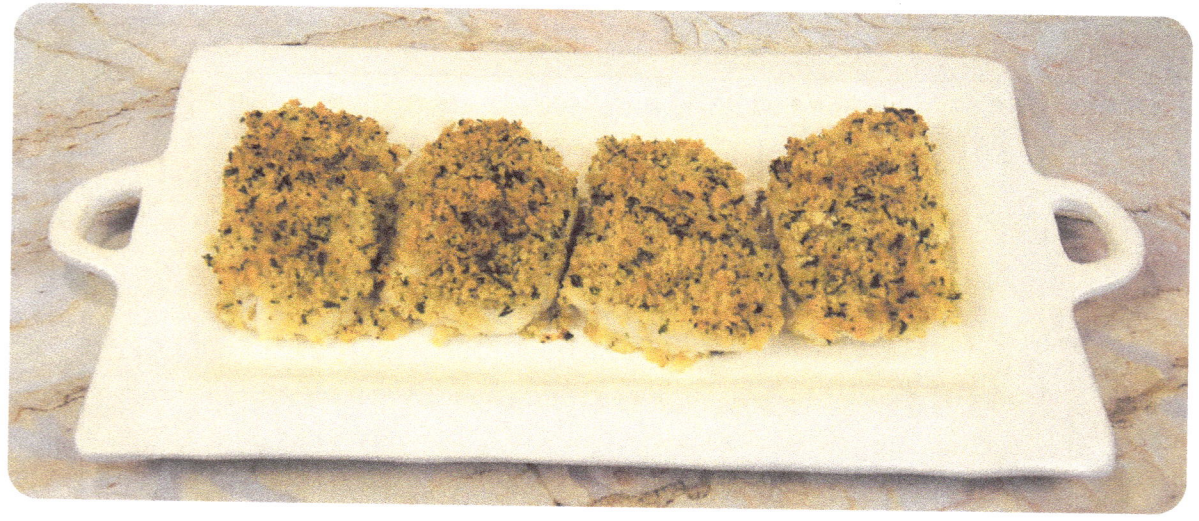

PROTEIN OTHER	Lentils del Sol^V Serves 2-4		Main
INGREDIENTS		**SUBSTITUTE**	
1½ C	Dry green lentils, rinsed	Any type of lentil	
4 C	Chicken stock	Water	
⅓ C	Sun dried tomatoes in oil, drained and diced	Dry sun dried tomatoes, soaked in hot water then finely sliced	
⅓ C	Olive tepanade, prefer with Kalamata olives	⅓ C Kalamata olives + 2 cloves of garlic + 1 Tbsp olive oil, minced and combined	
1-2 Tbsp	Extra Virgin Olive Oil		
2 tsp	Basil	Thyme or oregano	
1 tsp	Salt		
1-2 Tbsp	Pine nuts (optional)		
STEPS			
1	In a large pot, bring lentils and stock to a boil. Reduce heat and simmer until lentils are tender but not mushy; 25-45 minutes depending on the type of lentil (refer to package).		
2	Drain any excess liquid from lentils. If you prefer your lentils less dry, leave about ½ C liquid in the pot.		
3	In a small bowl, mix the tomatoes, oil, tepanade, basil and salt together. Stir tomato and tepanade mixture into lentils.		
4	Cook over low heat for 5-10 minutes before serving as a main or side dish. Garnish with pine nuts if desired. Serve warm or cold. Makes about 4 cups.		

AGILE RECIPES

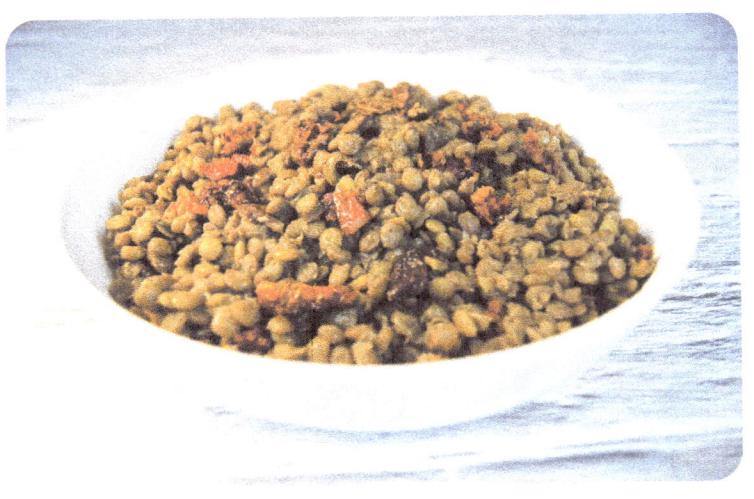

PROTEIN MEAT	Marinated Flank Steak Serves ~ 6		Main
INGREDIENTS		**SUBSTITUTE**	
1	Flank steak (1½ - 2 ibs)	Skirt steak	
½ C	Balsamic vinegar	Wine vinegar + 2 Tbsp sugar	
2 Tbsp	Brown sugar		
2 tsp	Garlic, minced (fresh is best)		
2 tsp	Herbs de Provence	1 tsp Rosemary + 1 tsp Thyme	
1 tsp	Salt		
½ tsp	Cracked black pepper		
STEPS			
1	Use a large fork to perforate steak on each side. This allow the marinade to penetrate the meat more effectively.		
2	Place meat in a gallon Ziploc bag (preferred) or a flat glass dish that may be covered.		
3	Mix marinade in a small bowl and then pour over the meat. Turn to ensure meat is covered.		
4	Allow to marinate over night, turning a few times to ensure even flavor.		
5	Take meat out of refrigerator an hour prior to cooking.		
6	GRILL METHOD: Preheat grill to Medium High. Grill steak on each side for 4-6 minutes. Internal temperature of 125 - 130°F will result in medium rare as temp will continue to rise.		
7	OVEN METHOD: Preheat oven to 425°F. Use a broiling pan and roast for 4-6 minutes per side. Internal temperature of 125-130°F will result in medium rare. Temp will continue to rise.		
8	Allow meat to rest for at least 5 minutes before carving.		
9	Cut meat into thin strips, slicing against the grain of the meat.		

AGILE RECIPES

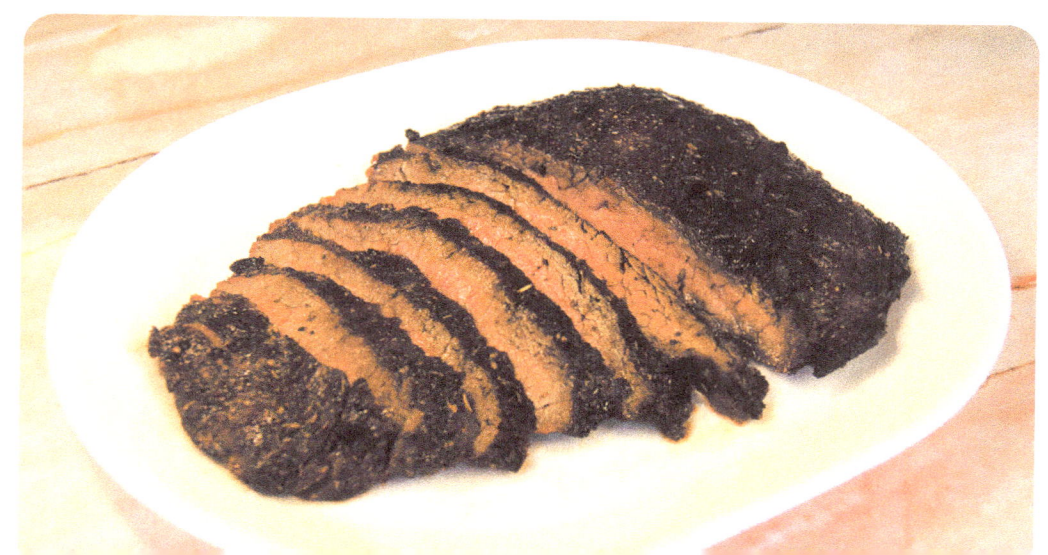

PROTEIN MEAT	Meatballs – Italian Makes 8 - 12 meat balls		Main
INGREDIENTS		**SUBSTITUTE**	
1 lb	Ground beef	Ground pork, chicken, turkey, or lamb	
2	Slices of bread, torn into pieces	½ C dried bread crumbs	
3	Cloves garlic	1½ tsp minced jarred garlic	
1	Egg, large or XL		
2 Tbsp	Milk		
¼ C	Grated Parmesan cheese		
2 tsp	Italian seasoning	Oregano or basil	
STEPS			
1	Preheat oven to 400°F.		
2	Chop bread into crumbs using a blender or immersion blender. Add garlic cloves and blend until it is minced finely.		
3	In a bowl, mix all ingredients together until thoroughly incorporated. Can be done with hands, a large fork or a mixer.		
4	Form into uniform balls about 1½ inch diameter and place on baking sheet. An ice cream scoop works well to get a uniform shape and size.		
5	Bake for 15 minutes or until brown and cooked through (internal temperature of 160°F).		
6	Serve with you favorite sauce and pasta or to make meatball subs.		

AGILE RECIPES

Everyone, Almost Everywhere, Love Meatballs!

The first known reference to meatballs is in an ancient Roman collection of recipes, titled Apicius, which dates back to the 4th or 5th century CE.

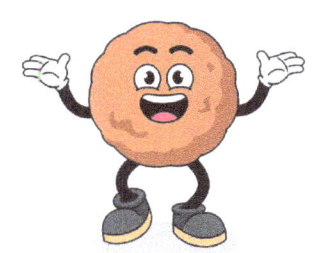

Meatballs are popular around the world - Europe, the Middle East, China, Japan, Southeast Asia, and the Americas. There are thousands of recipes using a large variety of meats, cheeses, grains, nuts, and local spices. Meatballs can be fried, baked, or steamed.

Experiment with your options and enjoy!

PROTEIN MEAT	Meatloaf Serves ~ 8		Main

INGREDIENTS		SUBSTITUTE
2 lb	Ground beef or beef-pork mixture	Any ground meat including chicken, turkey, pork, veal or lamb.
2	Medium onions, diced	⅓ C dried onions, soaked in 2 Tbsp hot water.
2	Eggs, large or XL	
2	Slices of bread, diced	½ C dry bread crumbs or rolled oats or crushed crackers or corn flakes
3 Tbsp	Worcestershire sauce	
2 Tbsp	Tomato paste	Ketchup
1 tsp	Salt and pepper, each	
1 tsp	Thyme or Herbs de Provence	Poutry seasoning may be used for ground chicken or turkey.
¼ C	Beef broth or bouillon	Use chicken broth for poultry.
½ C	Ketchup (can add some hot sauce if desired)	BBQ sauce or steak sauce

STEPS	
1	Preheat oven to 350°F.
2	In a large mixing bowl, combine all ingredients except ketchup. Mix well but avoid compressing the mixture.
3	Cover a sheet pan with foil or parchment paper for easier clean up (optional).
4	Gently form the meat mixture into a rectangular loaf on the sheet pan. A 9 x 13 baking dish can be used but leave room around the loaf.
5	Spread ketchup over the top of the loaf.
6	Bake for 45-60 minutes, until the internal temperature reaches 165°F.

OPTIONS	
A	**BBQ**: Substitute 1 tsp cumin and 1 tsp chili powder for thyme. Use BBQ sauce instead of ketchup on top. Add bacon crumbles if desired.
B	**Italian**: Replace onions with 4-6 cloves of minced garlic and replace thyme with oregano. Spread marinara sauce on top instead of ketchup.
C	**Mushroom**: Sauté 8-16 oz of sliced, fresh mushrooms then add to the meat mixture.
D	**Cheeseburger**: Stir in 8 oz of diced or grated cheddar cheese. Use half steak sauce and half ketchup for the glaze.

AGILE RECIPES

PROTEIN MEAT	Oven-Fried Chicken Serves 4-6		Main

INGREDIENTS / SUBSTITUTE

INGREDIENTS		SUBSTITUTE
2 -3	Boneless chicken breast (1-1½ lb)	Chicken tenders or cutlets
¼ C	Mayonnaise	Any type, including reduced fat
½ tsp	Seasoning salt	
½ tsp	Black pepper	
1 tsp	Poultry seasoning	
½ tsp	Paprika	
1¼ C	Panko bread crumbs	Any dry bread crumbs, crushed corn flakes or crackers

STEPS

STEPS	
1	Preheat oven to 400°F. Line sheet pan with parchment paper if desired.
2	Slice chicken breasts into cutlets, medallions or strips which are ½ - ¾ inches thick.
3	In a medium bowl, mix mayonnaise and spices. Add chicken pieces and turn to coat thoroughly.
4	Put crumbs in a shallow bowl. Place one or two pieces of chicken at a time into the bread crumbs.
5	Place breaded chicken pieces onto the sheet pan, leaving space between.
6	For a crispier crust, lightly spray chicken with oil using an oil mister (optional).
7	Bake for 20-25 minutes until chicken is cooked through (165°F internal temperature). Avoid overcooking as chicken will dry out.

OPTIONS

OPTIONS	
A	**Gluten Free**: Replace bread crumbs with almond meal or any unsweetened crispy crushed gluten free cereal made from corn, oats or rice.
B	**Italian**: Use Italian seasoned bread crumbs and replace poultry seasoning with oregano or Italian seasoning.
C	**Cajun Spicy**: Replace poultry seasoning and seasoning salt with a cajun spice blend. Add ¼ tsp red pepper flakes for extra heat.
D	**Crispy Garnish**: Instead of discarding, stir remaining crumbs and mayo together then bake on the sheet pan along with the chicken. Use as a tasty crispy topping for a side dish.

Photo on page 273

AGILE RECIPES

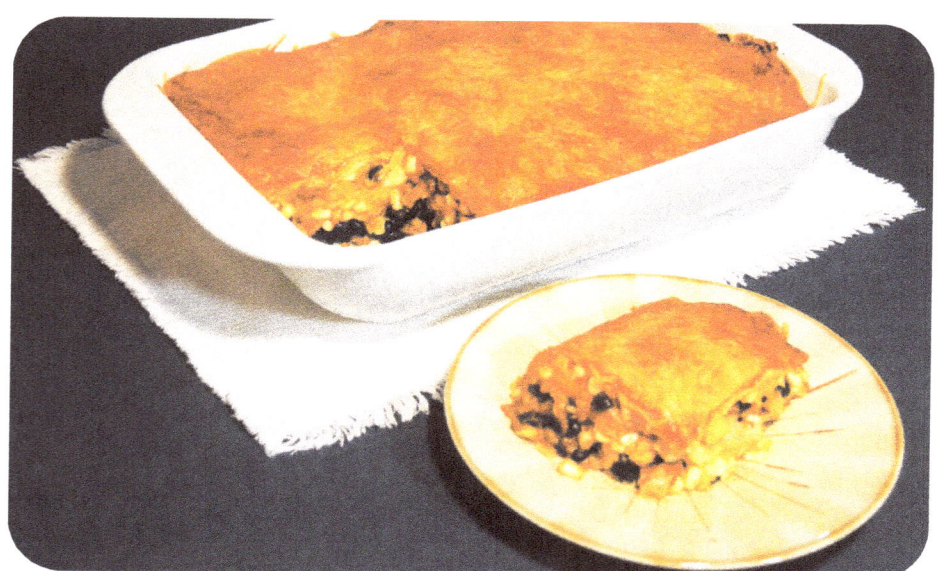

Enchilada Surprise

Recipe on page 247

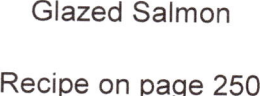

Glazed Salmon

Recipe on page 250

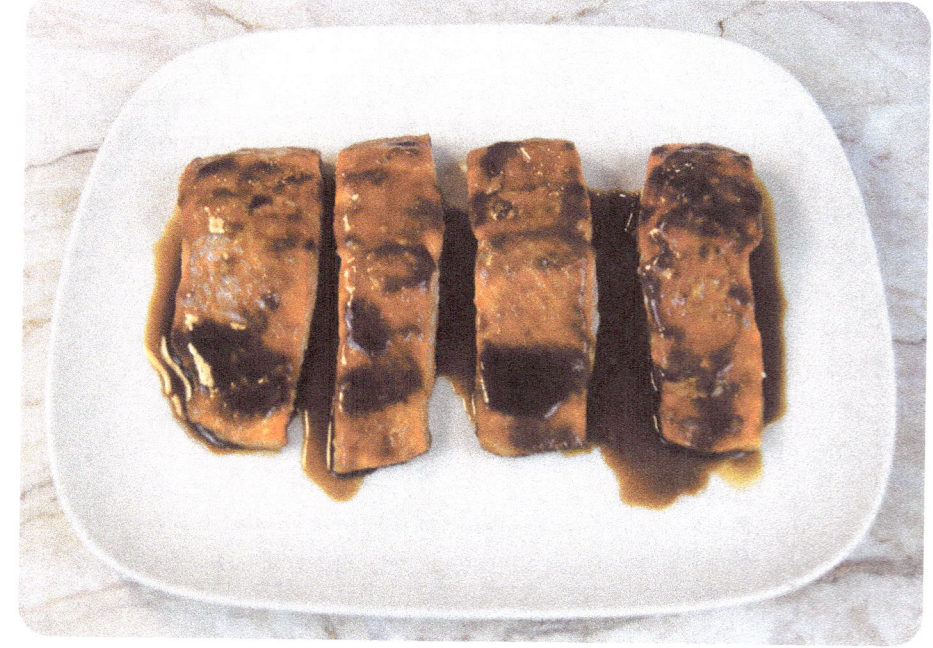

PROTEIN MEAT	Picadillo Serves 4-6		Main
INGREDIENTS		**SUBSTITUTE**	
1 lb	Ground beef	Half ground pork + half ground beef	
2	Onions, medium, chopped		
2	Cloves garlic, minced		
2 Tbsp	Extra Virgin Olive Oil	Any olive oil or light cooking oil	
1	15 oz can of tomatoes, diced or crushed		
1 tsp	Oregano		
1 Tbsp	Vinegar		
½ C	Raisins, chopped		
1 Tbsp	Tomato paste	2 Tbsp ketchup (omit vinegar)	
½ C	Green olives with pimento, sliced or whole		
STEPS			
1	In a large heavy bottomed pot, sauté onion in oil until soft then add the garlic and cook for an additional two minutes.		
2	Add ground beef and brown. Drain excess oil if necessary.		
3	Add remaining ingredients and bring to a boil.		
4	Reduce heat, cover and simmer for about an hour. Stir occasionally.		
5	Serve with white rice and black beans, or moro (recipe on page 298).		

AGILE RECIPES

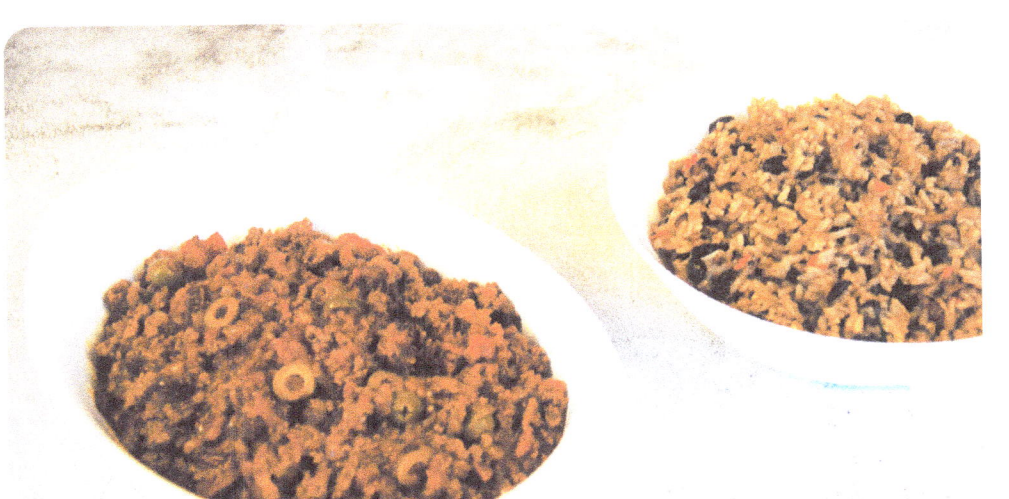

Shown with Cuban
Moro Beans & Rice

Recipe on page 298

PROTEIN MEAT	Poached Chicken Serves ~ 2		Main
INGREDIENTS		**SUBSTITUTE**	
2-4	Chicken breast, whole, boneless	Fish fillets, shellfish	
	Water	Chicken broth	
	Lemon (optional)	Garlic	
	Herbs de Provence (optional)	Rosemary, Italian seasoning	
STEPS			
1	Select a pot with a tight-fitting lid, large enough that the chicken breast fit snugly in a single layer.		
2	Place the chicken breasts in the pot and add any desired flavorings such as lemon, garlic or herbs.		
3	Cover chicken breast with enough water to cover the chicken breast plus two inches.		
4	Bring the liquid to a boil over medium high heat. Immediately turn the heat down to a simmer and cover the pot.		
5	Simmer for 10-15 minutes, until the internal temperature reaches 165°F. Start checking the temperature after about 10 minutes. For seafood, reduce time as needed.		
6	Remove chicken from the liquid and allow to stand for five minutes prior to slicing. If not using immediately, store chicken uncut to maintain moisture.		
7	Poached chicken is great in salads, casseroles, sliced for sandwiches or served sliced with a complimentary sauce.		

AGILE RECIPES

Why poach?

Poaching is a great way to cook chicken, fish or shellfish so that it stays moist and tender with a delicate flavor. It is ideal for serving chicken or seafood cold; in salads, sandwiches or just with a flavorful sauce. Poaching is also a great way to quickly cook an item before it spoils!

PROTEIN MEAT	Roast Pork Tenderloin Serves 6-10		Main
INGREDIENTS		**SUBSTITUTE**	
2	Pork tenderloins, about 2½ lbs		
1 recipe	Apple Cider Vinegar Marinade (page 274)	Dry rub, BBQ sauce	
STEPS			
1	Make the marinade in a gallon Ziploc bag and add the pork. Allow pork to marinate overnight in the refrigerator, turning occasionally.		
2	Preheat oven to 400°F.		
3	Place tenderloins on a broiling pan or roasting pan, preferably with grates or a rack.		
4	Roast for 30-40 minutes. Test for doneness with an instant read thermometer inserted in the thickest part of the meat. An internal temperature of at least 145°F is recommended.		
5	Allow the pork to rest for at least 5 minutes before slicing and serving.		
OPTIONS			
A	**Dry Rub**: Instead of marinating the pork, simply coat the exterior with your favorite spice blend or dry rub.		
B	**BBQ**: Instead of marinating the pork, brush the top with your favorite BBQ sauce once before putting it in the oven and again after 20 minutes.		

AGILE RECIPES

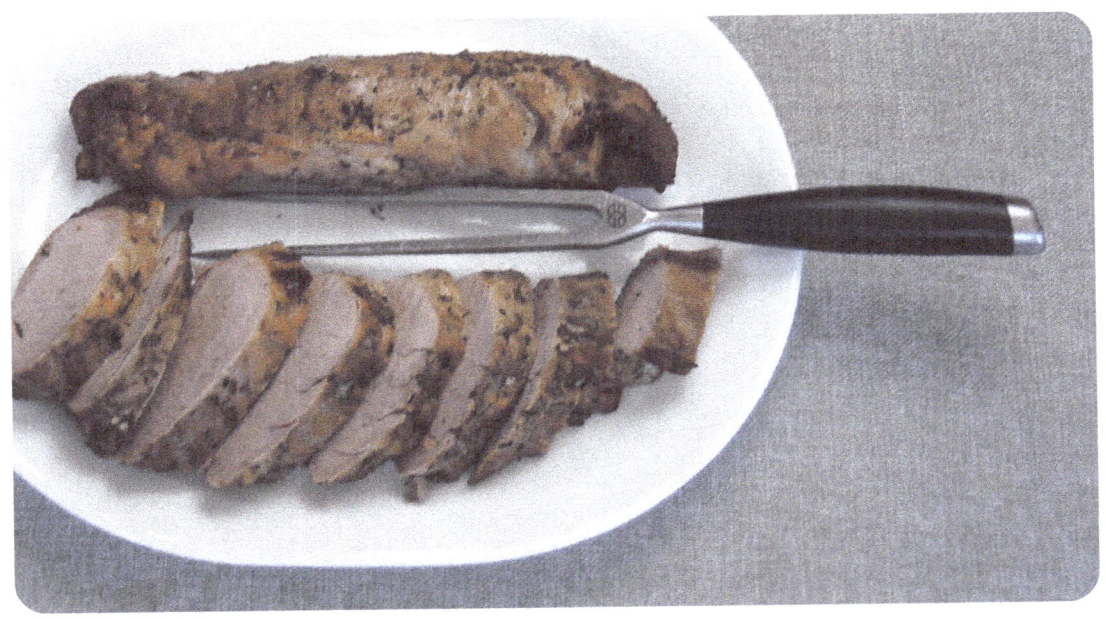

AGILE RECIPES

PROTEIN MEAT	Shrimp Scampi Serves 4		Main
INGREDIENTS		**SUBSTITUTE**	
12 oz	Angel hair pasta	Linguini	
1 lb	Shrimp, cleaned and deveined		
4	Cloves garlic, minced	2 tsp jarred minced garlic	
2 Tbsp	Extra Virgin Olive Oil		
1 C	Dry white wine		
3 Tbsp	Lemon juice		
5 Tbsp	Butter		
1 tsp	Salt		
¼ tsp	Red pepper flakes (optional)		
½ C	Grated parmesan cheese		
2 Tbsp	Fresh parsley, garnish (optional)		
STEPS			
1	Cook the pasta to slightly less than al dente. It will cook more later. Reserve 1 C of the pasta water.		
2	In a large pan, heat the olive oil and add the garlic. Cook for about one minute.		
3	Cook the shrimp until it is just cooked through, about two minutes per side. Using a slotted spoon, remove the shrimp to a plate.		
4	Add the wine, lemon juice, salt, and red pepper flakes to the pan and cook for three minutes to allow sauce to thicken slightly.		
5	Add the shrimp back to the pan, along with the pasta, butter and ¼ C pasta water. Cook while turning in the pan to coat the pasta and melt the butter.		
6	Add more pasta water in 2 Tbsp increments if needed.		
7	Serve topped with parmesan cheese and a garnish of chopped fresh parsley.		

Photo on page 273

PROTEIN MEAT	Sloppy Joes Serves ~ 4		Main
INGREDIENTS		**SUBSTITUTE**	
1-1¼ lb	Ground beef	Ground turkey or ground chicken	
½	Onion, medium diced	1½ Tbsp dried onion or ½ Tbsp onion powder	
1	Red bell pepper	Green or yellow pepper	
1 tsp	Garlic, minced	½ tsp garlic powder or granules	
¾ C	Ketchup	[1/2 C tomato paste + 1 tsp sugar + 1 Tbsp vinegar + ¼ C water] or [8 oz tomato sauce + 1 tsp sugar + 1 Tbsp vinegar]	
2 Tbsp	Brown sugar	Any sweetener	
1 tsp	Mustard, yellow or Dijon	1 tsp dry mustard powder	
½ C	Water		
1 tsp	Corn starch		
½ tsp	Salt and pepper, each		
STEPS			
1	Brown meat, onion and garlic in large frying pan. Drain excess oil if necessary.		
2	Add ¼ C water, ketchup, sugar, and mustard to the pan then bring to a boil.		
3	Reduce heat and simmer for 5-10 minutes, stirring occasionally.		
4	Mix corn starch and ¼ C cool water together. Add to pan over low heat and stir until thickened. Salt and pepper to taste.		
5	Serve on hamburger buns, dinner rolls for sliders or over rice or cauliflower rice.		

AGILE RECIPES

PROTEIN MEAT	Spaghetti Sauce Serves 6-10		Main
INGREDIENTS		**SUBSTITUTE**	
1 lb	Ground beef, lean	Ground turkey, chicken or pork	
2 Tbsp	Extra Virgin Olive Oil	Any olive or light oil	
1	Onion, diced		
2	Cloves garlic, minced	1 tsp minced jarred garlic	
1 Tbsp	Flour		
1 C	Dry red wine	Any dry wine	
28 oz	Can crushed tomatoes	Diced tomatoes or whole tomatoes cut up	
6 oz	Tomato paste		
1 C	Beef broth	Water + bouillon powder	
2 tsp	Oregano	Basil or Italian Seasoning	
1 C	Mushrooms, fresh sliced (optional)	Canned mushrooms	
STEPS			
1	In a stock pot, sauté onion in the oil until soft. Add the garlic and cook for an additional minute.		
2	Stir the flour into the ground beef and then add it to the pot and cook until crumbly.		
3	Add the wine and cook over medium high heat for two minutes.		
4	Add remaining ingredients and simmer over low heat, stirring occasionally. If you are in a rush, simmer for a half hour but simmering for 1½ hours will produce a better flavor.		
5	Serve with pasta or any dish calling for a tomato based Italian sauce. Freezes well.		

AGILE RECIPES

PROTEIN OTHER	Stuffed Shells^V Serves 4-6		Main

INGREDIENTS | SUBSTITUTE

INGREDIENTS		SUBSTITUTE
16 oz	Ricotta cheese	
2	Eggs, large or XL	
3 Tbsp	Grated Parmesan cheese	Grated mozzarella, Romano, or Swiss cheese
1 box	Jumbo shells, uncooked	
6 C	Chicken broth or vegetable stock	6 C water + 6 tsp bullion powder
	Olive oil and grated cheese for serving	Alfredo sauce, marinara sauce, or sour cream

STEPS

1	In a medium sized bowl, mix the ricotta cheese, eggs and grated Parmesan well.
2	Fill uncooked shells with the ricotta mixture. Set the filled shells aside on plates or a cookie sheet. You will use about 24 shells.
3	Place two large (10 inch diameter) skillets or stock pots with tight-fitting lids on the stove and put half of the broth in each one. Bring liquid to a boil.
4	Turn off heat and carefully place half of the shells in each of the pots, open side facing up. A large spoon or tongs work well. Shells should be almost submerged.
5	Turn heat back on to a gentle simmer and place the lids on the pots. Check that the liquid does not boil too vigorously as this will dislodge the cheese from the shells.
6	Cook for 15-20 minutes, until shells are cooked to al dente.
7	Remove cooked shells to a serving dish with a slotted spoon, gently draining any residual liquid.
8	Serve plain or with your choice of topping such as butter or olive oil and grated cheese, sour cream, Alfredo sauce, or Marinara sauce.

AGILE RECIPES

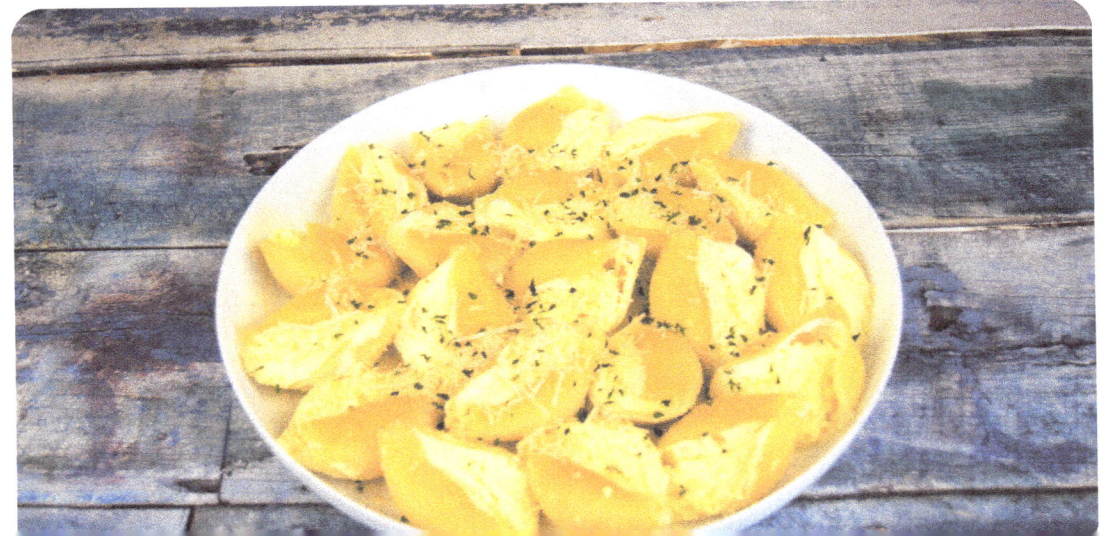

AGILE RECIPES

PROTEIN MEAT	Tacos Serves 3-4		Main
INGREDIENTS		**SUBSTITUTE**	
1	Medium onion, diced	2 Tbsp dehydrated onion	
1 lb	Ground beef	Any ground or diced meat: chicken or turkey	
2	Cloves garlic, minced	1 tsp jarred garlic or ⅔ tsp garlic powder	
1½ Tbsp	Chili powder		
1 Tbsp	Cumin		
½ tsp	Oregano		
½ tsp	Paprika		
1 tsp	Salt		
1 tsp	Sugar		
2 Tbsp	Tomato paste	Ketchup (eliminate sugar)	
2 tsp	Corn starch		
½ C	Beef broth (cold)	Chicken broth or just water	
STEPS			
1	Sauté onion in an oiled pan until soft. (If using dehydrated onion, just add it to meat.)		
2	Add garlic and ground meat to pan. Brown over medium heat.		
3	Skim off excess fat if necessary.		
4	Add all spices and tomato paste, then mix well. Allow to cook for about 5 minutes.		
5	Mix corn starch into broth until smooth. Add to meat & stir over medium heat until thickened.		
OPTIONS			
A	**Tacos:** Serve in corn or flour tortillas with cheese, lettuce, tomato, salsa, sour cream, etc.		
B	**Burritos**: Roll meat in flour tortilla with your choice of refried beans, rice, cheese, salsa, etc.		
C	**Taco Pie** - Mix meat with 1 bag of cooked frozen corn and place in the bottom of a baking dish. Top with 1 package of corn bread dough made to package instructions and then bake for 15-20 minutes at 350°F or until corn bread is done.		
D	**Nachos**: Spread a layer of corn chips on a baking pan. Top chips with meat mixture and choice of refried beans, peppers, salsa and cheese. Toast under broiler to melt cheese (or 400°F oven for 5 minutes).		
E	**Stuffed Peppers**: Fill any clean pepper with meat mixture and bake at 350°F for 45 minutes. Meat mixture can include up 50% cooked rice, drained beans, or corn.		

PROTEIN MEAT	Teriyaki for All Serves 4-6		Main
INGREDIENTS		**SUBSTITUTE**	
2 lb	Chicken breast or thighs, boneless, skinless	Steak or pork, boneless	
1 C	Teriyaki Marinade (recipe on page 275)		
⅓ C	Water (cold)		
2 tsp	Corn starch		
1 Tbsp	Canola oil		
1 tsp	Sesame oil (optional)		
	Green onions and sesame seeds for serving		
STEPS			
1	Cut meat into one inch pieces and put into Ziploc bag or covered dish.		
2	Pour ⅔ C of the teriyaki marinade over the meat and refrigerate for two to six hours. Reserve the remaining ⅓ C marinade for later.		
3	After the meat has marinated, remove it from the marinade and discard the used liquid.		
4	In a large skillet, heat the canola oil to shimmering and add the meat. Cook the meat quickly over medium high heat.		
5	Mix the reserved marinade with the water, corn starch and sesame oil (if using), stirring to form a smooth slurry.		
6	When the meat is thoroughly cooked, add the marinade/cornstarch mixture and cook for 3-5 minutes while stirring. The sauce should thicken and coat the meat.		
7	Serve with rice and veggies, garnished with sliced green onions and sesame seeds as desired.		

AGILE RECIPES

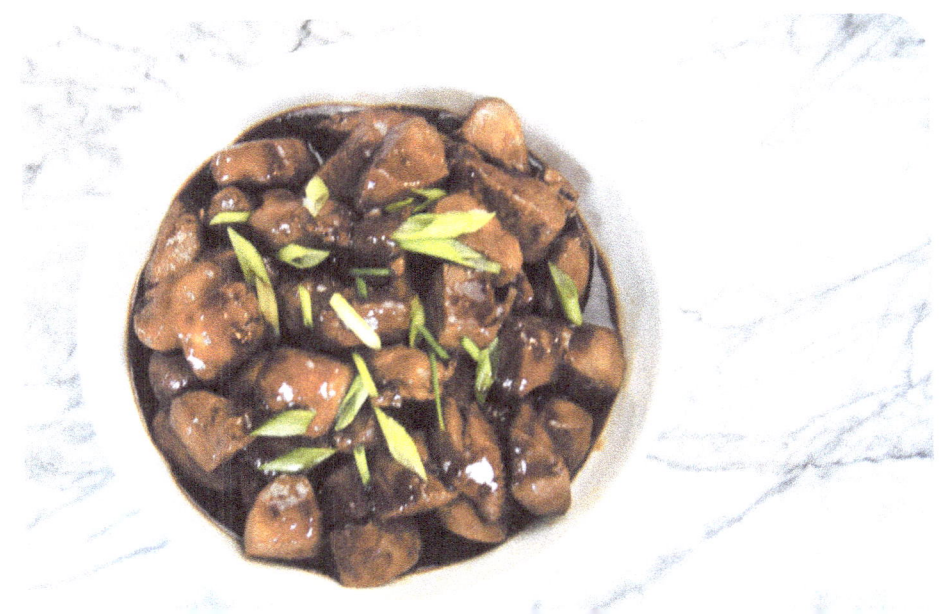

PROTEIN MEAT	Tuna Cake Serves 4-6 patties		Main
INGREDIENTS		**SUBSTITUTE**	
2	5 oz cans of tuna	Canned salmon	
¼ C	Mayonnaise		
2 Tbsp	Onion, finely diced	1 Tbsp dehydrated onion +1 Tbsp water	
2 Tbsp	Red pepper, finely diced	Diced celery or olives or capers	
1 tsp	Chili sauce (optional)	½ tsp red pepper flakes	
1 Tbsp	Dijon mustard	½ Tbsp Worcestershire sauce	
2	Eggs, large or XL		
¼ C	Bread crumbs, Panko	Any bread crumb or crushed cracker	
2 Tbsp	Extra Virgin Olive Oil	Any olive oil light oil for pan frying	
STEPS			
1	Drain tuna and break apart in a bowl.		
2	Mix in mayonnaise, onion, pepper, chili sauce, mustard and eggs.		
3	Add bread crumbs and mix gently. Mixture should hold together. Add more crumbs if needed.		
4	Form mixture into patties about ¾ inch thick. Makes about four large or six small patties. Chill patties briefly to help them hold their shape.		
5	Pan fry the patties in oil over medium high heat until golden brown and crispy – about four minutes per side.		
6	Serve alone or on a sandwich with a condiment such as mayo, dijonnaise, rémoulade, tartar sauce or a lemon wedge.		

AGILE RECIPES

PROTEIN MEAT	Tuna Salad Serves 2-4		Main
INGREDIENTS		**SUBSTITUTE**	
2	5 oz cans of tuna		
2 Tbsp	Pickle relish, sweet	Diced dill pickle or olives or capers	
2	Green onion, sliced	2 Tbsp red onion, diced	
2	Ribs celery, diced	Red bell pepper, diced	
½ C	Mayonnaise		
1 tsp	Dijon mustard (optional)		
STEPS			
1	Drain tuna well and break apart in a bowl.		
2	Add all remaining ingredients and mix well.		
3	Serve on bread, crackers, lettuce cups, tomato or cucumber slices or on salad greens.		
OPTIONS			
A	**Mediterranean**: Replace sweet pickle relish with capers or sliced olives. Replace celery with red pepper. Use 2-3 Tbsp diced red onion in place of green onion. Replace mayonnaise with 2 Tbsp Extra Virgin Olive Oil and 1 Tbsp lemon juice.		

AGILE RECIPES

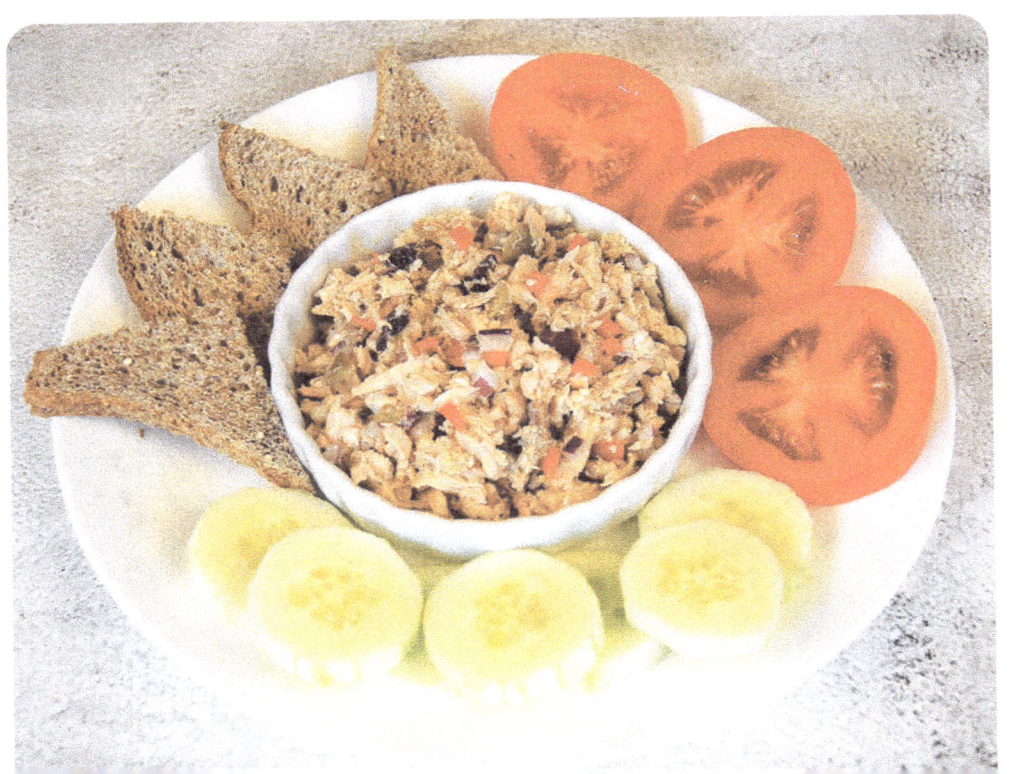

Mediterranean
Tuna Salad

PROTEIN MEAT	Yogurt Marinated Chicken Serves 4-6		Main
INGREDIENTS		**SUBSTITUTE**	
1-1½ lb	Chicken breast – whole, fillets or kabobs	Cut up chicken pieces or thighs (double weight if on the bone w/ skin)	
1 C	Yogurt, plain Greek	Plain yogurt	
1 Tbsp	Lemon juice	Lime juice or orange juice	
2	Garlic cloves, minced	1 tsp minced jarred garlic	
1 tsp	Paprika		
2 tsp	Cumin		
½ tsp	Oregano	1 tsp ginger paste	
	Salt and pepper to taste		
STEPS			
1	Mix yogurt, lemon juice and spices together in a large Ziploc bag.		
2	Add chicken to the bag and turn to coat all surfaces.		
3	Press air from the bag, seal it and refrigerate for four hours to overnight.		
4	Remove chicken from the marinade and shake off any excess. Discard leftover marinade.		
5	Cook chicken over high heat. This can be on the grill, pan fried on the stove top, or roasted in a 400°F oven. Chicken is done when it reaches 165°F internal temperature.		
6	Goes well with any rice, bread, naan or pita.		
OPTIONS			
A	**Greek:** Omit the paprika and cumin, then double the amount of lemon, garlic and oregano.		
B	**Middle East Kabob:** Omit the paprika and cumin. Double the garlic and oregano, and add 2 tsp tomato paste, and ¼ tsp each cinnamon and allspice.		
C	**Tandoori:** Omit the oregano, reduce the cumin to 1 tsp and double the paprika. Add 1 tsp ginger paste, ½ tsp each cinnamon and coriander.		

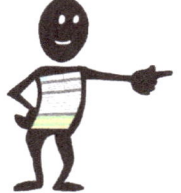

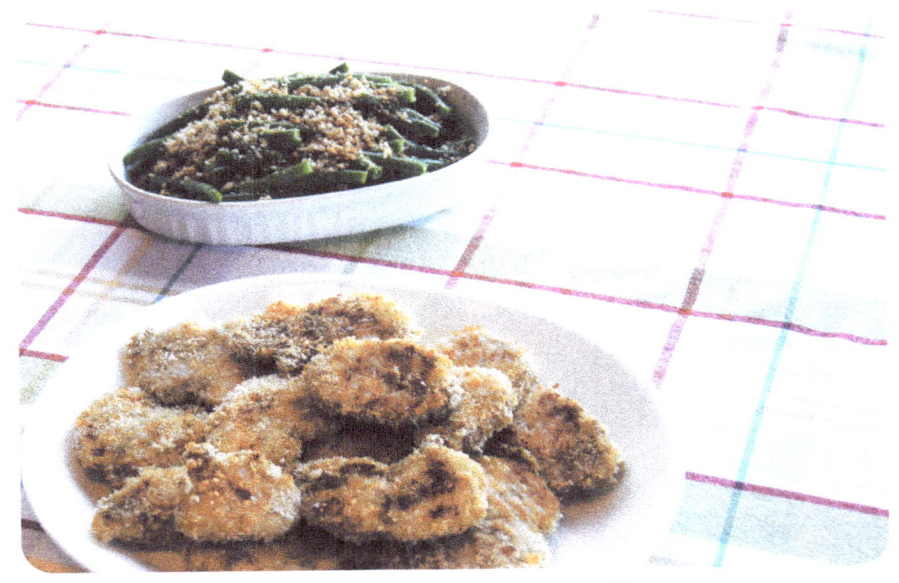

Oven-Fried Chicken

Recipe on page 259

AGILE RECIPES

Shrimp Scampi

Recipe on page 264

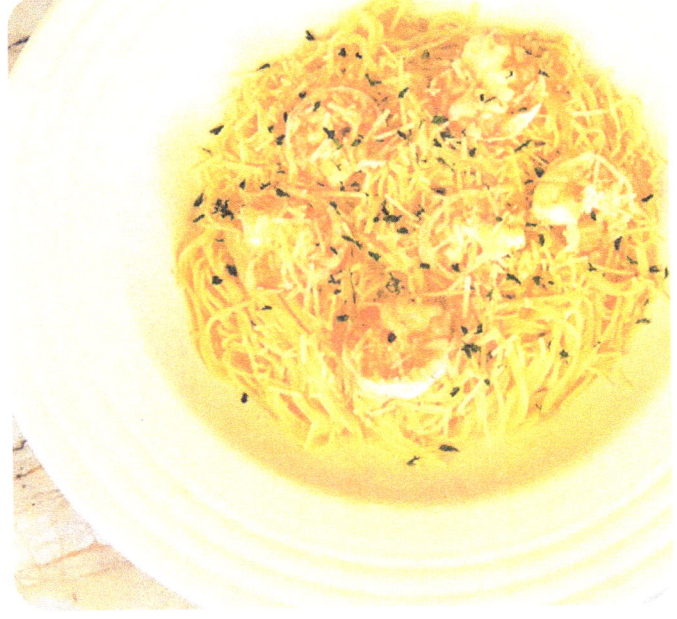

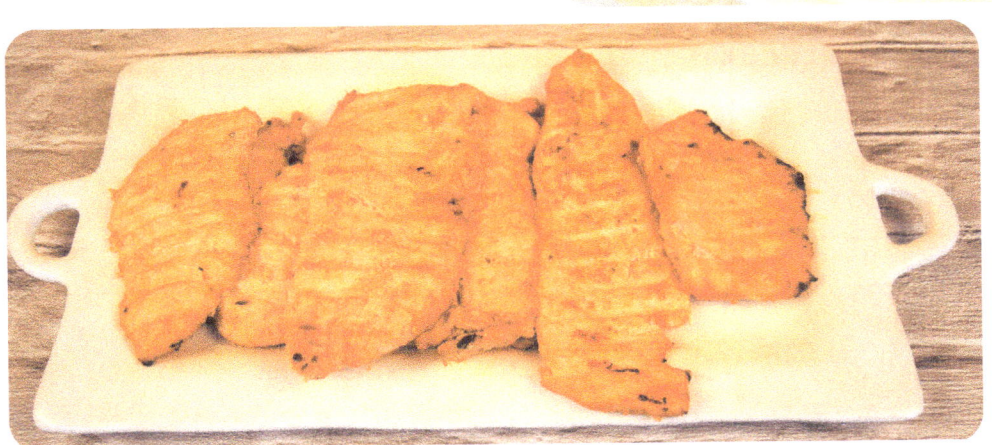

Yogurt Marinated

Chicken

Previous page

Marinades & Brines

Marinades and brines are great ways to create delicious meat dishes with minimum effort. You can always buy prepared marinades in the grocery store, but making your own is quick, easy and inexpensive. Additionally, you have more control over the ingredients and volume.

Marinades and brines often tenderize the meat and help keep it from drying out during cooking, in addition to imparting flavor. Thinly sliced meat and fish can get by with a quick marinate of 1-2 hours. However, I always prefer several hours to overnight if possible. If I am adding this step, I want to make it count!

You will notice that most marinades follow a simple pattern, making them ideal to put in a tabular form. You can easily adapt the recipes to meet your tastes and ingredients on hand. It is probably safe to say that you always have ingredients on hand to make a marinade.

Below are several easy recipes to expand your meat preparation repertoire. Each recipe is for about 3 lb of meat. In general, if you need a bit more volume, you can add an additional ¼- ½ C water or wine.

Type	Liquid	Flavor	For
Apple Cider Vinegar Marinade	1 C Worcestershire 1 C Apple cider vinegar	½ C brown sugar 1 Tbsp garlic, minced 1 Tbsp thyme or other herb	Pork tenderloin, loin roast, or pork chops
Balsamic Vinegar Marinade	1 C Balsamic vinegar	2 Tbsp brown sugar 1 Tbsp minced garlic 1 tsp salt 1 tsp ground pepper	For any steak, especially skirt or flank steak. Pierce meat with fork prior to putting in marinade.
Brown Sugar Brine	1 qt water	¼ C salt ½ C brown sugar 2 tsp garlic, minced Herbs de Provence or other spice blend	Poultry or pork. Soak overnight and then pat dry before cooking.

Type	Liquid	Flavor	For
Citrus Marinade	1 C orange juice ¼ C EVOO	1 Tbsp honey 1 tsp salt 2 tsp basil ½ tsp white pepper	Chicken (4-24 hours) or fish (2 hours)
Fajita Marinade	¼ C Orange Juice ¼ C Lime Juice ¼ C EVOO	1 tsp garlic, minced 2 tsp chili powder 1 tsp cumin 1 Tbsp cilantro (opt) 1 tsp salt	Marinate chicken or steak for 2-24 hours before grilling.
Greek Marinade	½ C EVOO ¼ C vinegar 2 Tbsp lemon juice	2 Tbsp garlic, minced 1 Tbsp sugar 2 tsp basil 2 tsp oregano 1 tsp rosemary 1 tsp salt ½ tsp black pepper ½ tsp red pepper flakes	Chicken or lamb. Great for kabobs. Marinade can be blended for a more intense flavor.
Italian Marinade	1 C EVOO ½ C vinegar (wine)	2 tsp salt 2 tsp garlic, minced 2 tsp oregano or Italian seasoning ½ tsp black pepper	Chicken, beef or lamb
Red Wine Marinade	1 C red wine ¼ C EVOO	2 tsp salt 2 Tsp rosemary 2 tsp garlic, minced 1 tsp black pepper ½ tsp red pepper flakes	Any steak, marinate over night
Teriyaki Marinade	½ C soy sauce ¼ C water 1 Tbsp vinegar (rice) 2 tsp sesame oil (opt)	1 Tbsp garlic, minced 1 Tbsp ginger, minced 4 Tbsp honey or sugar	Beef, pork, chicken, fish or tofu. Grill or pan fry, or use in stir fry.
Thyme Chicken Marinade	½ C EVOO 2 Tbsp lemon juice	2 Tbsp thyme (fresh) 1 Tbsp lemon zest 1 Tbsp parsley	Coat thin chicken cutlets with paste. Rest for 4-24 hours.
Yogurt Marinade	1 C yogurt 1 Tbsp lemon juice	1 tsp salt 1 tsp garlic, minced 2 tsp cumin 1 tsp paprika ½ tsp oregano	Chicken, marinate for 6–24 hours.

AGILE RECIPES

VEGGIE	Bean Salad[V] Serves 8-10		Salad
INGREDIENTS		**SUBSTITUTE**	
1	14.5 oz can, kidney beans	Black beans	
1	14.5 oz can, white navy beans	Cannellini beans, black eyed peas	
1	14.5 oz can, wax beans		
1	14.5 oz can, green beans	Fresh or frozen green beans, cooked	
½	Onion, diced		
½	Bell pepper, diced, red or green		
1	Rib, celery, diced		
½ C	Canola oil	Any light, neutral oil	
½ C	Apple cider vinegar	Any vinegar	
¼ C	White sugar		
	Salt and pepper to taste		
STEPS			
1	Rinse and drain all of the canned beans.		
2	Whisk the oil, vinegar and sugar (or other dressing) together.		
3	Mix all ingredients. Cover and chill for several hours before serving.		
OPTIONS			
A	**Classic**: Recipe above with green bell peppers. Add ½ C chopped jarred pimento peppers if desired.		
B	**Southern**: Replace all of the beans with four cans of black eyed peas. Add 12 oz of cherry tomatoes, halved. Use 1 C of Dijon Vinaigrette dressing (page 286) instead of oil, vinegar and sugar.		
C	**Tex-Mex**: Use one can each of black beans and black eyed peas. Add 8 oz of halved cherry tomatoes and a 14.5 oz can corn (drained). Replace sugar with 1 tsp each chili powder and cumin.		
D	**Greek**: Replace green and wax beans with one can of chickpeas. Add 1 C diced cucumber and 8 oz halved cherry tomatoes. Use 1 C of the Greek salad dressing (page 287) in place of the oil, vinegar and sugar. Garnish with crumbled feta.		

AGILE RECIPES

VEGGIE	Brussels Sprouts Salad^V Serves 6-8		Salad
INGREDIENTS		**SUBSTITUTE**	
1½ lb	Brussels sprouts, fresh		
2	Apples	Pears	
¾ C	Cherries, dried	Dried cranberries	
¾ C	Almonds, sliced	Sunflower seeds, pumpkin seeds or toasted, chopped walnuts	
¾ C	Parmesan cheese, grated	Sharp cheddar cheese	
1 C	Honey Mustard Salad Dressing (page 287)	Lemon, Orange or Raspberry Vinaigrette dressing (page 287)	
STEPS			
1	Cut Brussels sprouts into thin slices with knife or mandolin.		
2	Toss the Brussels sprouts with the dressing and allow to stand while preparing the other ingredients to allow the sprouts to soften.		
3	Peel apples if desired and then dice into small pieces. May be grated.		
4	Toss remaining ingredients with the Brussels sprouts and serve.		
Copyright © 2024 Alin E. Steele May be copied for personal use only. www.ReEngineeringtheKitchen.com			

AGILE RECIPES

For a change of pace, try purple Brussels sprouts:

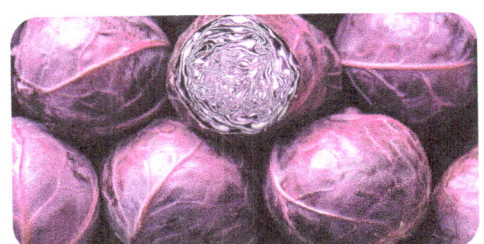

- » Typically harvested in the fall.
- » Milder and sweeter flavor than green Brussels sprouts.
- » Flavor and color makes them great in salads.

VEGGIE	Carrot Salad w/ Fruit^V Serves 4-6		Salad
INGREDIENTS		**SUBSTITUTE**	
1 lb	Carrots, grated	Bagged grated or matchstick carrots	
¾ C	Mayonnaise	Yogurt, plain or vanilla. Omit honey if using sweetened.	
1 Tbsp	Lemon juice	Apple cider vinegar	
2 Tbsp	Honey		
1	20 oz can crushed pineapple, drained	1 apple, diced	
½ C	Raisins, separated	Dried cranberries or cherries	
½ C	Pecans, chopped	Walnuts or ¼ C sunflower seeds	
STEPS			
1	In a good size bowl, mix the mayonnaise, lemon juice and honey until smooth.		
2	Add remaining ingredients and toss until combined. Refrigerate until ready to serve.		

AGILE RECIPES

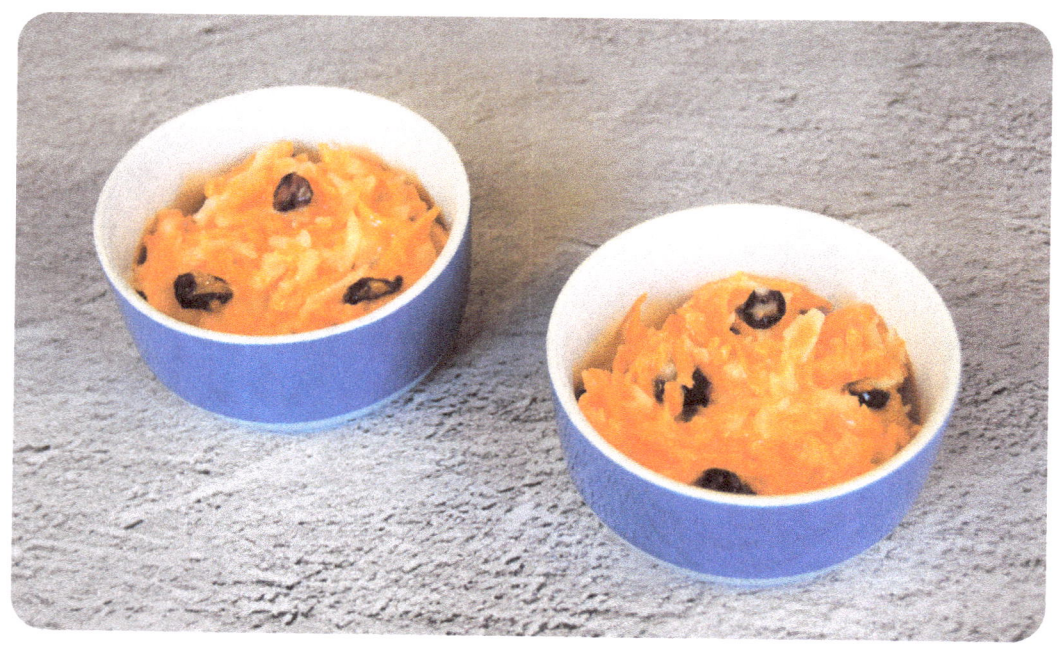

VEGGIE	Cucumber Salads^V Serves 4-6		Salad
INGREDIENTS		**SUBSTITUTE**	
2	Cucumbers, (about 2 pounds)	Hot house or English	
½	Red onion, medium, sliced thinly	White, yellow or green onions	
3 Tbsp	Dill, fresh	2 tsp dried dill, fresh basil or parsley	
2 Tbsp	Extra Virgin Olive Oil		
½ C	Apple cider vinegar	Any vinegar, lemon juice	
1 Tbsp	Sugar		
	Salt and pepper to taste		
STEPS			
1	Cucumbers may be peeled or not, depending on your preference. Slice cucumbers into disks.		
2	Mix all ingredients in a bowl, cover and chill.		
OPTIONS			
A	**Creamy:** Omit the sugar, oil and vinegar. Add ¼ C each of mayonnaise and sour cream (or Greek yogurt).		
B	**Greek:** Omit the sugar and apple cider vinegar. Replace the dill with 2 tsp oregano. Increase the Extra Virgin Olive Oil to ¼ C and add 2 Tbsp of lemon juice. Add 2 diced tomatoes, ½ C of black or Kalamata olives, and 4 oz Feta cheese.		

AGILE RECIPES

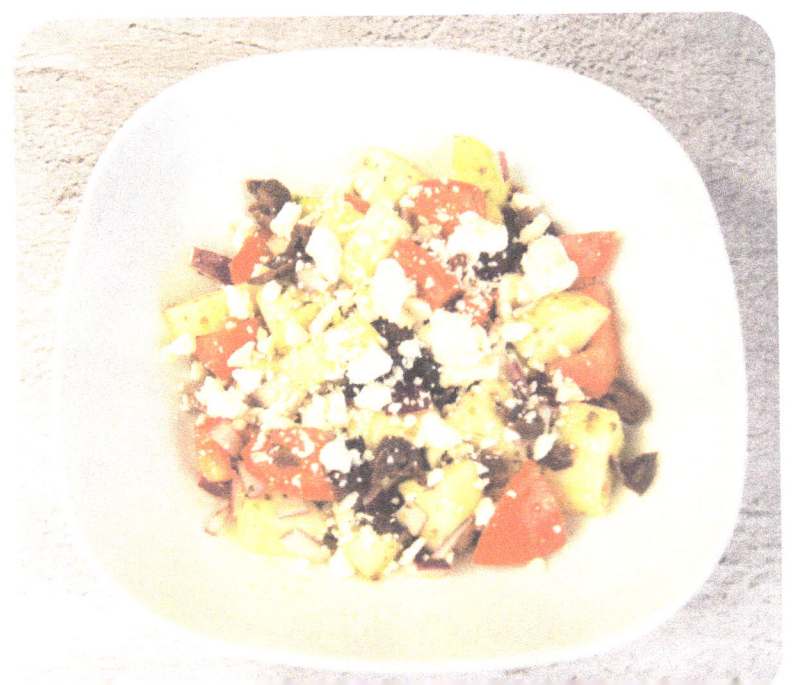

VEGGIE	Green Bean Salad w/ Goat Cheese^V Serves 4		Salad
INGREDIENTS		**SUBSTITUTE**	
2 lb	Fresh green beans	Frozen whole green beans	
½ C	Orange Basil Vinaigrette (recipe page 287)		
4 oz	Goat cheese, crumbled		
½ C	Walnuts, chopped	Pecans	
STEPS			
1	Steam green beans until they are tender crisp. Cool by putting them in ice water for five minutes or refrigerate for later use.		
2	Toss cool, drained green beans with the dressing.		
3	Garnish with crumbled goat cheese and chopped walnuts.		

AGILE RECIPES

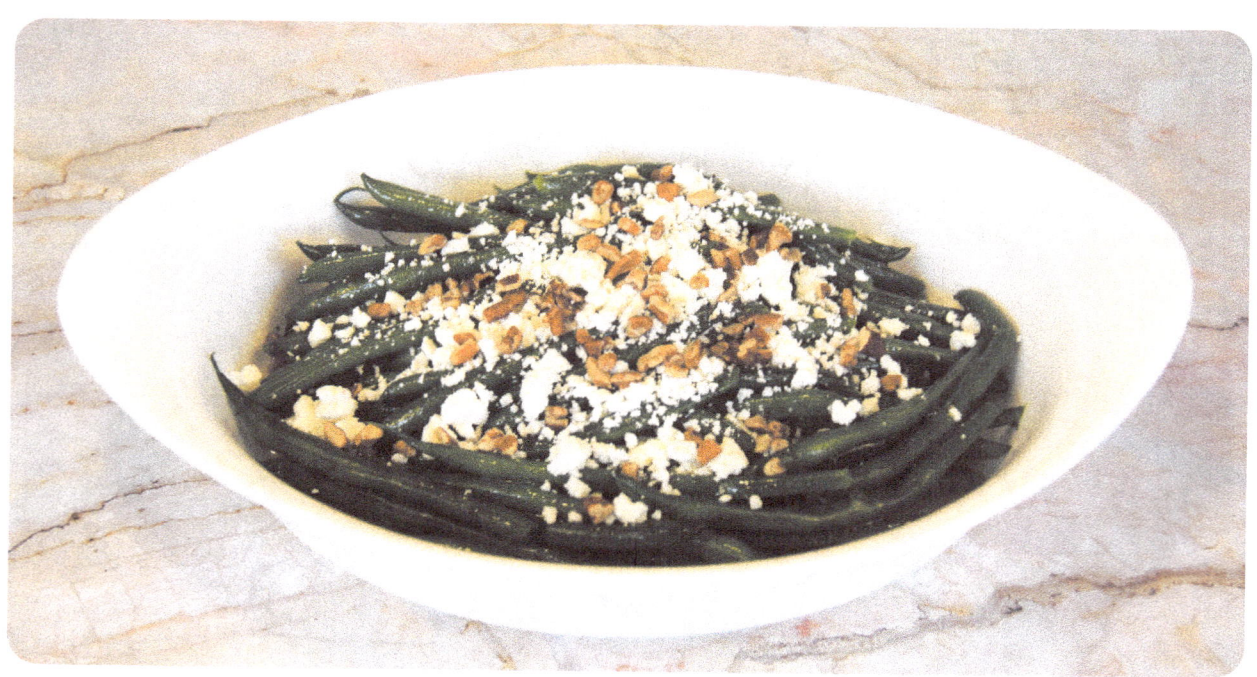

VEGGIE	Napa Cabbage Salad Makes 6 side salads		Salad

INGREDIENTS		SUBSTITUTE
1	Head napa cabbage (large)	
2-3	Carrots, grated or julienned	
6	Green onions, finely sliced	
1	Orange, peeled and cut	Mandarin orange sections, drained
½	Red bell pepper, finely sliced (optional)	
½ C	Sliced almonds	Peanuts
~ ½ C	Ginger Soy Salad Dressing (recipe pg 286)	

STEPS	
1	Finely slice the cabbage.
2	Combine all ingredients and toss.
3	Serve plain or top with grilled chicken and crispy wantons.

AGILE RECIPES

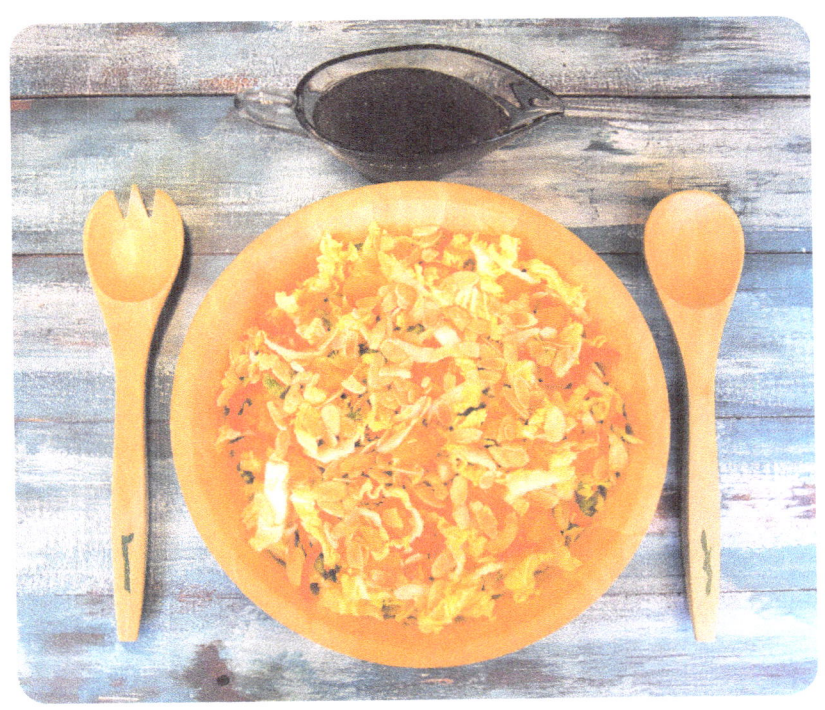

AGILE RECIPES

GRAIN	Pasta Salad^V Serves 10-12		Salad
INGREDIENTS		**SUBSTITUTE**	
1 lb	Pasta, any shape		
1	Onion, small, red, diced	Green, white or yellow onion	
1	Red bell pepper, diced	Green pepper	
1 pint	Tomatoes, cherry		
4 C	Broccoli, cut into bite sized florets		
8 oz	Cheddar cheese, grated		
1½ C	Ranch Salad Dressing (recipe on page 287)	Any salad dressing	
STEPS			
1	Cook pasta to al dente then rinse in cold water and drain well.		
2	Steam the broccoli until tender but still crisp. Rinse in cold water and drain well.		
3	Toss all ingredients together, chill and serve.		
OPTIONS			
A	**Greek:** Omit the broccoli and cheddar cheese. Add 1 diced cucumber, 1 C Kalamata or black olives, and 8 oz crumbled feta cheese. Use Greek salad dressing instead of Ranch (shown on page 287).		
B	**Italian:** Omit the broccoli and cheddar cheese. Add 6 oz salami in small pieces, 1 C sliced black olives and 8 oz of shredded mozzarella. Use Lemon or Balsamic Vinaigrette dressing (page 287).		
C	**Tuna:** Omit the tomato, broccoli and cheddar cheese. Add two 5 oz cans of tuna (drained), 3 diced hard boiled eggs and 2 C of cooked peas. Use 1½ C mayonnaise and ¼ C sweet pickle relish as the dressing.		

GRAIN	Rice Salad^V Serves 8-10	Salad

INGREDIENTS		SUBSTITUTE
4 C	Rice, cooked al dente (1⅓ C uncooked)	White or brown
1	Red bell pepper, diced	
1	Red onion, small, diced	Green onion
2	Celery stalks, diced	
2	Carrots, diced	
½ - ¾ C	Lemon Vinaigrette (see recipe on page 287)	Any salad dressing

STEPS	
1	Rice should be cooked so that it is no longer crunchy but not mushy. Chill before using.
2	Mix all ingredients and then chill prior to serving.

OPTIONS	
A	**Mediterranean:** Omit the carrot and celery. Add one 15 oz can of white beans or chickpeas, ½ C Kalamata or black olives and ½ C feta cheese. Use Greek salad dressing shown on page 287.
B	**Tex-Mex:** Omit the carrot and celery. Add one 15 oz can of black beans, one 15 oz can of corn, and two diced tomatoes. Dress with ½ C EVOO, ¼ C lime juice and ½ tsp each chili powder and cumin. Fresh cilantro and avocado are optional but nice additions.

AGILE RECIPES

PROTEIN MEAT	Tuna Salad Niçoise Serves ~ 2		Salad
INGREDIENTS		**SUBSTITUTE**	
1	Head of romaine	Any type of lettuce	
2 C	Green beans, fresh (12-16 oz)	Frozen, whole	
1	5 oz can of tuna (high quality)		
1	Potato, medium Russet, sliced	Any type of potato	
1	Tomato, cut into wedges		
2	Eggs, hard boiled, quartered		
¼ C	Olives, Kalamata	Any type of olive	
½ C	Dijon Vinaigrette Salad Dressing (page 286)	Lemon Vinaigrette, Greek or Caesar Dressings shown on pages 286 & 287	
STEPS			
1	Steam green beans to tender crisp. Cool under cold water, drain well and chill.		
2	Cook potato by boiling until just tender but not mushy. Drain well and chill.		
3	Assemble salad: bed of greens, topped with remaining ingredients. Drizzle with dressing.		

AGILE RECIPES

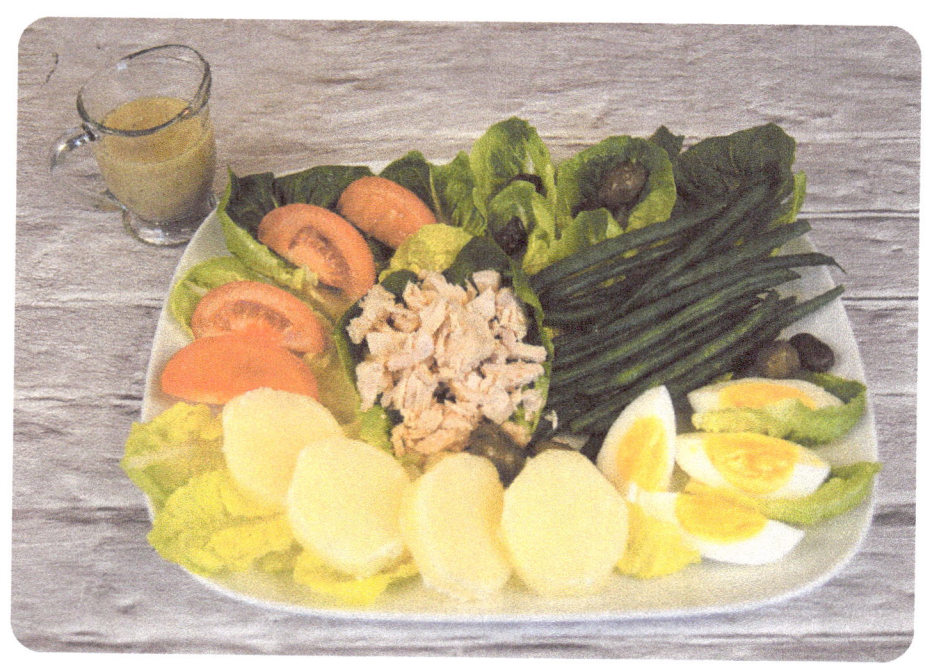

Salad Dressings

I like salads but I love salad dressings! There are many good, prepared salad dressings available in the grocery store. However, I no longer rely on them. This is an area where many people default to purchasing bottled dressings, assuming that making your own is complicated. It is not. On the following pages there are recipes for several common types of dressings. The creamy ones also serve well as dips. You should never feel that you can't make a salad because you are "out of dressing".

When you make your own dressing, you make the right volume and can control the ingredients. For example, you may choose to use high-quality olive oil and balsamic vinegar, avoiding seed oils, sugar, MSG, modified food starch, and preservatives. When you make your own dressing, you save money in two ways. **The first way you save is by reducing waste.** How many partial bottles of salad dressing have you discarded over the years? A certain percentage tends to be thrown out because it is hard to match use to the product size. On the other hand, staple ingredients like olive oil and vinegar are generally used completely. *The second way you save is that home-made dressing costs less than one-half per ounce to make vs. pre-made dressings – even using high quality ingredients!*

Salad Dressing Tips & Tricks:

- » Multiply the recipes to get the desired volume.
- » To mellow the flavor of fresh garlic, microwave the oil and garlic for 15 seconds on high, then allow to cool.
- » A few drops of water added to vinaigrettes help emulsify the oil and vinegar. Not essential, but helpful if serving dressing on the side.
- » Can substitute garlic powder for crushed garlic.
- » Can substitute dehydrated onion flakes for grated onion.
- » Types of vinegar can be interchanged with minimal effect.
- » Extra Virgin Olive Oil can be replaced with canola or any light vegetable oil.
- » Plain or Greek yogurt can be substituted for sour cream.
- » If you have a little prepared non-creamy dressing left but need a bit more, add equal amounts of oil and vinegar to the bottle to get the desired volume. If it is a creamy dressing, add a little mayo, sour cream, or yogurt, thinned with milk. Shake well.
- » Fresh Buttermilk substitute – for ¼ C
  - » Prepared powdered buttermilk per package directions
  - » Mix ¼ C milk with 1 tsp lemon juice or vinegar and sit 10 minutes
  - » Mix 3 Tbls yogurt or sour cream with 1 Tbls milk

Simple Salad Dressings
Makes ~ ½ C, enough for 2 entree or 4 side salads

AGILE RECIPES

Type	Oil	Acid	Sweet	Flavoring
Balsamic Vinaigrette	¼ C EVOO	¼ C Balsamic vinegar	N/A	½ tsp garlic ¼ tsp pepper ½ tsp salt ½ tsp basil (or any herb)
Blue Cheese	¼ C mayo	¼ C sour cream	⅛ tsp sugar	1 Tbsp blue cheese crumbles ⅛ tsp pepper 1 Tbsp milk
Caesar	⅓ C mayo 1 tsp EVOO	1 Tbsp lemon juice	N/A	½ tsp garlic ¼ tsp Dijon mustard 1 tsp Worcestershire 1 Tbsp grated Parmesan
Coleslaw - Classic	¼ C mayo	¼ C apple cider vinegar	1 tsp sugar	¼ tsp salt ¼ tsp pepper ¼ tsp celery seed (opt)
Coleslaw - Russian	¼ C mayo	¼ C sour cream	⅛ tsp sugar	1 Tbsp grated onion
Creamy Dill	¼ C mayo	¼ C sour cream	⅛ tsp sugar	1 tsp dill ⅛ tsp pepper ¼ tsp salt 1 Tbsp milk
Dijon Vinaigrette	6 Tbsp EVOO	2 Tbsp vinegar	N/A	2 tsp Dijon mustard ½ tsp dehydrated onion ½ tsp salt ¼ tsp pepper
French	⅓ C EVOO	1½ Tbsp wine vinegar	¾ tsp sugar	½ tsp garlic 1½Tbsp chili sauce 1 tsp Worcestershire
Ginger Soy	¼ C EVOO	2 Tbsp rice vinegar	1 Tbsp honey	1 tsp ginger paste 1 Tbsp soy sauce ½ tsp garlic

Simple Salad Dressings
Makes ~ ½ C, enough for 2 entree or 4 side salads

Type	Oil	Acid	Sweet	Flavoring
Greek	¼ C EVOO	¼ C wine vinegar	N/A	½ tsp garlic ¼ tsp Dijon mustard ¼ tsp oregano ¼ tsp basil ¼ tsp pepper ¼ tsp salt ¼ tsp onion powder Feta cheese on salad
Honey Mustard	¼ C EVOO	3 Tbsp apple cider vinegar	2 Tbsp honey	2 Tbsp Dijon mustard
Lemon Vinaigrette	¼ C EVOO	2 Tbsp lemon juice 2 Tbsp white wine vinegar	1 tsp honey	½ tsp oregano ¼ tsp pepper ¼ tsp salt ¼ tsp dehydrated onion (opt)
Orange Basil Vinaigrette	¼ C EVOO	1 Tbsp orange juice concentrate 3 Tbsp white vinegar	1 tsp honey	1 tsp basil ¼ tsp pepper ¼ tsp salt
Ranch	¼ C mayo	¼ C buttermilk 1 Tbsp sour cream (opt)	N/A	1 tsp parsley ½ tsp dill ¼ tsp dehydrated onion ⅛ tsp garlic powder ⅛ tsp onion powder ⅛ tsp pepper ¼ tsp salt
Raspberry Vinaigrette	¼ C EVOO	¼ C raspberry vinegar	1 Tbsp raspberry preserves	¼ tsp basil ⅛ tsp pepper ¼ tsp salt
Sweet Vinegar	¼ C EVOO	⅓ C apple cider vinegar	3 Tbsp sugar	½ tsp salt
Thousand Island	½ C mayo	N/A	1 tsp sweet pickle relish	1 tsp ketchup 1 tsp minced onion, fresh or dehydrated

Sauces

Sometimes even a simple little sauce can take a dish from "meh" to "mmm". Recipes for making lovely dishes with intricate sauces are readily available so we don't need to talk about them here. If you are making Veal Piccata or Eggs Benedict with scratch-made Hollandaise to impress the in-laws, the internet has you covered. What we include here are a few of the most basic, easy sauces and then some even easier short-cut sauces. These sauces exist for moments when you are thinking, "Gee, a little sauce would really help."

The line between sauce and gravy is only flavor, not technique. If it tastes like meat, we tend to call it gravy. For our purposes, a sauce is any thickened liquid that adds flavor, whether it be sweet or savory. The most common sauces use either flour or corn starch as a thickening agent, so we have included recipes for a basic Flour-Roux Sauce and a Corn Starch Sauce, each with several variations. There are also recipes for several cooking sauces that are commonly purchased. And then we have the short-cut sauces that are so quick and easy that it almost feels like cheating. These short-cut sauces may not win any culinary awards, but when you've conjured a sauce out of almost nothing, it seems like magic.

Sauce Type	Ingredients	Method
Caramel	2 Tbsp butter 2 Tbsp brown sugar 1 tsp milk or cream	Mix in microwave safe bowl. Microwave on 60% power in 15 second increments, stirring in between, until melted and fairly smooth (not perfect). Serve with ice cream or other desserts.
Cocktail	¼ C ketchup 1 tsp prepared horseradish 1 tsp Worcestershire sauce ½ tsp lemon juice	Mix all ingredients and serve with shrimp.
Dijonnaise	2 Tbsp mayo 1 tsp Dijon mustard	Mix. Use to jazz up your sandwiches or salads.
Fondue Cheat	1 C white wine 1 Tbsp corn starch 2 C grated cheese (mix of types)	Mix cold wine and corn starch in a small pan. Warm over very low heat until thickened. Mix in cheese and stir until melted. Serve as dip, can keep warm in a mini crock pot.
Fruit Dip	1 C Greek yogurt, plain 8 oz cream cheese 1/4 C honey, maple syrup, or fruit preserves 1 tsp vanilla extract	Combine all ingredients in a bowl and beat until smooth. Serve as a dip with fresh fruit or as a creamy topping for any dessert.

Sauce Type	Ingredients	Method
Fruit Sauce/Glaze	½ C fruit juice (any flavor) ½ Tbsp corn starch 2 Tbsp jam or preserves	Mix cold juice and corn starch in a small pan. Warm over low heat, stirring until thickened. Stir in jam or preserves until smooth. Serve as a glaze or sauce for meat or poultry, or as a topping for desserts, pancakes etc.
Instant Marinara	1 C tomato sauce 1 tsp oregano 1 tsp onion powder ½ tsp garlic powder ½ tsp basil ¼ tsp red pepper flakes (opt)	Mix together and warm. Use as a pizza sauce, dipping sauce, or to extend volume of any tomato-based sauce in cooking. Use to top vegetables, pasta or meat and then bake with cheese.
Magic Cheese	2 Tbsp sour cream 2 Tbls milk or cream 2 oz grated cheese Salt and pepper to taste	Mix in microwave safe bowl. Microwave on 60% power in 15 second increments, stirring in between, until melted and smooth. Serve with veggies, pasta, rice potatoes, etc.
Mayonnaise 1	1 large egg (pasteurized) ¾ C canola oil 1 Tbsp lemon juice or vinegar 1 tsp salt ¼ tsp pepper 1 tsp Dijon mustard (opt)	Mix all ingredients except oil. Add oil gradually, and whip until emulsified using whisk, immersion blender, blender or food processor
Mayonnaise 2	1 hard boiled egg – XL ¼ C canola oil 1 tsp lemon juice ¼ tsp salt 1 tsp Dijon mustard	Mix all ingredients and blend for several minutes until emulsified and creamy using immersion blender, blender or food processor.
Orange Honey Ginger Syrup	½ C water ½ C white sugar 2 Tbsp OJ concentrate 2 Tbsp honey 2 tsp ginger paste or crystallized ginger (minced)	Mix ingredients in a small saucepan and bring to a boil. Allow it to boil until it starts to thicken slightly then cool. Serve over fruit, desserts, pancakes or in drinks. Use as a glaze for chicken or fish.
Remoulade	½ C mayo 1 Tbsp Dijon or brown mustard 1 tsp lemon juice 1 tsp garlic powder ½ tsp paprika 1 tsp hot sauce 1 Tbsp ketchup 1 tsp chopped capers (opt)	Mix ingredients. Better if allowed to rest to meld flavors. Serve with fish, fries, chicken tenders, shrimp, asparagus or as a spread on a sandwich.

VEGGIE	Classic Marinara^V Makes about 2 cups		Sauce
INGREDIENTS		**SUBSTITUTE**	
28 oz	One can whole tomatoes, high quality	Crushed or diced tomatoes	
4 Tbsp	Extra Virgin Olive Oil		
½	Medium onion, finely diced		
8	Cloves fresh garlic, minced	4 tsp jarred minced garlic	
½ tsp	Salt		
1 tsp	Basil	Oregano	
⅛ tsp	Red pepper flakes (optional)		
STEPS			
1	Put tomatoes in a large bowl and crush into small pieces. May use hands but a pastry cutter or large fork work also.		
2	In a large, heavy bottomed pot, sauté the onion over medium heat until very soft – about five minutes.		
3	Add the garlic and continue cooking for another 1-2 minutes.		
4	Add all of the other ingredients to the pot. Bring to a boil and then reduce heat to simmer.		
5	Simmer uncovered for at least 20 minutes, stirring often. Sauce will thicken as it cooks.		
6	Serve over pasta or use in any recipe calling for a marinara-type sauce.		

(Sidebar, left margin: AGILE RECIPES)

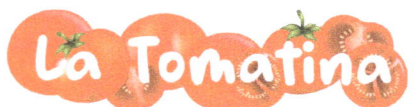

Bunol, Spain hosts the craziest tomato festival in the world each August. It is called La Tomatina and is said to be the world's largest food fight. About 20,000 participants pay to throw about 150,000 tomatoes at each other. In the end, they look like they are all swimming in Marinara sauce!

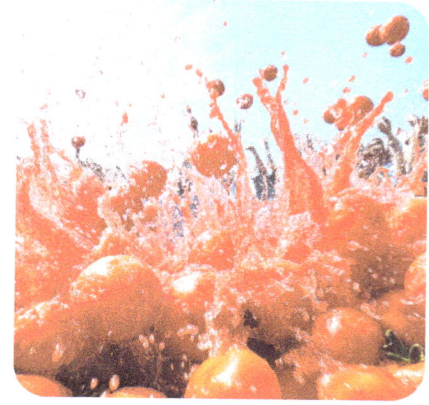

GRAIN	Corn Starch Sauces^V Makes 1 cup		Sauce
INGREDIENTS		**SUBSTITUTE**	
1 Tbsp	Corn starch		
1 C	Water, broth, juice, or wine - cool	Any clear liquid	
	Liquid flavoring: include in liquid measure	Worcestershire, soy sauce, chili sauce, vinegar, lemon juice	
	Seasoning additions	Salt, pepper, spices	
STEPS			
1	Measure cold liquid including any liquid flavoring. Stir in corn starch until well mixed.		
2	Warm the corn starch and liquid mixture over medium heat, stirring until thickened. The cold corn starch mixture may be added directly to a pan with cooked food (e.g. stir fry) and warmed together as sauce thickens.		
3	Add seasoning and flavor additions to sauce. Return to heat only as necessary to fully incorporate and/or to warm.		
OPTIONS			
A	**Lemon Sauce**: Include 2 Tbsp of lemon juice in liquid. Dissolve ¼ C sugar in liquid before heating. Add grated lemon zest at the end. Serve as a topping for spice cake, pancakes or desserts.		
B	**Cheese Fondue**: Use white wine as the liquid to make sauce. When thickened, add 2 C grated cheese (Swiss or Gruyere) to sauce and then stir over low heat until cheese melts.		
C	**Stir Fry**: Use ½ C each of water and soy sauce for the liquid. Add 2 tsp each ginger, garlic and sugar (or honey). Add 1 tsp chili sauce if desired. Mix well and add to pan with stir fry meat and/or veggies, stirring until thickened.		
D	**Mushroom Sauce**: Use wine or broth for liquid. Add 8-16 oz sautéed mushrooms to thickened sauce. Add salt, pepper, garlic and herbs if desired.		
E	**Fruit Compote**: Use fruit juice for liquid (may be drained from canned or frozen fruit or other juce). Add ¼ - ½ C sugar to thickened sauce if needed. Stir in drained fruit and warm thoroughly.		

AGILE RECIPES

VEGGIE	Enchilada Sauce^V Makes about 2½ cups		Sauce
INGREDIENTS		**SUBSTITUTE**	
1½ Tbsp	Extra Virgin Olive Oil	Any olive oil, cooking oil, or butter	
1 Tbsp	Flour		
1 C	Chicken stock	Beef or vegetable stock or water	
1 Tbsp	Onion powder or dehydrated onion	½ C diced onion, sautéed	
½ tsp	Garlic powder or granules	1 tsp minced garlic	
1	Can (15 oz) tomato sauce	Diced, crushed or pureed canned tomatos, blended	
1½ Tbsp	Chili powder		
1 Tbsp	Oregano		
½ Tbsp	Cumin		
1 Tbsp	Lemon juice		
½ tsp	Rosemary, ground		
¼ tsp	Pepper		
¼ tsp	Cayenne pepper (optional)		
STEPS			
1	In a medium suace pan, cook oil and flour over medium heat stirring often. Allow to bubble for for two to three minutes to make a light roux.		
2	Add stock to the roux and mix well. Cook over medium heat, stirring constantly to slightly thicken the stock mixture.		
3	Add all other ingredients to the sauce pan and simmer for at least 10 minutes (20 is better), stirring occasionally.		

GRAIN	Flour-Based Sauces^V Makes about 1 cup		Sauce

INGREDIENTS		SUBSTITUTE	
1½ Tbsp	Butter	Any oil or rendered meat fat.	
1 Tbsp	Flour		
1 C	Milk	Broth, wine or other liquid compatible with flavors.	
	Salt and pepper to taste		

STEPS	
1	Melt butter in small pan. Add flour.
2	Cook flour and butter over medium low heat for at least three minutes. Should gently bubble. Flour and oil mixture (roux) may cook longer and will develop a nutty flavor as it browns.
3	Remove pan from heat to cool slightly. Add all of the liquid, stirring to fully incorporate.
4	Return pan to medium low heat, stirring constantly until the sauce thickens. Do not allow to come to a boil. Remove from heat when thickened.
5	Add seasonings and additions to the sauce. Return to low heat only as necessary to fully incorporate and warm.

OPTIONS	
A	**White Sauce**: Cook flour in butter for minimum time, use milk and then season with salt and ⅛ tsp nutmeg. Mix with any cooked veggie for creamed peas, red cabbage, corn, etc.
B	**Cheese Sauce**: Use butter and milk. Stir in 2 C of grated cheese until melted. Add a little milk if sauce is too thick. A mixture of sharp and mild cheeses develop the best flavor. Season with salt, pepper, paprika. Serve over veggies like brocolli or 8 oz cooked pasta.
C	**Sausage Gravy**: Use butter and milk. Stir in 1 lb cooked, drained pork sausage. Add salt, pepper, red pepper flakes. Serve over toast or fresh biscuits.
D	**Roast Meat Gravy**: Use oil from pan drippings (just fat, no liquid!). Use strained, skimmed pan drippings and/or broth for the liquid. Salt and pepper to taste.
E	**Mushroom Sauce**: Use any oil and milk, broth or wine to make the basic sauce. Stir in 8-16 oz mushrooms, sauteed with garlic. Season with salt, pepper, and basil. Serve with meat, poutry, eggs, potatoes or veggies.
F	**Onion Gravy**: Use any oil and either milk or broth. Stir in 1 sliced onion which has been sauteéd to at least soft, preferably carmelized. Salt and pepper to taste. Great with pork.

AGILE RECIPES

VEGGIE	Mushroom Parmesan Cream Sauce[v] Makes 3 cups		Sauce
INGREDIENTS		**SUBSTITUTE**	
1-2 lb	Mushrooms, sliced (white or brown)	Any type or mix of mushrooms, frozen	
2 Tbsp	Extra Virgin Olive Oil		
4	Cloves garlic	2 tsp minced jarred garlic	
2 tsp	Basil	Parsley	
¾ C	Heavy cream	¾ C milk blended with 1½ tsp flour	
½ C	Parmesan cheese, grated		
½ tsp	Black pepper		
STEPS			
1	In a large sauté pan, cook the mushrooms and garlic in the oil until all of the moisture from the mushrooms has evaporated.		
2	Stir the basil and the heavy cream into the mushrooms, mixing well over low heat until it starts to thicken.		
3	Stir in the Parmesan cheese and pepper. Turn off heat and stir gently. The sauce should continue to thicken.		
4	Serve tossed with pasta or as a topping for grilled chicken, bruschetta, polenta or vegetables.		

AGILE RECIPES

TEMPERATURE

FAHRENHEIT	CELSIUS
100 °F	37 °C
150 °F	65 °C
200 °F	93 °C
250 °F	121 °C
300 °F	150 °C
325 °F	160 °C
350 °F	180 °C
375 °F	190 °C
400 °F	200 °C
425 °F	220 °C
450 °F	230 °C
500 °F	260 °C
525 °F	274 °C
550 °F	288 °C

GRAIN	$100 Macaroni & Cheese[V] Serves 8-10		Side
INGREDIENTS		**SUBSTITUTE**	
1 lb	Pasta, penne or spirals	Any shape that does not pack tightly	
3 Tbsp	Flour		
3 Tbsp	Butter	Extra Virgin Olive Oil	
3 C	Milk		
6 oz	Sharp cheddar cheese		
6 oz	Swiss cheese (preferably aged)		
4 oz	Asiago or Parmesan cheese		
4 oz	Colby or Co-Jack cheese		
½ tsp	Salt		
STEPS			
1	Preheat oven to 350°F. Prepare a 9" x13" pan or 2½ quart baking dish by coating with cooking spray.		
2	Grate all of the cheese and mix together in a bowl. Measure cheese, including pre-shredded cheese, by weight.		
3	Cook the pasta to slightly less done than al dente and drain. It will cook more in the oven later.		
4	In a heavy bottomed sauce pan, melt butter and mix in the flour. Cook over medium heat for three to five minutes to cook flour.		
5	Remove from heat and add the milk. Stir to fully incorporate and then return to heat.		
6	Heat milk/flour mixture over medium heat, stirring constantly. Sauce will thicken as it comes to almost a boil. Turn off the heat.		
7	Stir in ¾ of the cheese to the sauce, reserving the remainder for topping. Allow the cheese to melt, only adding enough heat as is necessary to get a smooth sauce.		
8	Mix the pasta and sauce together, then pour in the prepared pan. Top with the remining grated cheese.		
9	Bake for 30-45 minutes, until bubbly and golden brown on top.		

AGILE RECIPES

Photo on page 312

VEGGIE	Aloo Gobi^v Serves 6-8		Side

INGREDIENTS		SUBSTITUTE
1	Head cauliflower (about 2 lb)	
2-3	Potatoes (about 1½ lb)	
1 Tbsp	Ginger paste or grated ginger	
4	Cloves garlic	2 tsp minced garlic
2 Tbsp	Extra Virgin Olive Oil	Coconut oil, any olive or light oil
3 Tbsp	Curry powder or curry paste	1½ Tbsp coriander + 2 tsp cumin + ½ tsp turmeric + 2 tsp Garam Masala
½ tsp	Kashmiri chili powder (optional)	½ tsp red pepper flakes (optional)
1 C	Water	
1 tsp	Salt	

STEPS	
1	Cut cauliflower into one inch florets. Dice potatoes into similar size cubes.
2	In a large pot with a lid, heat oil and add ginger and garlic. Cook for 1-2 minutes. Add spices and cook for another minute.
3	Add potatoes, water and spices to the pot, stirring to coat potatoes. Put on the lid and cook over medium heat for about 10 minutes, stirring occasionally.
4	Add the cauliflower and stir to coat pieces. Replace lid and cook for another 12-15 minutes, stirring occasionally, until cauliflower and potatoes are tender. Adjust the salt.
5	Serve with rice or naan, and a garnish of cilantro leaves if desired.

AGILE RECIPES

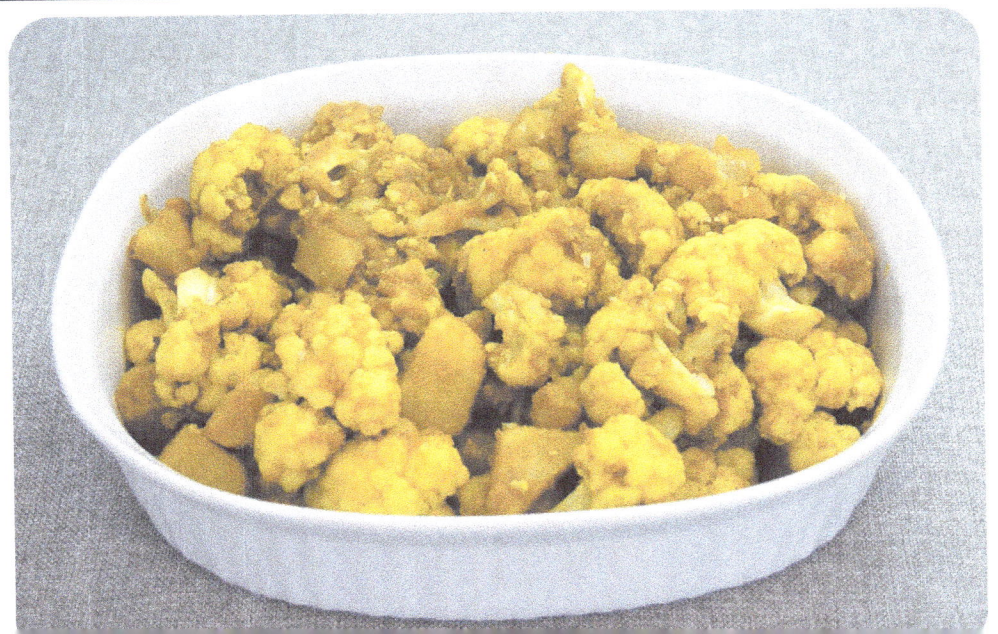

PROTEIN OTHER	Beans & Rice[v] Serves 4-6		Side
INGREDIENTS		**SUBSTITUTE**	
1 Tbsp	Extra Virgin Olive Oil		
1	Onion, diced		
½	Red or green bell pepper, diced		
2	Cloves garlic, minced	1 tsp jarred minced garlic	
1 C	White rice, uncooked		
1	15.5 oz can red kidney beans, drained	Black beans	
1	14.5 oz can diced tomatoes		
12 oz	Andouille sausage, diced	Smoked sausage, bacon	
1 C	Chicken or vegetable stock	1 C water + 1 tsp stock paste	
2 tsp	Cajun spice blend		
STEPS			
1	In a large pot with a lid, sauté the onion and pepper in the oil until it is soft. Add the garlic and cook for another minute.		
2	Stir sausage and spices in and cook over medium high heat for 3-4 minutes, stirring.		
3	Add tomatoes, rice, beans and stock and bring to a boil. Reduce heat to a simmer and cover pot.		
4	Simmer for 20 minutes with the lid in place and then stir. If rice is not yet done, return to heat for another five minutes.		
5	Remove from heat and allow to rest for five minutes with lid on. Salt to taste.		
OPTIONS			
A	**Dirty Rice**: Recipe above. Pairs well with fried okra, collard greens or cornbread.		
B	**Spanish Rice**: Omit the Andouille sausage. Replace the Cajun spice blend with 1 tsp paprika and ½ tsp each of cumin and oregano. Garnish with ¼ C sliced green olives.		
C	**Cuban Moro**: Replace sausage with four slices crumbled cooked bacon. Use black beans, omit the tomatoes, and add 1 C of water. Replace Cajun spice mix with ½ tsp each of cumin and oregano.		

AGILE RECIPES

Photo with Picadillo on page 261

VEGGIE	Braised Cabbage^V Makes ~ 8 cups		Side
INGREDIENTS		**SUBSTITUTE**	
1	Cabbage head, ~ 3 lb, cut into ½ inch slices	Red or green cabbage	
1	Onion, medium sliced	Any type	
3 - 5	Carrots, cut to ½ inch thick (optional)		
2 tsp	Stock paste, chicken	Bouillon powder or cubes, beef or vegetable	
½ C	Water		
½ tsp	Salt and pepper, each		
1 Tbsp	Balsamic vinegar	1 Tbsp vinegar + 2 tsp sugar	
2-3 Tbsp	Butter		
STEPS			
1	Layer cabbage, onion and carrots in the bottom of a large pot with a tight lid.		
2	Add water, stock paste, salt and pepper, then close lid.		
3	Cook over medium high heat for 10-15 minutes, stirring occasionally, until veggies are tender-crisp. Add a small amount of water only if necessary to keep pot from drying out.		
4	Stir in vinegar and butter. Cook uncovered for a few minutes, continuing to stir, until moisture is nearly gone.		
5	Serve plain or with a garnish of bread crumbs or bacon crumbles. Pairs nicely with cured or uncured pork, or sausage.		

AGILE RECIPES

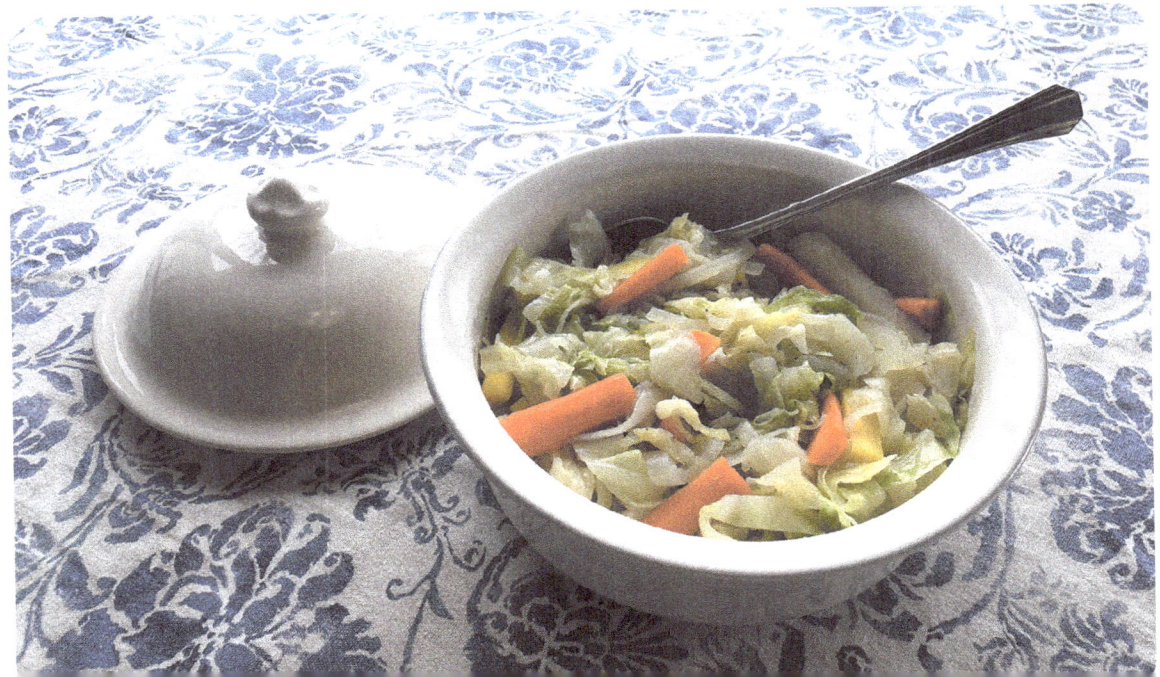

VEGGIE	Cauliflower Marinara^V Serves 4-6		Side
INGREDIENTS		**SUBSTITUTE**	
1	Head cauliflower		
3½ C	Marinara sauce (see Classic Marinara recipe on page 290)	Marinara sauce, one 24 oz jar	
1 C	Mozzarella, shredded	Fontina or Parmesan cheese	
1 C	Red bell pepper, sliced (optional)		
STEPS			
1	Preheat oven to 375°F. Spray 9" x 13" baking pan with cooking spray.		
2	Cut up cauliflower florets into pieces no thicker than 1½ inches. Arrange cauliflower and red pepper (if using) in pan in a single layer.		
3	Spread Marinara sauce over cauliflower evenly.		
4	Bake in oven for 20 minutes or until you can push a fork into the cauliflower with a little effort (undercooked).		
5	Spread grated cheese over the cauliflower and return to the oven for another 20 minutes.		

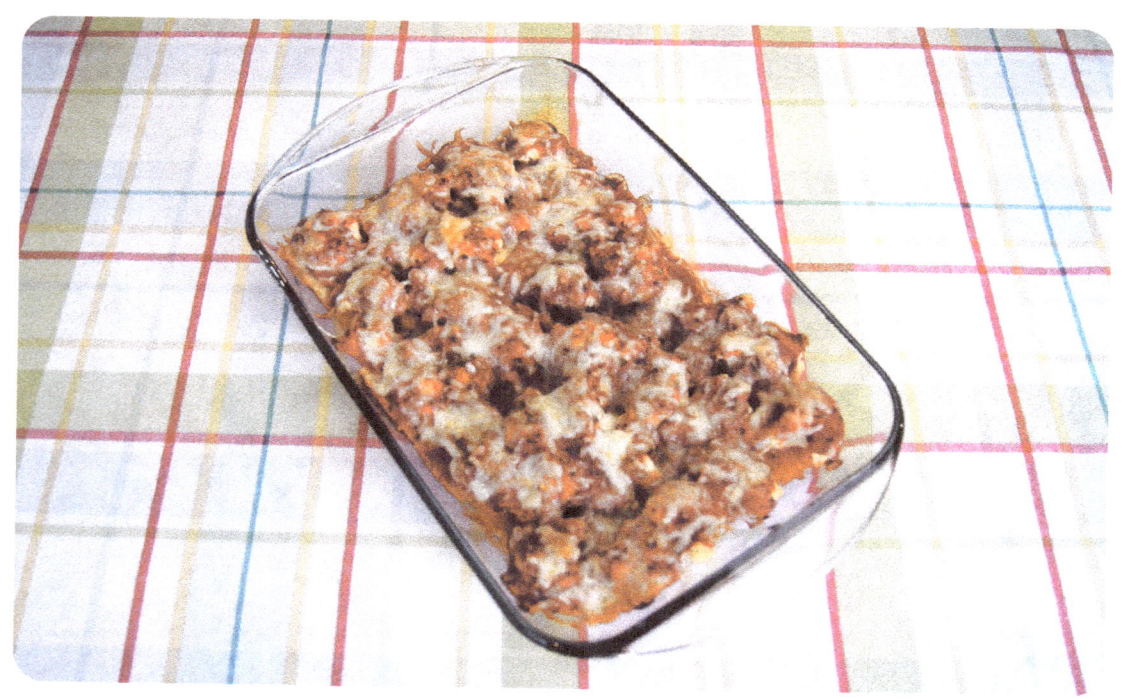

VEGGIE	Citrus Brussels Sprouts^V Serves 4		Side
INGREDIENTS		**SUBSTITUTE**	
1 lb	Brussels sprouts, fresh	Frozen Brussels sprouts	
2 Tbsp	Extra Virgin Olive Oil		
2 Tbsp	Butter		
2 Tbsp	Orange juice concentrate		
2 Tbsp	Brown sugar	White sugar or honey	
	Salt and pepper to taste		
STEPS			
1	Preheat oven to 400°F. Line a sheet pan with parchment if desired.		
2	Prepare fresh sprouts by cleaning well and cutting in half. If using frozen, leave them whole.		
3	In a bowl, toss the sprouts with the oil to coat them. Put them on the sheet pan in a single layer.		
4	Roast the sprouts for 30-40 minutes, stirring them once after about 20 minutes. Remove from the oven once they are tender.		
5	In a small sauce pan, bring the butter, orange juice concentrate and brown sugar to a boil.		
6	Combine the roasted sprouts and the sauce in a serving bowl, stirring to coat the Brussels sprouts.		

AGILE RECIPES

Brussels sprouts interesting facts:

» **A cup of Brussels sprouts has 35 calories, 3 g of fiber, and 3 g of protein.**
» **Contains four times more vitamin C than oranges.**
» **Stay fresh in the refrigerator vegetable drawer for up to 10 days.**
» **They contain sulforaphane that has been shown to help lower cancer risks.**
» **Contain zeaxanthine, an antioxidant, that is good for eye health.**

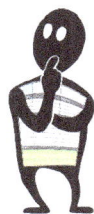

PROTEIN OTHER	Continental Beans^V Makes ~ 2 cups		Side
INGREDIENTS		**SUBSTITUTE**	
2 C	Cooked white beans, drained (15 oz can)	Any cooked or canned beans	
2 oz	Bacon, diced (optional)	Pancetta or ham, diced	
½	Onion, diced		
3 tsp	Garlic, minced		
1 Tbsp	Herbs de Provence	Rosemary + Thyme	
1 Tbsp	Lemon juice	Vinegar	
½ Tbsp	Dijon mustard		
2 Tbsp	Olive oil		
STEPS			
1	Cook bacon in a sauté pan until almost crisp, remove from pan for later.		
2	Remove all but 2 Tbsp of bacon grease from pan.		
3	Cook onion in fat from bacon (or add a little oil if you didn't use bacon) until onion is soft.		
4	Add garlic and herbs to the pan and cook another three minutes.		
5	Add beans and bacon to the pan and mix. Heat thoroughly.		
6	Mix lemon juice, mustard and olive oil together in small cup and drizzle over beans prior to serving.		

AGILE RECIPES

VEGGIE	Creamed Vegetables^V Serves 2-4		Side

INGREDIENTS / SUBSTITUTE

INGREDIENTS		SUBSTITUTE
3 Tbsp	Butter	
½	Onion, finely minced	
1¼ Tbsp	Flour	
1 C	Milk	Heavy cream or Half & Half
1 tsp	Salt	
1 lb	Vegetables, fresh or frozen	

STEPS

1	Cook vegetables by boiling on the stove top or microwave, per your preference. Drain well.
2	In a large skillet, melt the butter and cook the onion over medium heat until it is soft and there is no free moisture.
3	Add the flour to the pan and cook while stirring for two to three minutes to cook the flour.
4	Add the milk and stir or whisk vigorously to fully incorporate. Continue to heat while stirring until the mixture almost boils and the sauce thickens. Add salt.
5	Stir the cooked and drained vegetables into the sauce. Add a tablespoon of milk if the sauce is too thick.

OPTIONS

A	**Peas:** Make plain or add 2 oz of grated Parmesan cheese and a ¼ tsp of nutmeg to the sauce before combining with peas.
B	**Potatoes**: Use small red or fingerling potatoes, cut into halves. Multiply the sauce recipe by the number of pounds of potatoes. If desired, add 1 C grated cheese to the sauce.
C	**Cauliflower**: Cut one head of cauliflower (about 2 pounds) into florets before cooking. Double the amount of sauce and add 1 C grated cheese to the sauce if desired.
D	**Spinach**: After cooking the spinach, squeeze to remove as much water as possible. Add 2 oz of grated parmesan cheese and a ¼ tsp of nutmeg to the sauce before combining.
E	**Corn**: Start with fresh or frozen corn, cook and drain well. Add 1 tsp of sugar and ¼ tsp black pepper to the sauce before combining.
F	**Mixed**: Combine any two veggies (e.g. peas + cauliflower, peas + potatoes, corn + green beans). Multiply the sauce recipe by the number of pounds of veggies.

VEGGIE	Frizzled Cabbage^V Makes about 3-5 cups		Side
INGREDIENTS		**SUBSTITUTE**	
1-1½ lb	Cabbage, sliced finely	Red or green cabbage, fresh or bag	
1-2 Tbsp	Extra Virgin Olive Oil	Bacon fat or butter or any oil	
2 - 4	Slices of bacon, chopped (optional)	Finely chopped ham or pancetta	
½ C	Onion and/or red pepper, sliced (optional)		
½ - 1 C	Carrot, shredded (optional)		
1 tsp	Salt and pepper, each		
2 Tbsp	Butter, as dressing	2-3 Tbsp Tahini or 4-6 Tbsp sour cream	
STEPS			
1	If using bacon, cook in large skillet until crispy. Remove bacon and leave fat in pan.		
2	Sauté cabbage and any other veggies in the oil (or bacon fat) over medium high heat, stirring often, until tender and beginning to caramelize. About 15 minutes.		
3	Salt and pepper to taste. Toss with butter (or Tahini or sour cream) prior to serving.		
4	Top with crumbled bacon, if using.		
OPTIONS			
A	**Simply Savory**: Recipe above - plain red or green cabbage with salt, pepper and butter.		
B	**Colorful and Complex:** Cabbage, onions, pepper and carrots frizzled to a nice caramelized tenderness. Stir in Tahini prior to serving for a rich and satisfying taste.		
C	**Creamy:** Frizzle the cabbage then stir in sour cream prior to serving. Particularly good with a crispy pancetta or bacon garnish.		

AGILE RECIPES

VEGGIE	Glazed Carrots^V **Serves 4**		**Side**
INGREDIENTS		**SUBSTITUTE**	
1 lb	Carrots, any type		
2 Tbsp	Butter	Extra Virgin Olive Oil	
2 Tbsp	Brown sugar	Maple syrup, honey	
½ tsp	Cinnamon	Ginger	
STEPS			
1	Peel and cut carrots so that they are uniform in shape and thickness. Can be sticks or coins or can use bagged baby carrots.		
2	Boil carrots in water until tender – about 6-10 minutes depending on thickness.		
3	Drain carrots well and set aside. The serving bowl works well.		
4	Put remaining ingredients into the pan and heat over medium heat, stirring to combine.		
5	When the glaze is bubbly, return the carrots to the pan. Stir over medium heat for several minutes to glaze the carrots.		
OPTIONS			
A	**Orange Ginger**: Add 1 Tbsp orange juice concentrate to the glaze mixture and replace the cinnamon with 1 tsp ginger paste or ½ tsp dried ginger.		
B	**Maple Bourbon**: Add 1 Tbsp bourbon to the glaze mixture and replace brown sugar with maple syrup.		
C	**Sweet & Spicy**: Replace cinnamon with ½ tsp red pepper flakes and ¼ tsp salt.		

AGILE RECIPES

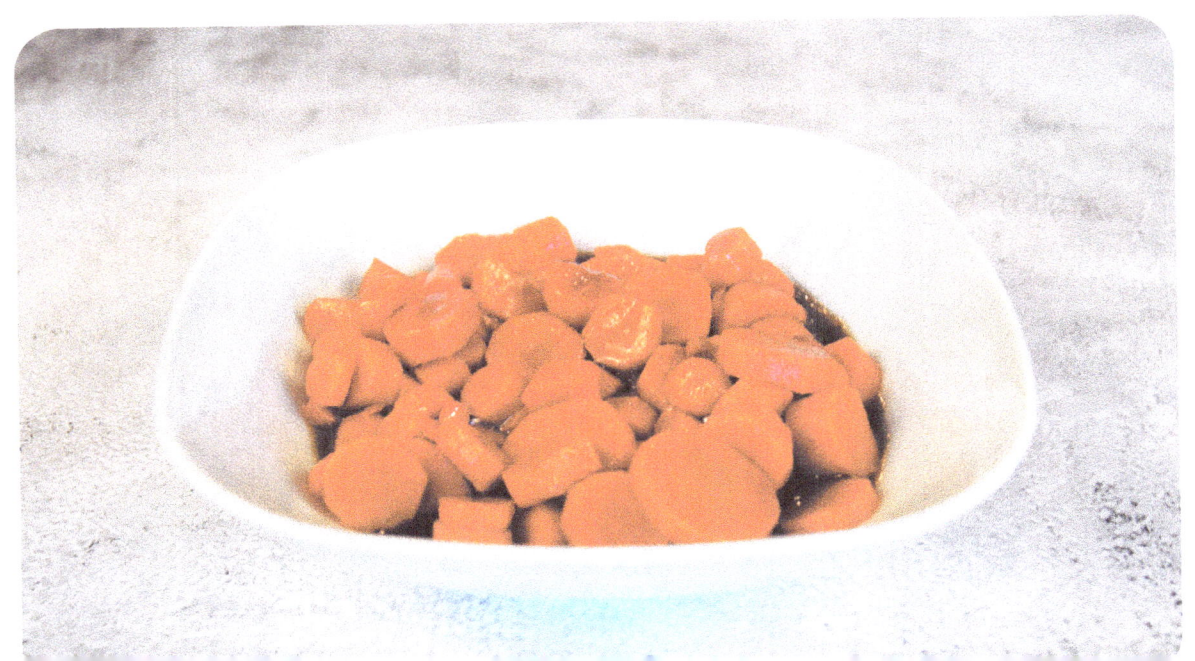

VEGGIE	Green Beans^V Serves 2-4		Side
INGREDIENTS		**SUBSTITUTE**	
1 lb	Green beans, whole	Frozen green beans	
2 Tbsp	Extra Virgin Olive Oil	Butter	
4	Cloves garlic, minced	2 tsp jarred minced garlic	
¼ tsp	Red pepper flakes		
STEPS			
1	Steam or microwave green beans until they are tender-crisp, slightly less than done. Drain.		
2	In a sauté pan, cook the garlic and pepper flakes in the oil or butter for 1-2 minutes.		
3	Add the cooked green beans to the pan and toss over medium heat to thoroughly coat the green beans. Salt to taste and serve.		
OPTIONS			
A	**Almondine**: Garnish with ½ C sliced almonds.		
B	**Mushroom**: Add 8 oz of sautéed mushrooms to the garlic and oil, then toss with the green beans.		
C	**Italian**: Add ½ of a sautéed sliced red pepper and ½ tsp oregano or basil to the garlic and oil, then toss with the green beans.		
D	**Asian**: Sauté 1 tsp ginger paste with the garlic. Add 2 Tbsp soy sauce and 1 Tbsp honey when tossing the green beans.		

AGILE RECIPES

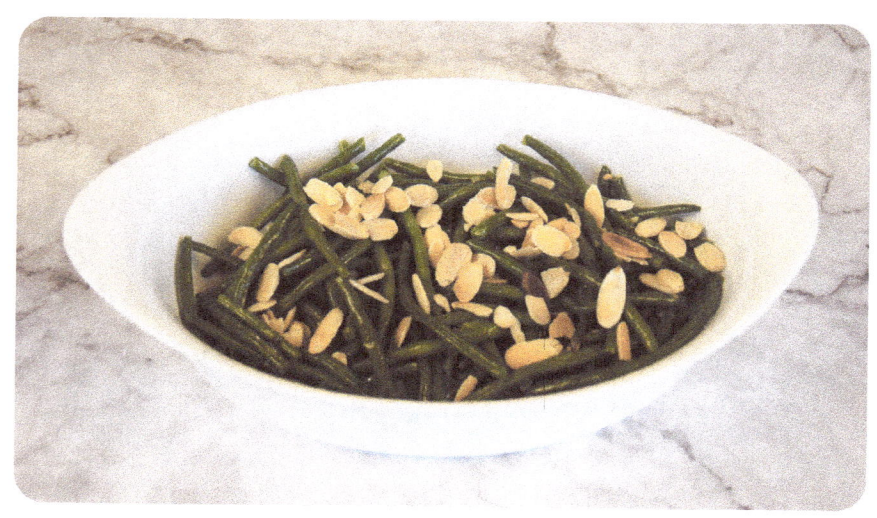

VEGGIE	Green Bean Succotash^v Serves 4-6		Side
INGREDIENTS		**SUBSTITUTE**	
1 lb	Green beans, whole fresh	Frozen	
12 oz	Sweet corn, cut from cob	Frozen	
2 Tbsp	Butter	Extra Virgin Olive Oil	
½	Red bell pepper, thinly sliced (optional)		
1 C	Cherry tomatoes, halved (optional)		
STEPS			
1	Put green beans and corn in a pot together and add 1 cup of water. Bring water to a boil then cook for about eight minutes or until desired doneness. Drain.		
2	If including bell pepper, sauté it in the butter for about four minutes.		
3	Add the cooked green beans, corn, and cherry tomatoes (if using) to the pan and stir together over medium heat for 1-2 minutes to thoroughly mix. Salt to taste and serve.		
Copyright © 2024 Alin E. Steele May be copied for personal use only. www.ReEngineeringtheKitchen.com			

AGILE RECIPES

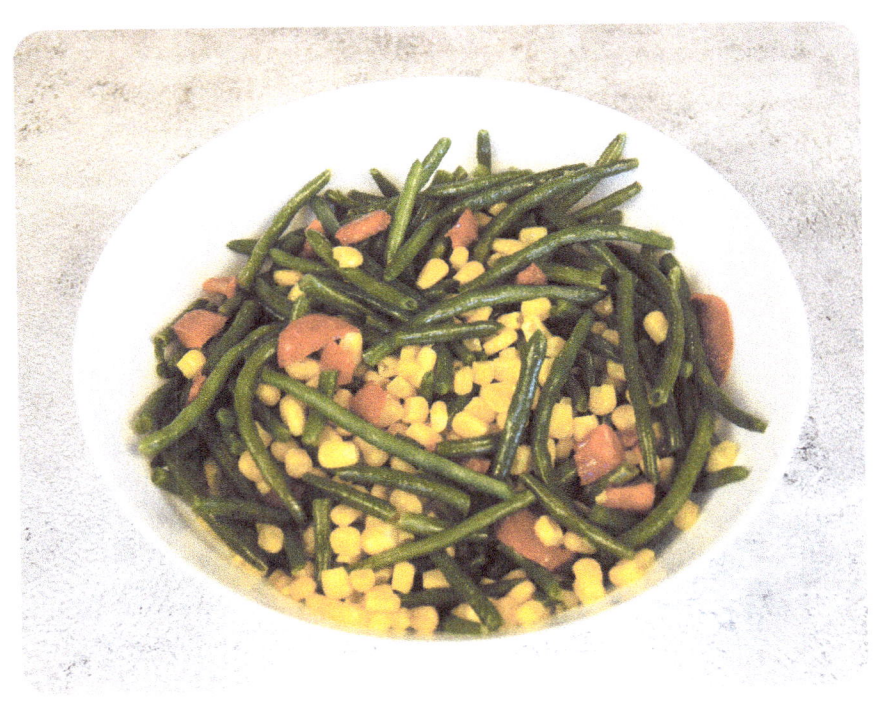

VEGGIE	Green Bean Un-Casserole^V Makes 4 cups		Side
INGREDIENTS		**SUBSTITUTE**	
1 lb	Green beans, trimmed	Frozen green beans	
1½ Tbsp	Butter	Extra Virgin Olive Oil, olive or other light oil	
1 Tbsp	Flour		
1 C	Milk		
½ Tbsp	Dehydrated onion flakes	2 Tbsp diced onion + 2 tsp oil microwaved together for 20 seconds on high (covered)	
1 Tbsp	Mushroom or Umami seasoning	1 Tbsp mushroom powder + 1 tsp salt	
½ C	Bread crumbs (optional)		
STEPS			
1	Put green beans in a sauce pan with one cup of water and cover. Bring to a boil and then cook for five to seven minutes to desired tenderness. Drain and set aside.		
2	In a sauté pan, melt butter and add flour. Cook over medium heat and allow to bubble while stirring for two to three minutes to make a light roux.		
3	Add milk to pan, stirring continuously. Bring mixture to almost a boil so that the sauce thckens.		
4	Remove from heat and add onion flakes and mushroom seasoning.		
5	Toss green beans with the onion / mushroom sauce.		
6	Top with bread crumbs (optional) then serve.		

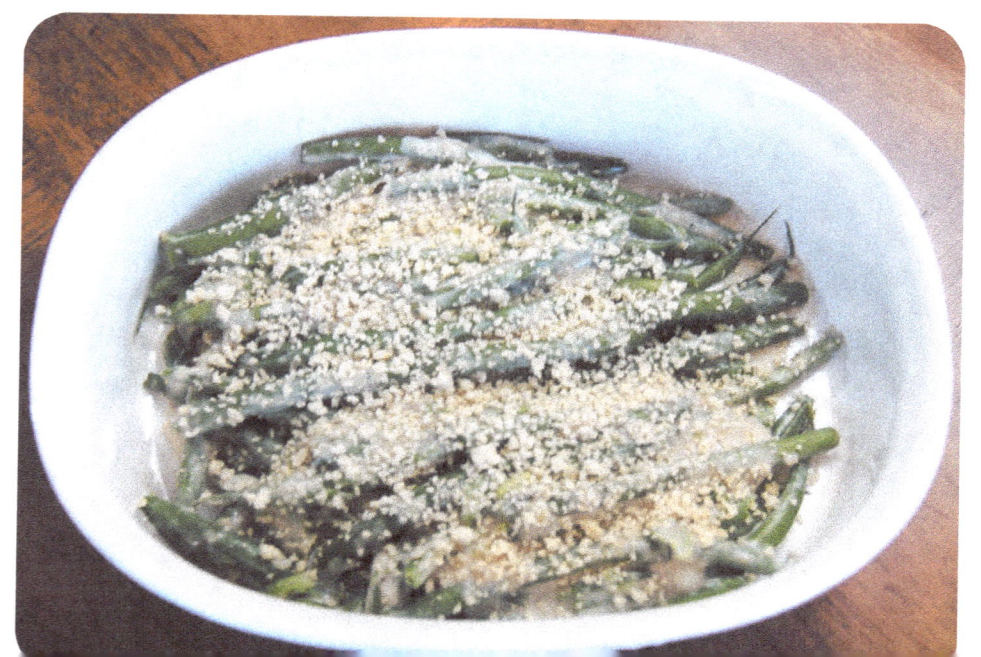

VEGGIE	Lemon Bacon Brussels Sprouts^V Serves 4-6		Side
INGREDIENTS		**SUBSTITUTE**	
1½ ibs	Brussels sprouts		
3-4 slices	Bacon, diced		
1	Lemon, cut into ¼ inch thick slices		
1 tsp	Salt		
STEPS			
1	Preheat oven to 400°F.		
2	Prepare Brussels sprouts by cleaning and cutting into halves.		
3	In an large oven proof skillet, sauteé bacon until crispy and fat has rendered.		
4	Add sprouts to the pan with the bacon and fat. Allow them to brown over medium high heat for three to four minutes, then stir/turn them to brown on the other side for another three to four minutes.		
5	Add salt and lemon slices, stirring just enough to evenly distribute through the sprouts.		
6	Bake for 10-15 minutes, or to desired tenderness.		

AGILE RECIPES

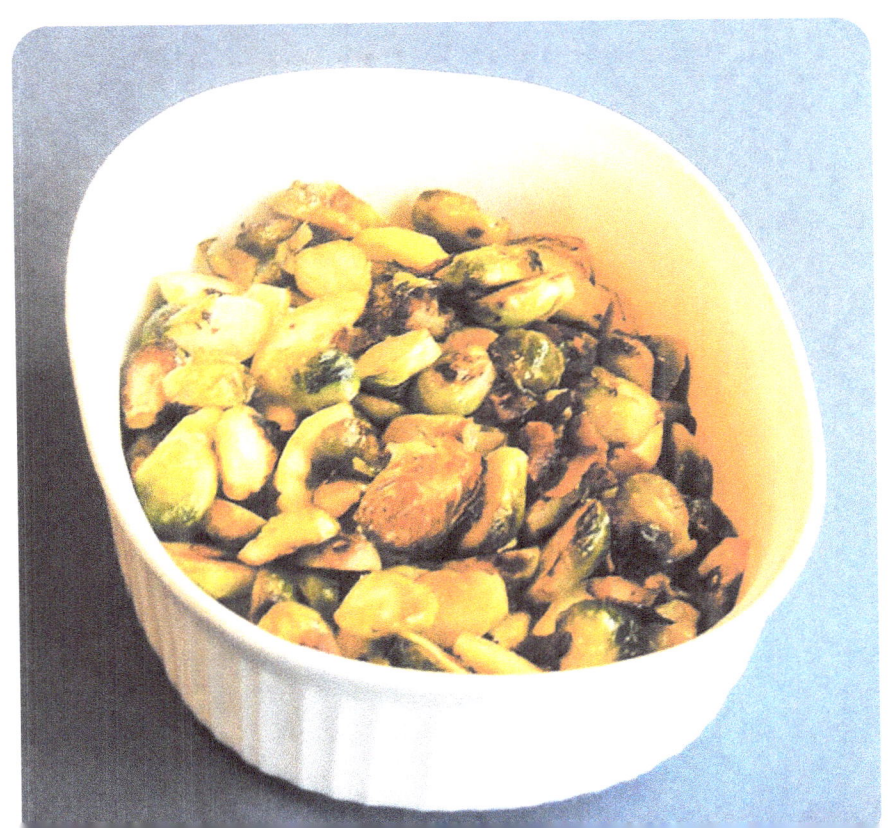

VEGGIE	Lemon Garlic Kale^V Serves 2-4		Side
INGREDIENTS		**SUBSTITUTE**	
1 bunch	Fresh kale (about 9 oz)		
2 Tbsp	Extra Virgin Olive Oil	Any olive or light cooking oil	
3 - 4	Garlic cloves, minced	Jarred minced garlic	
1 tsp	Stock paste or bouillon powder		
½ C	Water		
1 Tbsp	Lemon juice		
1 Tbsp	Butter	Margarine	
1 Tbsp	Grated Paremesan cheese (optional)		
STEPS			
1	Prepare kale by washing well in cold water and then remove stems and slice leaves.		
2	In a large sauce pan, sauté garlic in olive oil for two minutes.		
3	Add water and stock paste to the pan and then stir in kale.		
4	Cover the pan and cook over medium heat for about six minutes until kale leaves are tender.		
5	Stir in the lemon juice and butter, and continue to cook uncovered until liquid is mostly gone.		
6	Serve plain or with a garnish of grated parmesan cheese.		

AGILE RECIPES

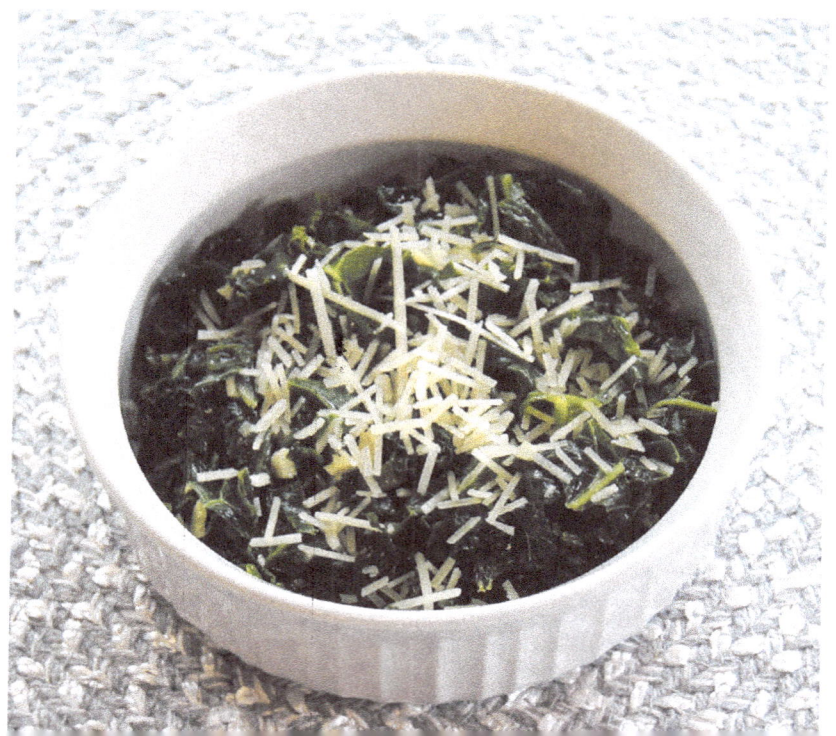

VEGGIE	Mediterranean Spaghetti Squash^V Serves 4-6		Side
INGREDIENTS		**SUBSTITUTE**	
1	Spaghetti squash (about 1½ lbs)	Summer squash, julienne cut	
2 Tbsp	Extra Virgin Olive Oil	Olive oil, butter, or any light cooking oil	
1	Onion, sliced (red)	Any onion	
1	Red bell pepper, sliced		
1	Medium tomato, diced	Cherry tomatoes, halved	
1 Tbsp	Oregano		
1 tsp	Salt		
2-4 oz	Feta, crumbled		
STEPS			
1	Remove the stem and cut the squash in half long wise. Scrape out and dispose of the seeds and associated strings.		
2	Place one half squash face down on a flat microwave safe plate or pan. Depending on the size of your microwave and available pans, you may need to cook the halves sequentially.		
3	For one half squash, microwave on high for seven minutes. Test for doneness by pressing on the outside (with an oven glove): if you can easily form a dent, the scuash is done.		
4	If not done yet, continue to cook on high in two minute increments until the flesh is tender and readily gives when pressed.		
5	Carefully scrape the squash fibers out of the shell using a fork, separating and fluffing them as you go. The cooked squash can be held at this point for later use.		
6	If you are using summer squash, steam briefly until tender crisp.		
7	In a large sauté pan, cook the onion and bell pepper until tender. Add the tomatoes and cook for another one to two minutes.		
8	Add the cooked squash, oregano and salt to the pan and toss together over medium heat for a two minutes to combine and warm.		
9	Serve with the crumbled feta on top.		

AGILE RECIPES

Photo on page 312

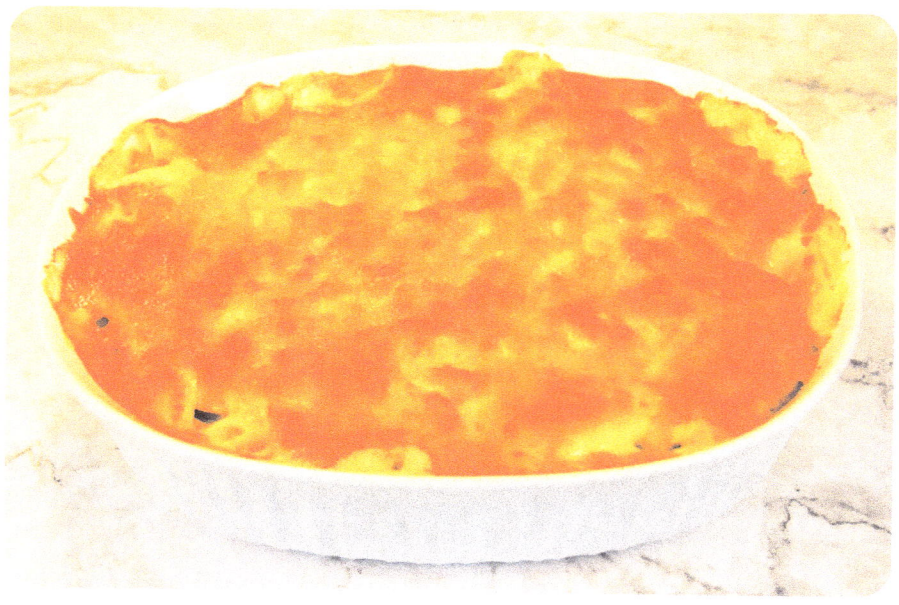

$100 Mac & Cheese

Recipe on page 296

Mediterranean Spaghetti
Squash

Recipe on page 311

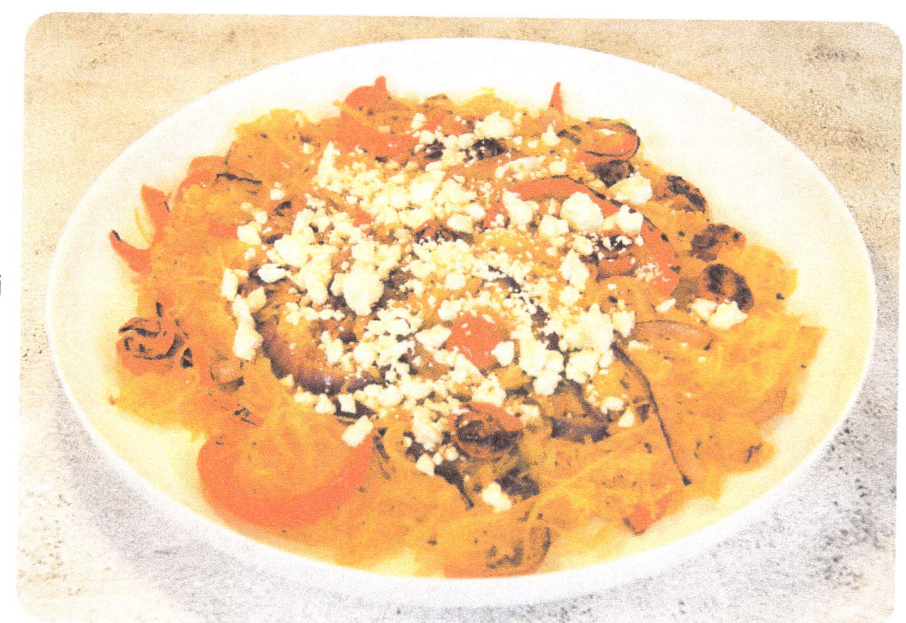

VEGGIE	Moroccan Cauliflower^V Serves 2-4		Side
INGREDIENTS		**SUBSTITUTE**	
1	Head cauliflower		
3 Tbsp	Extra Virgin Olive Oil	Olive oil, coconut oil, or avocado oil	
½ tsp	Turmeric		
1 tsp	Cumin		
1 tsp	Paprika		
1 tsp	Salt		
1 tsp	Cinnamon		
½ tsp	Clove		
2 Tbsp	Tahini (optional)		
STEPS			
1	Preheat oven to 400°F. Line sheet pan with parchment paper if desired.		
2	Cut cauliflower into florets approximately one to two inches in size.		
3	In a bowel, toss the cauliflower pieces with oil to coat.		
4	Mix spices together in a small bowel.		
5	Sprinkle spices over cauliflower pieces and turn to evenly distribute.		
6	Spread cauliflower onto sheet pan in a single layer.		
7	Roast for 20-30 minutes, until tender-crisp.		
8	Drizzle with Tahini if desired.		

AGILE RECIPES

VEGGIE	Quick Creamed Spinach^V Serves 2-4		Side

INGREDIENTS		SUBSTITUTE
1 lb	Frozen chopped spinach	Fresh spinach
4 oz	Cream cheese	Neufchatel or goat cheese
½ tsp	Dehydrated onion	¼ tsp onion powder
⅛ tsp	Nutmeg (optional)	
½ tsp	Salt (optional)	
1 Tbsp	Grated Parmesan cheese (optional)	

STEPS	
1	Cook frozen spinach according to package directions. If using fresh spinach, saute in olive oil until wilted.
2	Press excess water out of spinach by pressing it against the side of the pan with a fork. Drain water.
3	Add onion and cream cheese to cooked spinach. Allow to melt in warm pan.
4	Stir to incorporate the melting cream cheese. Use low heat if necessary.
5	Add nutmeg and salt if desired. Garnish with grated Parmasean.

OPTIONS	
A	**Side Dish**: Creamed spinach is always an elegant side dish served alone.
B	**Pasta Florentine**: Toss with 8 oz cooked pasta and ½ C pasta water. Serve with a generous garnish of Parmesan cheese.
C	**Chicken Florentine**: Dress up pan-sautéed chicken breast with a few tablespoons of creamed spinach on top.
D	**Cauliflower and Spinach**: Stir into lightly steamed and drained cauliflower florets.

Photo on page 318

VEGGIE	**Quick Spaghetti Squash**^{V} **Serves 4-6**	**Side**

INGREDIENTS		SUBSTITUTE
1	Spaghetti squash (about 1½ lbs)	
2 Tbsp	Butter	Extra Virgin Olive Oil
2 Tbsp	Orange juice concentrate	1 Tbsp lemon or lime juice
2 Tbsp	Sugar, white	Honey, brown sugar
1 tsp	Salt	
1 Tbsp	Parsley (optional)	

STEPS	
1	Remove the stem and cut the squash in half long wise. Scrape out and dispose of the seeds and associated strings.
2	Place one half squash face down on a flat microwave safe plate or pan. Depending on the size of your microwave and available pans, you may need to cook the halves sequentially.
3	For one half squash, microwave on high for seven minutes. Test for doneness by pressing on the outside (with an oven glove): if you can easily form a dent, the squash is done.
4	If not done yet, continue to cook on high in two minute increments until the flesh is tender and readily gives when pressed.
5	Carefully scrape the squash fibers out of the shell using a fork, separating and fluffing them as you go. The cooked squash can be held at this point for later use.
6	In a large sauté pan, stir the butter, orange juice concentrate, sugar and salt together over medium heat.
7	Add the cooked squash to the pan and toss to warm and coat it. Serve with a garnish of parsley if desired.

AGILE RECIPES

AGILE RECIPES

GRAIN	Rice Pilaf^V Serves 2-4		Side
INGREDIENTS		**SUBSTITUTE**	
4 C	Cooked rice		
2 Tbsp	Extra Virgin Olive Oil	Butter, any light oil	
1	Onion, diced		
2	Cloves garlic	1 tsp minced jarred garlic	
8-16 oz	Mushrooms, sliced	Peas, spinach, broccoli	
1 Tbsp	Basil	Thyme, oregano	
1 tsp	Salt		
1 C	Grated cheese (optional)		

STEPS	
1	In a large pot, sauté the onion in the oil until soft. Add the garlic and cook an additional minute.
2	Add the mushrooms and cook until the moisture is nearly gone. Stir in the salt and spices.
3	Add the cooked rice to the pot and stir to incorporate. If the rice is cold, you can add 2 Tbsp of water to the pot, cover over low heat for three to five minutes to warm it.
4	When the rice is hot, you can serve it directly or topped with grated cheese.
5	If desired, the pilaf can be put in a casserole dish with cheese on top and then baked for 10-15 minutes at 350°F, until the cheese is melted and golden.

OPTIONS	
A	**Mushroom Pilaf**: Recipe as above. Swiss cheese goes well with the mushrooms.
B	**Risi Bisi**: Replace the mushrooms with two cups cooked peas. Top with Parmesan cheese.
C	**Tuscan Pilaf**: Replace the mushrooms with 16 oz spinach, cooked and squeezed dry. Add ½ C diced sun dried tomatoes (in oil) and ½ C of pine nuts. Top with Parmesan cheese.
D	**Broccoli Cheddar**: Replace the mushrooms with two cups of cooked broccoli florets. Stir in one cup of sharp cheddar cheese and then top with another cup of cheese.

Photo on page 318

VEGGIE	Roasted Vegetables^V Serves 4-8		Side
INGREDIENTS		**SUBSTITUTE**	
2 lb	Mixed vegetables: Carrots, potatoes, onions, cauliflower, broccoli, peppers, sweet potatoes	Butternut squash, Brussels sprouts, summer squash, beets	
2 Tbsp	Extra Virgin Olive Oil	Melted butter	
1 tsp	Salt		
½ tsp	Cracked black pepper		
STEPS			
1	Preheat oven to 400°F.		
2	Prepare the vegetables by cutting them into uniform size pieces, no thicker than one inch.		
3	Place the more dense veggies (carrots, cauliflower, potatoes, etc.) in a large bowl and toss with olive oil and spices.		
4	Spread these veggies on a large sheet pan and put in the oven for 25 minutes.		
5	Place the less dense veggies (broccoli, onions, peppers, etc.) in a large bowl and toss with the remaining olive oil and spices.		
6	Remove the sheet pan from the oven and stir. Add the less dense veggies and roast for an additional 20-30 minutes, or until desired level of doneness.		
7	If you increase the recipe, use additional sheet pans so that the veggies can roast in a single layer.		
OPTIONS			
A	**Savory**: Mix 1 tsp minced garlic and 2 tsp Herbs de Provence or rosemary into the olive oil before tossing with the veggies.		
B	**Sweet**: Mix 2 Tbsp brown sugar and 1 tsp cinnamon into the oil before tossing with carrots, sweet potatoes or butternut squash.		
C	**Spicy**: Mix 1 tsp minced garlic and ½ tsp each cumin, coriander, paprika and red pepper flakes into the oil before tossing with the veggies.		
D	**Balsamic Glazed**: Mix 1 tsp minced garlic, 1 tsp thyme and ¼ C Balsamic vinegar with the oil before tossing with the veggies.		

AGILE RECIPES

Photo on page 318

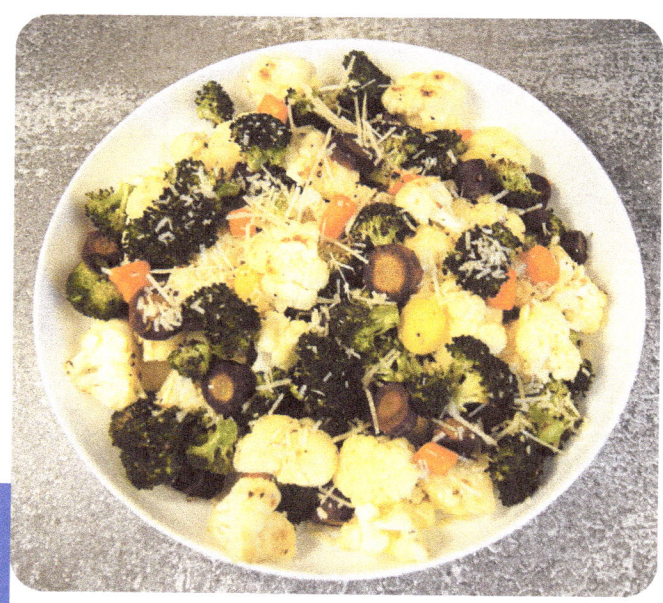

Roasted Vegetables

Recipe on page 317

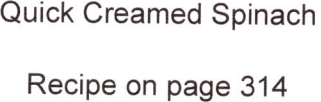

Quick Creamed Spinach

Recipe on page 314

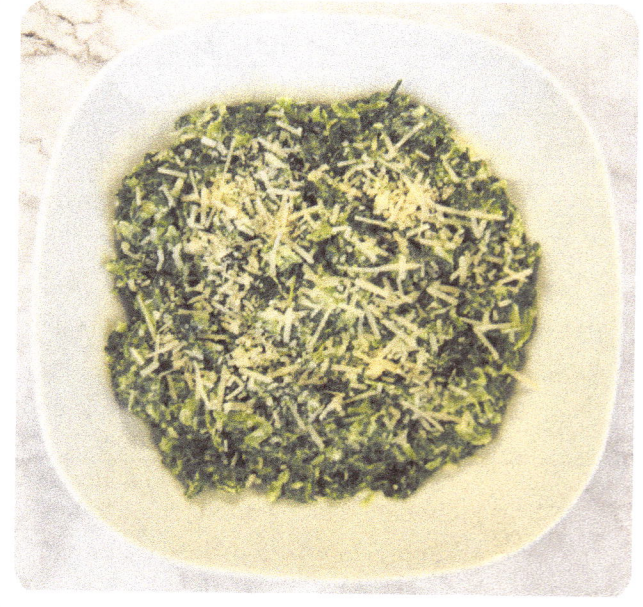

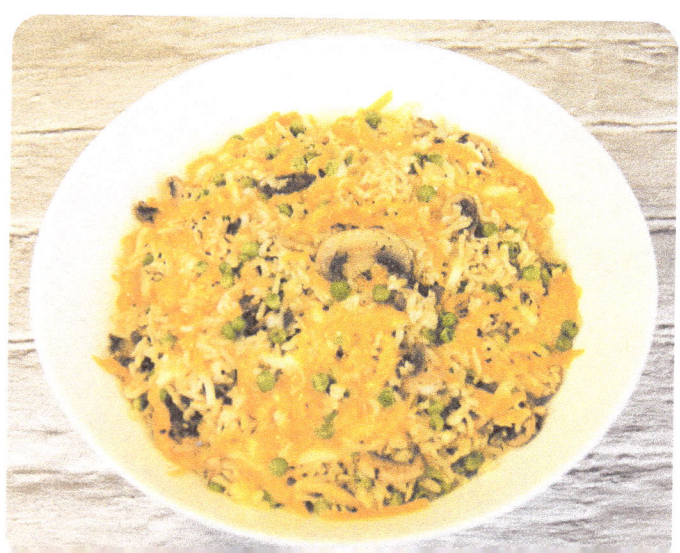

Rice Pilaf w/ Mushrooms and Peas

Recipe on page 316

VEGGIE	Sautéed Baby Bok Choy^V Serves 2-4		Side
INGREDIENTS		**SUBSTITUTE**	
4-6	Heads baby bok choy, halved longways		
2 Tbsp	Canola oil	Any light oil	
2	Cloves garlic	1 tsp minced jarred garlic	
2	Green onions, sliced		
2 Tbsp	Soy sauce		
1 tsp	Sesame oil		
1 tsp	Honey		
2 Tbsp	Water		
STEPS			
1	In a large fry pan with a lid, heat the oil and garlic and cook for one minute.		
2	Place the bok choy halves, face down in the pan in the hot oil. Cook over medium high heat for two minutes with out stirring so that the face starts to caramelize.		
3	Mix the remaining ingredients and add to pan. Shake the pan to coat the bok choy.		
4	Reduce heat to simmer and cover the pan. Allow to coot for an additional three to five minutes until tender.		

AGILE RECIPES

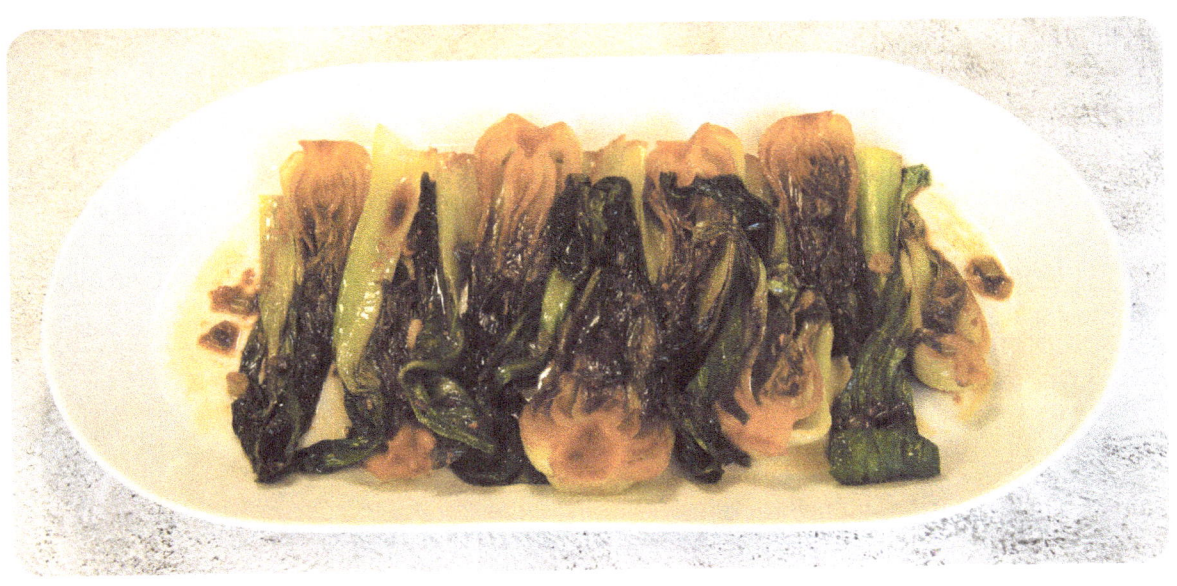

PROTEIN OTHER	Savory White Beans^V Makes about 2 cups		Side
INGREDIENTS		**SUBSTITUTE**	
2	15 oz cans Great Northern Beans, drained	Any canned beans or 4 C of any cooked beans	
1	Onion, chopped		
1 tsp	Minced garlic		
3	Carrots, diced		
1 Tbsp	Tomato paste	Ketchup (omit sugar)	
1 tsp	Chicken broth base or boullion powder	Vegetable broth base	
1 tsp	Herbs de Provence	Thyme + Sage	
1 tsp	Salt and black pepper, each		
1 tsp	Sugar	Any sweetener	
¼ C	Water	Add more if a thinner consistency is desired	
¼ C	Bread crumbs (optional)	Cracker, corn flake, or potato chip crumbs	
STEPS			
1	Sauté onion in a sauce pan with a little oil until soft		
2	Add garlic and cook for another few minutes.		
3	Add carrots and water to pan and cook for 8-10 minutes.		
4	Add all remaining ingredients except bread crumbs and simmer for 10 minutes. Add ¼ C water if beans become too dry.		
5	Serve with bread crumbs sprinkled on top.		
OPTIONS			
A	**Casserole**: Make recipe through step 3. Layer beans with 1 lb cooked pork or sausage in a 9" x 9" pan or 1-2 quart casserole dish. Top with crumbs and bake for 30 minutes.		
B	**Soup**: Make recipe through step 3. Add 2 C chicken broth and simmer for 30-60 minutes.		

Photo on page 329

VEGGIE	Simple Greens^v Serves 2-4	Side
INGREDIENTS		**SUBSTITUTE**
2 lb	Fresh collard greens	Kale, Swiss chard, turnip greens
2 Tbsp	Extra Virgin Olive Oil	Butter, bacon fat, any oil
1	Onion, medium, minced	
2	Cloves garlic	1 tsp minced jarred garlic
2 C	Vegetable or chicken stock	2 C water + 2 tsp stock paste
1 Tbsp	Apple cider vinegar	Any vinegar or lemon juice
1 Tbsp	Sugar, white	Honey, maple syrup
¼ tsp	Red pepper flakes	
STEPS		
1	Prepare greens by thoroughly washing them in cold water. Remove the central stem of each leaf and then slice the leaves into about one inch strips.	
2	In the bottom of a large pan with a lid, sauté the onion in the oil until soft then add the garlic and cook for an additional minute.	
3	Add remaining ingredients and bring to a boil, stirring occasionally.	
4	Reduce heat and simmer covered for 20-45 minutes or until greens are tender. Young, tender greens will cook faster than older, tougher ones.	

AGILE RECIPES

Besides being delicious, dark leafy greens like collard greens, kale, Swiss chard, and turnip greens are rich in iron, calcium, magnesium, potassium, and vitamins C, E, and K. They are also an excellent source of fiber and antioxidants.

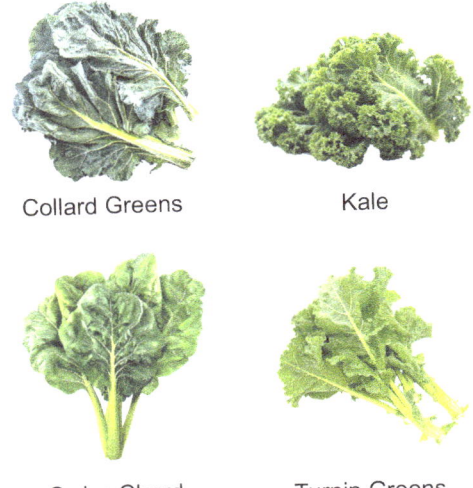

Collard Greens

Kale

Swiss Chard

Turnip Greens

VEGGIE	Spinach – Flash Sautéed^V Serves 2-4		Side
INGREDIENTS		**SUBSTITUTE**	
6 oz	Fresh spinach leaves		
3 Tbsp	Extra Virgin Olive Oil	Butter	
4	Cloves garlic, minced	2 tsp jarred minced garlic	
2 Tbsp	Grated Parmesan cheese		
STEPS			
1	Sort and rinse fresh spinach leaves. Dry to remove most of the residual water.		
2	In a large sauté pan, heat the oil and cook the garlic for two to three minutes over medium heat.		
3	Increase heat to medium high and start adding handfuls of spinach leaves. As they wilt, push to the side and add more until all of the spinach is in the pan.		
4	Stir the spinach gently, lifting from below so that it does not become compacted. Cook for about two minutes or until the spinach is uniformly cooked. Salt to taste.		
5	Serve with the parmesan sprinkled on top.		

AGILE RECIPES

Spinach and Popeye:

Everyone knows that spinach was Popeye's go to food for strength whenever he got in trouble. Ever wonder why?

The creator of Popeye read that spinach had a huge amount of iron, 35mg per 100g, so he ran with that and made spinach the symbol of strength in the series. It turns out that there was a typo in the article he read and the actual amount of iron is 3.5mg per 100gm of spinach, or about 20% of the daily recommended amount per serving. Ooops!

During the first four years that the Popeye series ran in the 1930's, spinach sales in the US increased more than 30%.

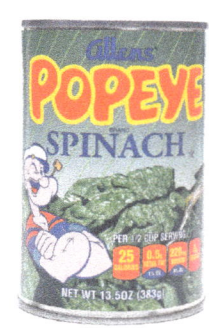

VEGGIE	Sweet Potato Casserole^V Make 8-10 servings		Side
INGREDIENTS		**SUBSTITUTE**	
3 lb	Sweet potatoes		
2	Eggs, large or XL		
2 tsp	Vanilla extract		
1 tsp	Cinnamon		
½ tsp	Salt		
1½ C	Brown sugar	White sugar	
¼ C	Flour (30 g)		
4 Tbsp	Butter, melted		
¾ C	Chopped pecans or walnuts (optional)		
STEPS			
1	Bake sweet potatoes on a parchment paper lined baking sheet until soft, about one hour at 350°F. Allow sweet potatoes to cool. This step can be done ahead of time.		
2	Preheat oven to 350°F. Generously grease a 9 x 9 inch baking pan or 2½ quart casserole dish.		
3	Scoop out cooked sweet potato meat into a large bowl.		
4	Mix eggs, vanilla extract, salt, cinnamon and ¾ C brown sugar into the sweet potatoes then turn into the prepared pan.		
5	In a small bowl, mix the flour, remaining ¾ C brown sugar, butter and chopped nuts. Spread topping over the sweet potato mixture.		
6	Bake for 35-45 minutes until bubbly and crisp on top. Allow to rest for at least 15 minutes prior to serving.		

AGILE RECIPES

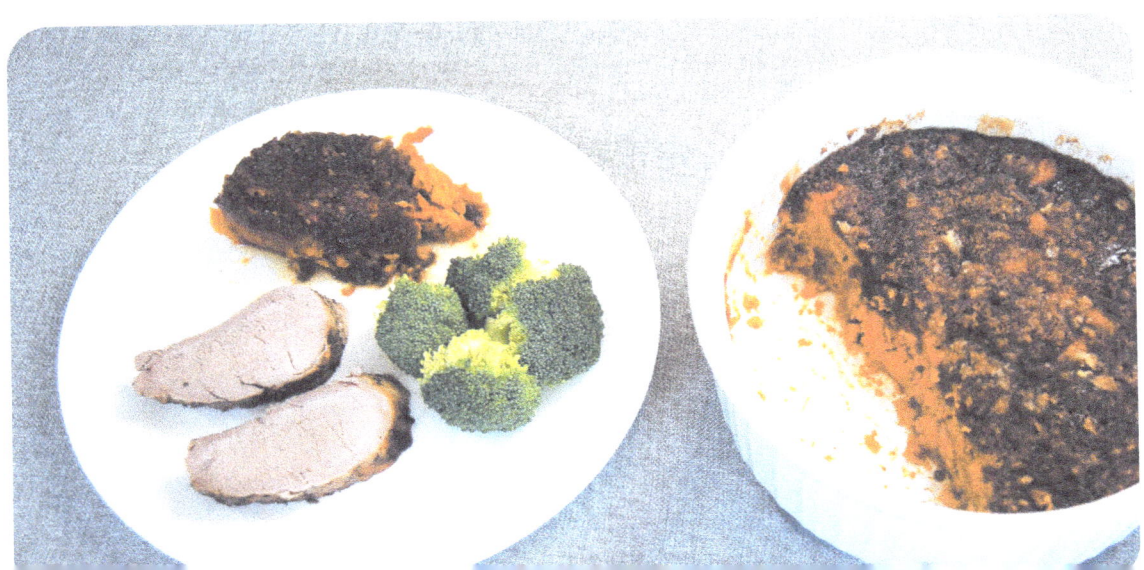

AGILE RECIPES

VEGGIE	Vegetables au Gratin^V Serves 4-6		Side

INGREDIENTS		SUBSTITUTE
2½ ib	Potatoes or other vegetable	Carrots, sweet potato, fennel, broccoli, or cauliflower
1	Onion, sliced thin and separated	
1 C	Cheese sauce (see recipe on page 293)	
¼ C	Heavy cream	Half & Half or milk
½ C	Grated cheese (optional)	
	Salt and pepperto taste	

STEPS	
1	Preheat oven to 350°F. Grease a 2 quart baking dish or 9 x 13 pan.
2	Prepare potatoes or other vegetables by peeling and cutting into thin slices. For root vegetables, slices should be ¼ inch or less.
3	Prepare cheese sauce as shown on page 293. Cheddar, Swiss, gruyere and parmesan cheeses are all good choices. Salt and pepper to taste.
4	Stir in an extra ¼ C of cream into the cheese sauce to thin it slightly.
5	Arrange one layer of vegetables in the pan using ¼ of the vegetables, forming a uniform pattern. Spread ¼ of the onion pieces and top with ¼ of the cheese sauce.
6	Repeat making layers until the veggies, onion and cheese sauce are used up.
7	Cover with foil and bake for 30 minutes. Uncover and bake for an additional 20-30 minutes or until the vegetables are tender.
8	If desired, add a layer of grated cheese on top for the last 10 minutes in the oven.

OPTIONS	
A	**Potatoes au Gratin**: For best results use Russet potatoes and slice very thin.
B	**Root Medley**: Use a mix of root vegetables of similar density. Carrots, sweet and white potatoes, fennel bulb are ideas. Use Gruyere, Asiago, Swiss or Parmesan cheese.
C	**Broccoli Cauliflower au Gratin**: Use one or both for a lighter side dish. Cut into larger slices and make fewer layers. Reduce covered cook time to 15 minutes.

PROTEIN OTHER	Bean Soup Express^V **Makes about 6 cups**	Soup

INGREDIENTS		SUBSTITUTE
4 C	Navy beans (two 15 oz cans) drained	Great northern or cannellini beans
1-2	Onions, chopped	
1-2 tsp	Minced garlic	
5	Carrots, diced	
3 Tbsp	Tomato paste	Ketchup
1 Tbsp	Diced parsley	
1 tsp	Thyme	
½ -1 C	Diced ham or pork sausage (optional)	Diced pancetta or cooked bacon: up to ¼ C
1	Potato, diced (optional)	
4 C	Chicken stock	Vegetable stock
	Salt and black pepper to taste	

STEPS	
1	Sauté onion, garlic and carrots in a large sauce pan with a little oil until onion is soft
2	Add all other ingredients, bring to a boil then simmer for at least 20 minutes. Flavors will develop further if cooked longer.
3	Meat is optional, but it will add a rich and salty flavor. The optional potato will thicken the soup.

AGILE RECIPES

VEGGIE	Cream of Mushroom Soup^V Serves 4-6	Soup

INGREDIENTS		SUBSTITUTE
4 Tbsp	Extra Virgin Olive Oil	Butter
2 lb	Mushrooms, sliced or chopped (white or cremini)	Wild mushroom blend
½	Onion, medium, finely diced	Shallots
4	Cloves garlic, minced	2 tsp jarred minced garlic
4 C	Chicken stock (1 qt box)	Vegetable stock
1 tsp	Salt	
½ tsp	Thyme	
½ C	Heavy cream	½ C milk + 2 tsp flour, mixed to a smooth slurry

STEPS	
1	In a large heavy bottomed stock pot, sauté mushrooms and onion until most of the moisture has evaporated.
2	Stir in the garlic and cook for another two minutes.
3	Add stock, salt and thyme and simmer for 20-30 minutes.
4	Remove from heat and blend the soup using a heat resistant immersion blender. A counter top blender could be used, exercising great care in handling the hot liquid.
5	Return to low heat and stir in the heavy cream. If you are using the milk/flour slurry, continue stirring over low heat until the soup thickens slightly.
6	Serve plain or garnished with chives or croutons.

AGILE RECIPES

VEGGIE	French Onion Soup^V Serves 4		Soup
INGREDIENTS		**SUBSTITUTE**	
4 Tbsp	Butter	Extra Virgin Olive Oil	
3	Onions, medium, sliced thin	Sweet or yellow onions preferred	
½ tsp	Salt and pepper, each		
2 tsp	Sugar		
1 C	White wine, dry	Dry red wine	
4 C	Beef stock (one 32 oz box)	Vegetable or mushroom stock	
1 tsp	Herbs de Provence	Thyme	
½	Baguette, sliced into 8 discs	Any bread, sliced	
4 oz	Aged Swiss cheese, grated	Gruyere or Emmentaler or Parmesan cheese	
STEPS			
1	In a large, heavy bottomed pot, sauté onions in the butter over medium heat until soft.		
2	Add salt, pepper and sugar to the onions and reduce heat to medium low. Continue to cook until onions are caramelized, stirring occasionally – about a half hour.		
3	Add wine to onions and cook over medium heat to reduce liquid by half.		
4	Add stock and herbs. Simmer for at least 20 minutes.		
5	Place bread slices on a cookie sheet and top with grated cheese.		
6	Broil bread and cheese until melty and crisp.		
7	Serve soup in four bowls, each with two to three cheese toasts floating on top.		

Agile Recipes

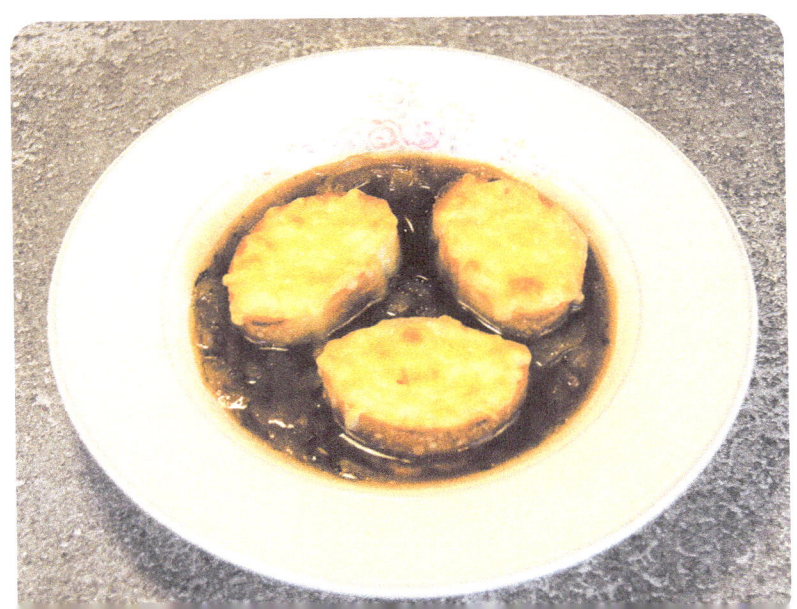

PROTEIN OTHER	Lentil Soup^V Makes about 6 cups		SOUP
INGREDIENTS		**SUBSTITUTE**	
1⅓ C	Lentils, brown, red or green		
1 Tbsp	Extra Virgin Olive Oil	Any olive or light cooking oil	
1	Onion, small, diced		
1 tsp	Garlic, minced		
2 tsp	Ginger paste	Grated fresh ginger root	
32 oz	Chicken broth (one 32 oz box)	Vegetable broth, water + 4 tsp bullion	
1 C	Water		
2 C	Chopped spinach or kale (optional)	Fresh or frozen	
8 oz	Tomato sauce	2 Tbsp tomato paste + 7 oz water	
2 tsp	Cumin		
3	Carrots, cut into coins (optional)		
1 tsp	Salt		
STEPS			
1	Rinse and sort lentils per package directions.		
2	Sauté onion in olive oil over medium heat until soft. Add garlic and ginger paste and cook for another minute or two.		
3	Add remaining ingredients and bring to a boil.		
4	Reduce heat to simmer and cover. Cook over low heat until lentils are tender, about 45 minutes. If soup seems too thick, add one cup of water.		
5	If you prefer a creamier texture, smash some the of the lentils. A few bursts with an immersion blender works well or you can smash some lentils with a spoon.		
6	Serve plain or with a dollop of sour cream or yogurt and chopped cilantro.		
OPTIONS			
A	**Curry**: Replace cumin with 1 Tbsp curry powder or curry paste.		
B	**Creamy**: Add one 15 oz can of coconut milk to the basic or curry recipe.		
C	**Spicy Tomato**: Omit tomato sauce and add one 15.5 oz can of diced tomatoes and 1 tsp red pepper flakes. Can be added to basic, curry or creamy recipes.		
D	**Meaty**: Brown a few ounces of bacon, ham, or pork sausage. Replace ginger and cumin with thyme and rosemary. Serve with a sprinkle of Parmesan cheese.		

AGILE RECIPES

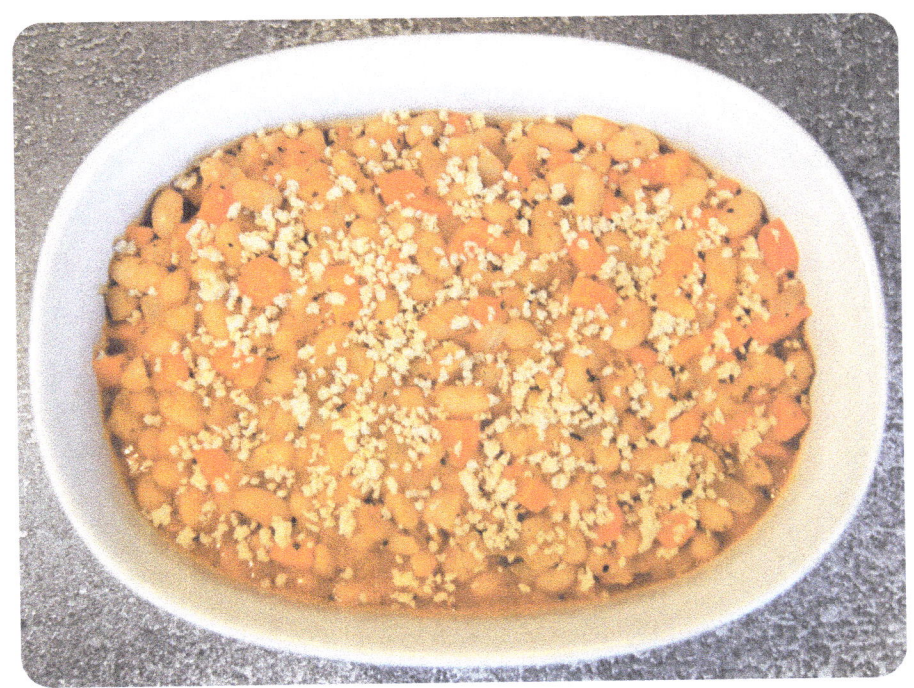

Savory White Beans

Recipe on page 320

Lentil Soup

Recipe on page 328

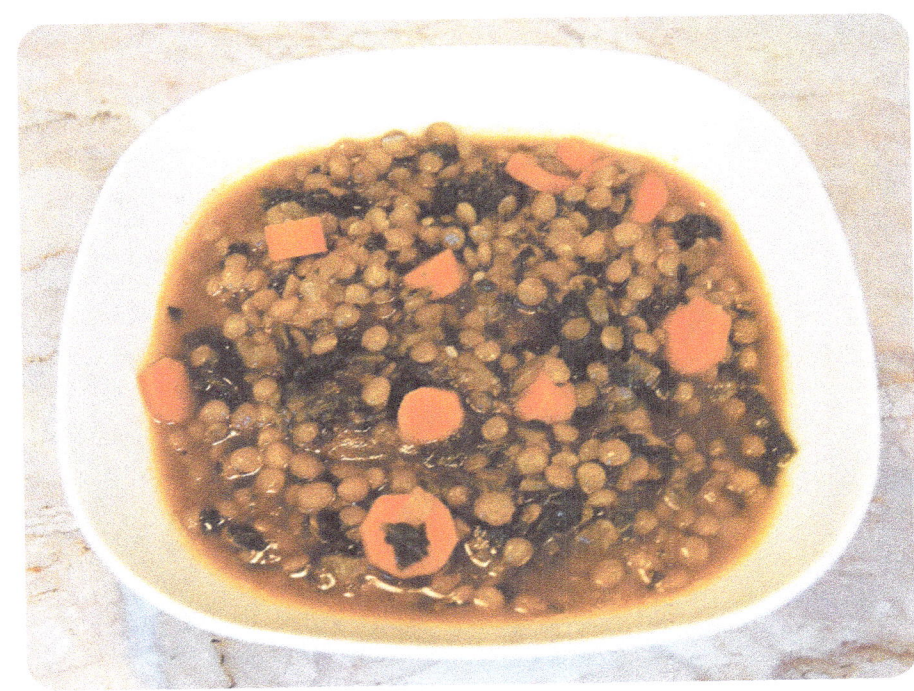

VEGGIE	Potato Broccoli Soup^V Serves 4-6		Soup
INGREDIENTS		**SUBSTITUTE**	
2 Tbsp	Butter	Light cooking oil	
1	Onion, finely diced		
4	Cloves garlic, minced	2 tsp minced jarred garlic	
1 lb	Potatoes, diced		
4-5 C	Broccoli florets (about 2 stalks)	Frozen broccoli florets	
32 oz	Chicken or vegetable broth		
2 C	Grated cheese, cheddar or Co-Jack		
STEPS			
1	In a stock pot, melt the butter and sauté the onion until soft. Add the garlic and cook another two minutes.		
2	Add the diced potatoes and broth to the pot and bring to a boil. Reduce heat and simmer for about six minutes.		
3	Add the broccoli florets and cook for another 5-10 minutes, until both broccoli and potatoes are soft.		
4	Remove from the stove and use a heat-resistant immersion blender to puree the soup. This can be done in a blender, handling the hot soup with great care.		
5	Stir in the grated cheese and allow to melt. Return to low heat if necessary to melt the cheese. Salt and pepper to taste.		
6	Serve plain or garnished with more grated cheese, crumbled bacon or croutons.		

AGILE RECIPES

VEGGIE	Vegetable Soup^V Serves 4-6	Soup
INGREDIENTS		**SUBSTITUTE**
1	Onion, diced	
2 Tbsp	Butter	Extra Virgin Olive Oil or any light cooking oil
4-8 oz	Beef, diced (delete for vegetarian soup)	Any leftover beef steak or roast
32 oz	Beef broth	Vegetable broth
14.5 oz	Canned tomatoes, crushed	
¼ Head	Cabbage, finely sliced (about 2 C)	
2	Carrots, diced	
1 C	Corn, frozen or canned	
2	Potatoes, diced	
1 C	Green beans	Peas or lima beans
2 tsp	Italian seasoning	Basil or parsley
STEPS		
1	In a large stock pot, sauté the onion in the butter until it is soft.	
2	If using meat, uncooked meat may be browned with the onions. If using leftover meat (e.g. steak or roast), simply add it.	
3	Add all other ingredients and bring to a boil. Reduce heat and simmer for at least a half hour, longer if time allows. Salt and pepper to taste	

AGILE RECIPES

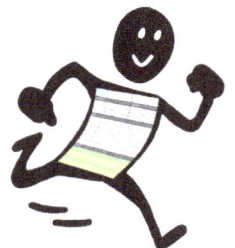

For more information and to download PDFs of Agile Recipes™
visit www.ReEngineeringtheKitchen.com.

PHASE IV

RE-ENGINEERING THE KITCHEN®

EFFICIENT KITCHEN MANAGEMENT

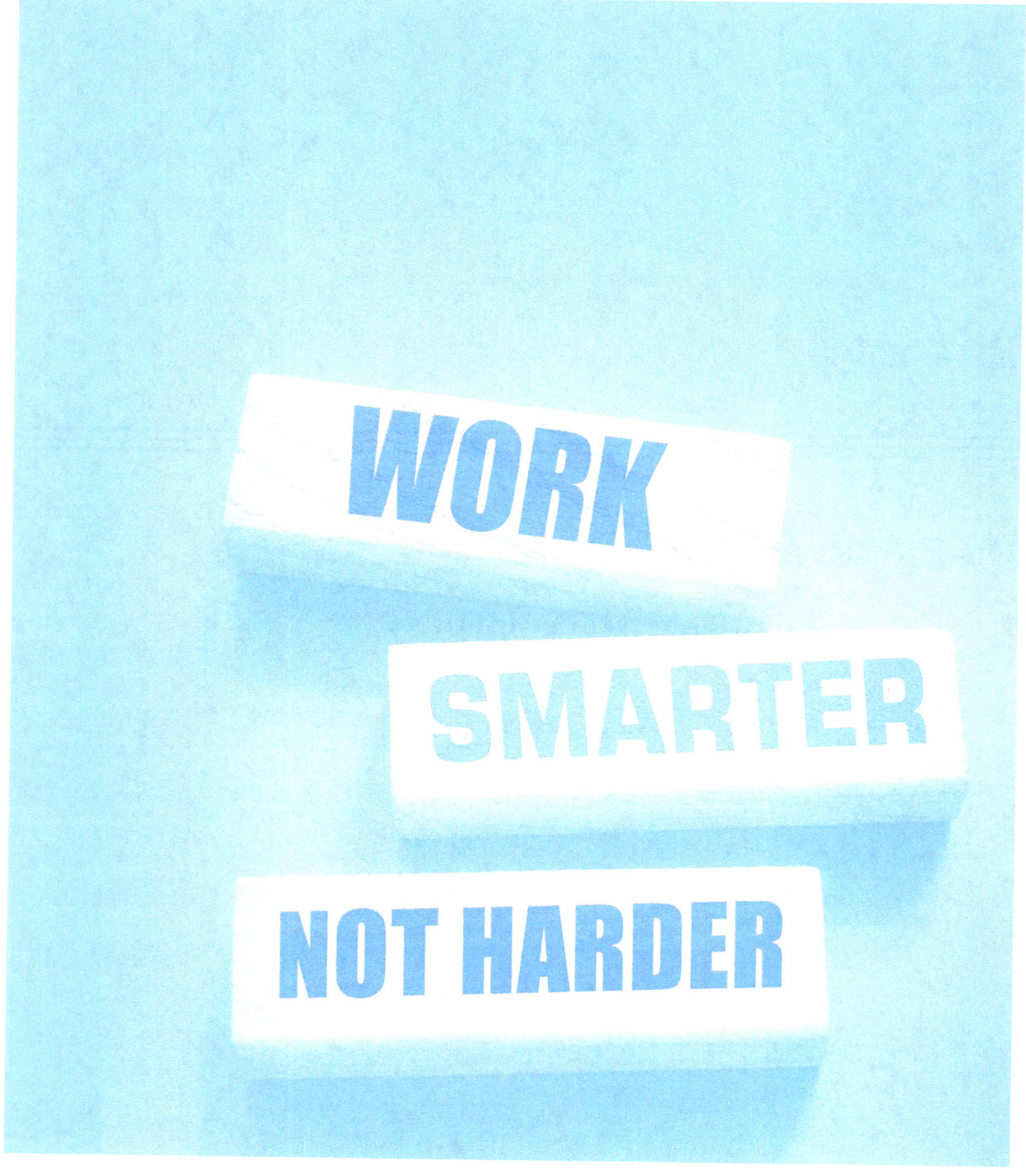

CHAPTER 21

A MORE PRODUCTIVE KITCHEN

You have many resources available to improve your cooking skills: family, books, magazines, TV, and the Internet. Every skill you hone and technique you acquire will improve your cooking efficiency and results. However, what we are discussing here is not cooking skill but rather strategies to make your kitchen more productive. In this chapter we will look at tips to save you time and effort at every turn. If you can work in the kitchen with ruthless efficiency, it will be easier to make better home-prepared food more often.

Who doesn't love watching cooking shows? The chefs are truly amazing in their skill and creativity. The on-set kitchens are idyllic, with vast spotless counters, veggies that are beautiful, and clean-up that magically occurs off-screen. However, this bears little resemblance to getting a family dinner on the table. Professional chefs are trained to work in professional kitchens, in concert with a staff of professionals from dishwashers to procurement managers. Many cooking skills and techniques are obviously transferrable to a home, but that does not make their kitchen-management process the best for your kitchen. For most of us, cooking is just one of many priorities. It is not our vocation. It is certainly important, but so is earning a living, raising children, walking the dog, and taking out the trash. We often simply need the quickest, easiest way to prepare a nice meal and get on with life.

In economics, there is a concept of "Barrier to Entry" which refers to the fixed cost (time, resources, expertise) required to begin an endeavor. For example, starting a business as an Uber driver has a very low barrier to entry (a car and a cell phone) as opposed to starting a business to manufacture cars (hundreds of employees and a factory). Every meal in your kitchen has a "barrier to entry": the commitment of effort and resources to make it happen. The lower that barrier to entry is, the more likely you are to dive in and prepare the meal. Many of the strategies presented here are ways to reduce the barrier to entry: reducing the time and resource commitment per meal. Let's make it a little easier to cook a little more.

Optimize your Kitchen!

Take a few minutes to consider your kitchen:

- How is it laid out?
- How much counter space is there?
- What is on the counters?
- What activities occur in your kitchen?
- Do you have space to prepare and cook food?
- Do you have the equipment you need?

Saying that "The kitchen is the heart of the home" may just be a charming way to say that it is a chaotic, multi-purpose space. There are few things more discouraging than having to clean the kitchen before you even start cooking: talk about a major barrier to entry! If cooking in your kitchen is a priority, then you may need to bite the bullet and impose some order on this corner of your life.

Most homes have limited counter space, and the kitchen counters are the only place to set anything down: mail, groceries, purses/bags, lunch boxes, school and work papers, gym bags, dirty dishes, broken toys, and random items waiting to be put away. Unfortunately, you cannot wish the clutter away. (I've tried!) Not only does the stuff need to go somewhere now, but you also need to prevent it from coming back. Look for opportunities to change the daily process of how you handle categories of stuff, such as:

- Mail/papers – can it go into a basket on a buffet, shelf, small table or desk?
- Purses and bags – can you leave these on a coat rack or a hook by the door?
- Cookbooks and decorative items – can these go on a shelf?
- Kitchen equipment and appliances – only items you use often deserve a place on your counters; all others need to go into a cupboard or maybe even a closet elsewhere.
- Random items to be dealt with – can you put a bin in another place, laundry or work area perhaps, for those items waiting to be repaired or dispositioned?
- Pet food and supplies – can this go into another room? Can it go into a container that is easily accessed from a cupboard?
- Projects – if you need to work on projects on your counter, always have a drawer, box, or bin to stash these in so that you can quickly clear space for cooking.

Once you've decided what still needs to be accessible on the kitchen counter, the next step is to contain the spread and minimize the area that it occupies. You may be able to save counter area by going up and utilizing vertical space. For example, if you have nowhere else for mail and papers, consider a multi-level in/outbox so that it occupies the smallest footprint and does not spread out. Consider a free-standing shelf to get an extra bit of surface space for books or vitamins, or stacked bins/baskets to contain loose items like fruit or bread. Can you hang anything on a wall?

Now that you have the clutter under control, the next step is to ensure that your kitchen is always ready for cooking. This means cleaning up as you go, everything from the pots and pans to the incidental cereal bowls and coffee cups. You may need to reset expectations with your family that leaving trash and dirty dishes scattered about the kitchen is no longer acceptable. No one likes to have their workspace used as a community junkyard; the kitchen is no less important than a computer or desk. Everyone eats so everyone gets to pitch in. If your family doesn't want to help clean up, they might prefer to help with cooking. That is not a bad outcome either.

Supporting Actors: Staples

It is easier to decide to cook something when you are confident that you have all the ancillary ingredients on hand. You probably have a list of staples in your mind and keep an inventory of these automatically. However, I'd suggest you look at the list below and evaluate if it makes sense for you to expand your list of items that you always have on hand. These are all items that can be stored for a long time so you will likely use them up eventually.

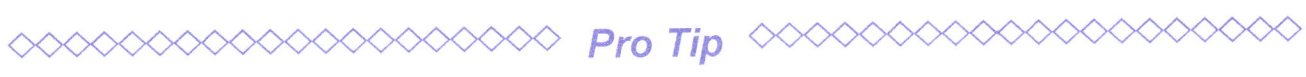

Pro Tip

Did you know you can freeze dairy products?

If you do not stock dairy products consistently, you may want to freeze small portions, so they are always available for cooking. Milk, buttermilk, sour cream, cream or yogurt may all be frozen, although they do tend to separate so may need to be mixed upon thawing.

Figure 64 – Suggested Essential Staples

Pantry	Fridge	Freezer	Spices
Baking Powder	BBQ Sauce	Butter	Basil
Baking Soda	Buttermilk Powder	Cream (for cooking)	Cardamon
Bouillon Powder *	Cream	Garlic *	Chili Powder
Breadcrumbs (Panko)	Curry Paste *	Ginger *	Cinnamon
Brown Sugar	Eggs	Milk (for cooking)	Cloves
Canola or Safflower Oil	Garlic – Minced Jar *	Nuts	Cumin
Coconut Oil	Ginger Paste *	OJ Concentrate	Curry *
Cooking Spray	Hot/Chili Sauce	Sour Cream (for cooking)	Dehydrated Onion
Corn Starch	Jam	Yogurt (for cooking)	Dill
Extra Virgin Olive Oil	Ketchup		Fennel Seeds
Flour	Lemon Juice		Garlic Powder
Honey	Mayonnaise		Ginger
Tomatoes and/or Sauce	Milk		Herbs de Provence
Tomato Paste – Can	Mustard – Dijon		Nutmeg
Vinegar – Apple Cider	Mustard – Yellow		Oregano
Vinegar – Balsamic	Onions		Paprika
Vinegar – White	Parmesan Cheese		Pepper
Vinegar – Wine	Sour Cream or Yogurt		Poultry Seasoning
White Sugar	Soy Sauce		Red Pepper Flakes
	Stock Paste *		Rosemary
	Syrup – Maple		Sage
	Tomato Paste – Tube		Salt
	Worcestershire Sauce		Thyme
			Vanilla

* Item is available in different formats; choose the one that you prefer.

Scale Up

We are going to apply another concept from economics to our Re-Engineered Kitchen: Economies of Scale. This is the idea that the cost per item goes down as the volume goes up. You deal with this every day as you evaluate buying the bigger container, which costs less per ounce, versus the smaller one that is easier to store and more likely to be fully used. The money spent purchasing food is an obvious "cost" and it pays to consider opportunities to purchase in quantities if discounts are available. When you do consider buying in bulk, remember to factor in the time and effort required to manage the food longevity, including repackaging, labeling, storing, and, in the case of meat, possibly freezing.

Now let's apply this Economies of Scale concept to the production process of cooking meals. An important "cost" is the time and effort you must spend to purchase, to store, and to prepare the food. Your time is precious, and you need to manage it as carefully as you do your money (if not more so). Look for ways to make every step in your food process more efficient by scaling up.

The Deep Freeze

When I met my husband in high school, his family had a big freezer. I'd never seen such a thing. Every so often, his extended family would buy a butchered side of beef and divide it up between several households. They always had a stock of really good quality angus beef. Still, it never occurred to me that I needed to have a separate storage freezer until we moved into a house with a tiny refrigerator with an even smaller freezer. It is almost like a toy fridge/freezer, with no room for a bigger one without tearing the kitchen apart. So, when our favorite warehouse retailer had a nice little freezer on sale for an improbably low price, I grudgingly agreed to buying one for the garage. Now I simply love it and wonder why we didn't do this decades ago.

I am surprised, however, by how we actually use our new-found freezer capacity. Of course, the freezer allows us to buy meat in bulk for a lower price. More importantly, it allows us to better manage other parts of our Food Process. One unexpected advantage is that we have reduced the overall number of shopping trips. For example, we can go to the aforementioned warehouse retailer every other month instead of every other week. Now there is enough room in the freezer for several prepared meals, bulky items like bread and storing those items that will simply last longer frozen. With two freezers, I have a chance to keep things organized better: high-frequency items in the house and longer term in the second freezer. I can actually find things. I have not had to discard a single unidentified, petrified, freezer-burnt lump since we bought the second freezer!

Choosing Where to Shop

First, let's optimize shopping. There are many constraints on the shopping process: mode of transport, choice of stores, distance and time to get to them, and storage capacity at home. If you live in a suburban or rural area, going to any grocery store is probably at least an hour expedition and probably uses a gallon of gas, so that's time and money. Home delivery has become available in many locations for both household items and for groceries. It can be a great option, but it comes with its own set of issues, including the delivery charge and then working your own schedule around the delivery window. Some stores will deliver household items like cleaners, vinegar and baking soda without the delivery charge, which lets you focus your grocery shopping efforts on food.

We all know that some stores have better quality or lower prices on certain items but who has time to go to several stores each week? This is where you can optimize your time and costs. If you can buy staples and non-food items in bulk, going to the bargain store infrequently, then perhaps you will have time to shop at the better store for fresh produce the rest of the time. The time and money you save on reduced trips can be shifted to better food preparation or better food quality. Maybe you would even have time to go to that farmer's market occasionally.

Scale Up Your Cooking

Next, let's consider ways to scale up your food-preparation efforts. I like to refer to it as "cook once, eat twice". The most obvious way to do this is to simply make meals in large batches. Things like spaghetti sauce, soup, stews, and chili are perfect for making a large amount and freezing it in meal-sized portions. When you are looking for a quick dinner after a long day, "shopping" in the freezer is a very welcome option!

For some reason, it feels like cheating if we plan to have the same meal twice a week. However, if it is a combination of dishes that keep well for a few days, then it makes sense to prepare a double batch and simply have it twice. I'd rather have the same nice meal a second time as opposed to fast food.

The real objective, though, is to look for every opportunity to prepare/cook any ingredient in larger batches, with a plan on using part today and storing the rest for use later. This reduces the time required to prepare food on a per-ounce, or per-meal basis. Take the process of peeling potatoes as an example. From grabbing the bag though clean-up it takes about 10 minutes to peel and cut 2.5 pounds of potatoes but it only takes an extra 5 minutes to prep the whole 5-pound bag, and almost no extra time to cook and mash. For those few extra invested minutes, there are mashed potatoes prepared for another day that stay good for several days in the fridge or can be frozen. We have reduced the average time per ounce of cooked potatoes. In addition, having a side dish already prepared makes cooking another day feel less daunting.

Opportunities to Double-Up

- Onions and peppers – if you need less than one in your recipe, chop the entire item and freeze the rest for later use. It takes barely more time to chop a whole onion vs half (or 2 vs 1) and then you have eliminated one clean-up cycle.
- Rice – if you are serving rice, make a large batch (2 or 3 times) of plain rice and refrigerate the extra. The leftover cooked rice can then be rewarmed or used in a rice pilaf, stir fry, or rice pudding. Cooked rice can be frozen in individual portions. This is a great way to ensure you always have time to prepare whole-grain brown rice.
- Meat – cook twice what you need for your meal. Leftover cooked meat can be used for sandwiches, salads, flatbreads, casseroles, and stir fry. It takes almost no additional time to prepare the larger amount of meat and, again, you only clean up once. In addition, you will likely save money per pound by buying the larger "family package" of meat.
- Fresh veggies – for broccoli, cauliflower, green beans, asparagus, cook (but don't overcook) twice the amount needed for your meal. Leftover veggies are great additions to cold salads, easy to rewarm for another meal, or cut up into a mixed dish.
- Baked potatoes – bake extra potatoes. Use them to make potato salad, or a green salad (Salad Niçoise). Or you can slice and fry the extra cooked potatoes for quick breakfast potatoes, make them twice baked, or use for quick Potato Frittata.
- Bacon or breakfast sausage – cook the entire package and refrigerate or freeze the uneaten portion. Save and freeze some of the rendered bacon fat if you like to cook with it. Clean up that greasy pan just once and avoid the messy raw meat storage.
- Cabbage – slice or shred the entire head to cook, make coleslaw, or add to salads. Sliced raw cabbage will keep for up to a week in the fridge.
- Mushrooms – sauté or roast double the amount you need. Use to serve with steak, omlettes, pizza/flatbread, or mix with peas or green beans.
- Oatmeal – make a big batch of oatmeal to enjoy on multiple days. Individual servings freeze nicely. This is a great way to make steel-cut oats, reducing the time per serving required.

These are just some suggestions. Every time you make something, ask yourself if it makes sense to double-up.

Emergency Meals

No matter how well you plan, there is always the chance that something unexpected will interrupt your shopping and cooking schedule. Life happens! Planes are delayed, people go to the hospital, natural disasters like earthquakes, ice storms and hurricanes occur. It could be anything from getting home late to coming down with the flu to storms and long-term power outages. Here are a few guidelines:

- Pantry meals – always have several meals in your pantry that are super-easy and do not require fresh food. Imagine getting home at midnight after unexpected delays and not having eaten all day. Spaghetti sauce and pasta, or masala sauce with chickpeas and rice, are a few ideas. Think about what works for your family.
- Illness – Covid has provided a stark reminder of the reality of being quarantined and unable to shop. Consider what you would want to have on hand if you got sick. Soup? Gatorade? Tea? Oatmeal? Crackers? Medicines? Next, consider how long you need to prepare for. If you live close to relatives in an urban area, maybe a few days is enough. If you are more remote, maybe you need to plan for a week or more.
- Emergency – the time to plan for an emergency is before it happens; by the time it's even anticipated, the store shelves are bare. If you suddenly had no power or water and could not buy anything – what would you do? How long could you last? There are a wide range of opinions about how long you should prepare for. The government website www.ready.org suggests having water and food for at least "several days". On the other end of the spectrum, the serious preppers are ready to go off-grid for the indefinite future. As you are planning out your panty, consider what additional items you need to meet your emergency preparedness goals. Drinking water is the highest priority but easy to overlook and at 6-8 cups (1.5-2 quarts) per day per person, the volume adds up quickly. As you are buying food and water, remember that you will have to manage expiration dates and rotate stock over time. Buying a lot during an emergency is hoarding: buying ahead of time is just good planning!

Faster Prep

Unlike those TV chefs, most of us are our own prep-chef. Let's be honest, cleaning and chopping produce, trimming, and prepping meat and fish can take a lot of time and is not particularly fun. Let's look for ways to make this part of the process faster and more efficient:

- Focus – the first step is to pay attention. It is easy to let your mind wander when you are peeling potatoes or trimming meat. Try to focus on doing it quickly. Time wasted here will have you feeling rushed later.

- Veggies – don't peel unless you need to. Wash your veggies with a brush, or even a clean dish scrubby, and leave the skin on whenever possible (more nutrients too). Use a swivel-blade type peeler and work on your speed. You can use that peeler to quickly clean up blemishes on any hard veggie like cauliflower, too. If you don't like your paring knife and peeler, try new ones. These are inexpensive but get a lot of use: it pays to have ones you like to work with.
- Scissors – kitchen scissors can be much faster than using a knife and can often complete the task without a cutting board, especially for small jobs.
  - Meat: trim fat, skin, and gristle from meat. Use it to cut up a whole chicken or remove back from the breast, cutting through bone and joints. Dice up bacon or other sliced meat such as salami.
  - Produce: scissors are great for prepping and chopping fresh herbs and some veggies. Use to trim ends of green bean or asparagus. Chop up green onions.
  - Sticky: cut up marshmallows, candies, and dried fruit.
- Knife skills – this is an area where it is worth investing the time to improve your skills and your tools. Obtaining a quality set of knives (or even just a few essential ones) and learning to keep them sharp will help improve ease of preparation. If you need to, learn basic knife skills – particularly how to keep your fingers out of the way of these sharp knives. It takes a bit of practice (see box on page 344). Having used dull, small knives for so long, many people frequently have bad habits to overcome.
- Clean up – minimize collateral damage as you go along and limit the number of items to wash:
  - Use one pan or bowl when feasible, for example, the pot used for steaming a veggie can then be used for making the sauce.
  - Use one cutting board sequentially with a quick clean in between: 1) dry food, 2) water wet, 3) gooey wet. (For food safety, anything that touched raw meat must be washed thoroughly in hot water.)
  - Store leftovers directly in a glass or ceramic dish to be used to reheat and serve.
  - Use parchment paper on baking pans to minimize scrubbing.
  - Perform messy chores next to the sink to expedite clean up.
  - Put a sheet pan with parchment under any casserole that may bubble over.
- Scale down for small jobs – use the bottom of a glass to press out a few cookies rather than a rolling pin and pastry sheet; use a potato peeler to shred a carrot for a salad; and use a whisk rather than the electric mixer to mash a few potatoes.

Knife Skills

We used cheap knives in our kitchen for decades; we simply didn't know any better. One year my husband splurged and gave me a nice set of quality knives as a birthday gift. WOW – I could not believe the difference! Suddenly the cutting tasks I dreaded were so much easier and quicker. Potatoes and cabbage sliced with little effort! Raw meat cut easily with no sawing back and forth! Buying that whole N.Y. Strip and cutting it into perfect steaks to freeze suddenly seemed like a great idea. It was like opening a glorious new window on cooking.

However, my poor knife habits had been born of ignorance and deeply ingrained from years of using crappy knives, using the wrong knife for the job, and then employing the wrong technique. Within a week of getting my beautiful new knives, I nearly cut off the pad of one finger. I was lucky that the cut, while deep, caused no permanent damage.

I used my forced vacation from cooking to research basic knife skills and commit to improvement, especially regarding safety. When I started trying to use proper techniques, it was like trying to write with my left hand. I was slow and awkward, and it just did not feel right. It certainly wasn't faster! Eventually, it got easier (and faster), and better techniques became my new habit. My meager skills still pale in comparison to professional chefs everywhere but at least I have not sliced any fingers lately!

A More Productive Kitchen – Key Points

Optimize kitchen space
   » **Clear the clutter and keep it clean**

Optimize shopping and consolidate trips
   » **Go to the best store for the types of food and non-food items**
   » **Go less often to save time**

Cook once/eat twice – cook two to three times what you need

Manage your staples – have essentials on hand

Emergency food – plan for the unexpected

Faster prep

Minimize clean-up – work smarter and streamline

For more information about kitchen productivity tips, visit
www.ReEngineeringtheKitchen.com.

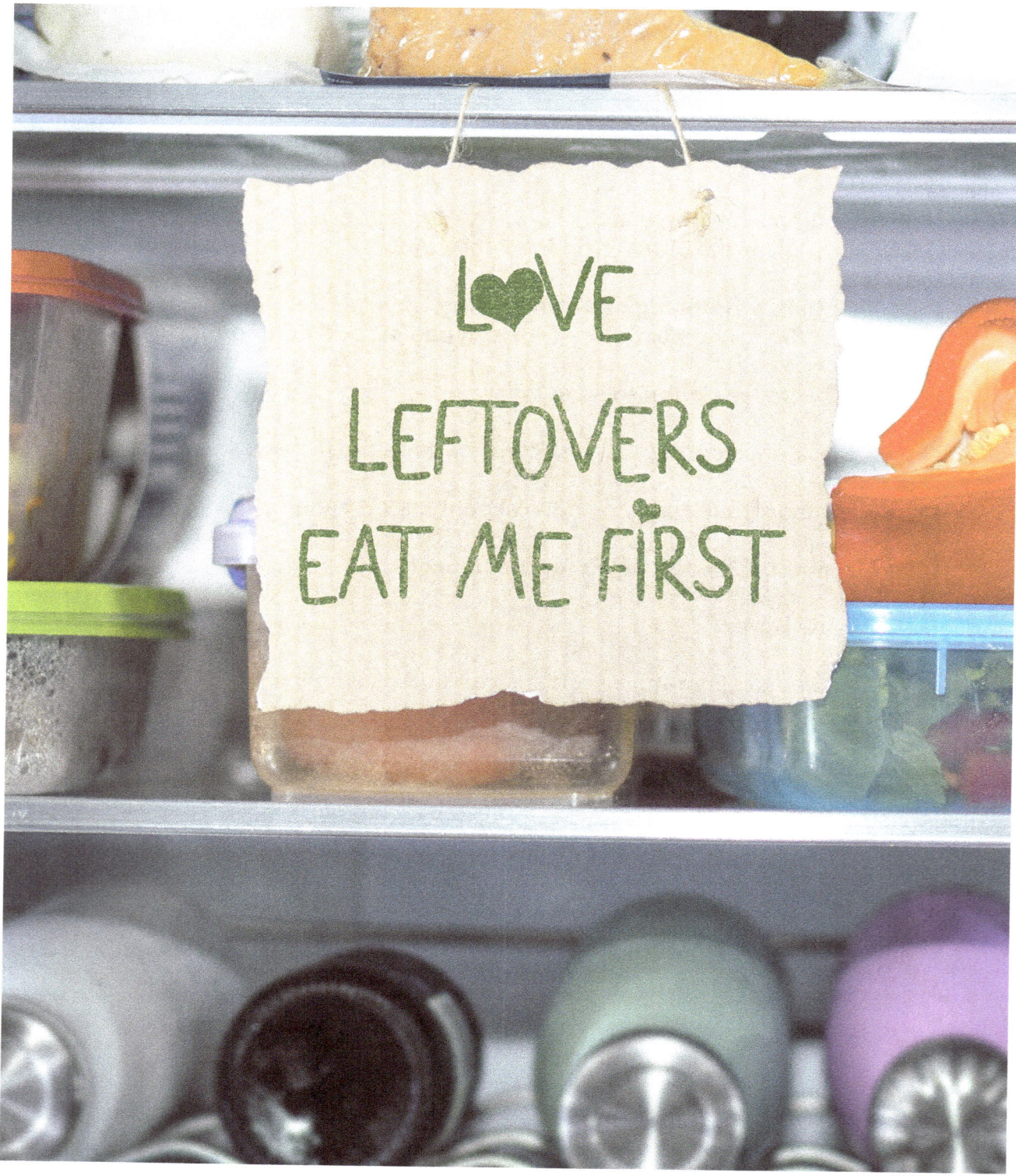

CHAPTER 22

STRATEGIES FOR REDUCING FOOD WASTE

Let's start by evaluating what food you are throwing out most often. Is it that little bit of leftover casserole or is it whole packages of fresh meat or yogurt that have spoiled? When food goes bad, it often creates a cascade of poor outcomes. First, the item itself is discarded. Often, the expired product is only discovered once cooking has started. Now the entire dish, or even meal, is in jeopardy if a suitable substitution is not readily available. The collateral damage can easily include additional time and money due to an emergency run to the store or ordering takeout.

Better Buying

Food-waste reduction starts with what you buy. If you are buying the right amount of your Priority Foods, you are off to a good start. If you find that you are routinely throwing away produce and protein because it has spoiled, go back to your Baseline Food Plan. You may need to shift to a more forgiving longevity ratio.

When shopping, there are so many things competing for your attention that it is hard to closely inspect every item. However, it is terribly disappointing to realize that an item you just bought is already half-way to the garbage can. It is seldom worth a trip back to the store to return it. This seems obvious but remember to check the "best by" dates and look closely at the produce. This is particularly important for the high-risk fresh items. Focus on selecting your Priority Foods first when you shop, while your mind is fresh and you're not yet tired of shopping.

There are those items that go bad before you can use them up: your rate of consumption does not match up nicely with package sizes and longevity. For example, if you only use a bit of cream in your coffee, you may end up wasting a lot of it. If you travel routinely, having cream for your coffee could seem hopeless. A better solution might be to buy a box of individual creamers that will stay good for months.

If you are frequently discarding half loaves of bread, consider either freezing half of each loaf right away or substituting tortillas, which last longer in the fridge. For these slow-use items, the key is to consolidate products where possible and focus on longevity.

Reduce the number of unique items you buy. For example, buy one big plain yogurt instead of multiple small, flavored yogurt containers, plus sour cream. Plain yogurt is more versatile and can be used in more applications. Also, it is simply easier to keep track of one item with an expiration date than several. Be cautious of variety packs as they invariably have varieties that no one wants.

Buy ketchup and prepared horseradish so you can make the right amount of your own cocktail sauce, instead of buying pre-made. (How many jars of various sauces have you ever completely used up?)

Buy the plain canned tomatoes or beans rather than seasoned so that they will work in any recipe. Buy the unsalted, unsweetened, unflavored version of everything possible as these are most versatile. You can always add sugar, salt, or spice, but cannot take it out.

Stick to the plan: Don't be seduced by the pretty produce or bargain fish – or anything that will expire quickly. Unless you truly have a plan to use it quickly, let it go. It is not a deal if you end up tossing it.

Enhanced Storage

Getting the food home from the store is only half the job. The other half is storing it to ensure it lasts long enough to use. Most foods have standard directions about how to store them, either on the package or readily available with a quick Internet search. However, the best way to store a given food depends on many factors, including how quickly it will be consumed, and your home environment. For example, dry goods storage in a humid region might be a little different than in arid areas. Below are some ideas for extending the life of foods that go beyond the basics. Consider what items you tend to throw away most and consider whether these enhanced storage techniques fit your situation. For most fresh foods, an ounce of prevention is worth a pound of cure. This includes being strategic about storage – doing everything you can to optimize the product's life:

Leafy greens: These precious nutrient-rich veggies can be most unforgiving to store. They require cold (but not freezing) temperatures and a moisture level that is neither too high nor too low. Plastic containers of ready-to-eat greens are very susceptible to condensation and moisture, leading to rapid degradation. If there is visible moisture inside the packaging, dry it with paper towels or a clean cloth, and maybe even leave a paper towel inside. You can extend the useful life of your greens by punching several holes in the plastic container to allow ventilation. For delicate greens, be sure to rinse with really cold water (under 70 degrees or less – you may need ice) to prevent wilting.

Berries: Delicious and fragile. Avoid condensation and moisture in the container, as above. If you plan to keep them for more than a couple of days, rinse with dilute vinegar/water (3 parts water to 1 part vinegar, then rinse with water) to retard mold growth. However, be sure to dry well before re-storing in the refrigerator.

Fruit: Apples, pears, stone fruits, citrus, and grapes all stay good longer in a refrigerator crisper than in the pretty fruit bowl on your counter. Remove any decaying items promptly as the gases they emit will cause nearby items to quickly overripen.

Nuts, seeds, peanut butter, oils, grains and whole-grain flours: These items degrade when the oil within them oxidizes and becomes rancid. While rancid food is not dangerous, the taste and smell can be unpleasant. If something has been sitting around for a while, you may notice an "off", stale or musty odor. Typical directions are to store these products in a "cool dry place". Most often these items end up in a kitchen pantry or cupboard, which is probably dry but not necessarily cool. If you are not eating these items quickly enough for the pantry, they will stay fresh longer in the fridge. However, cold storage will cause some oils and peanut butter to solidify. Also, be sure to protect any flour from moisture. Finally, if you use items like seeds, nuts or specialty flours very infrequently, these can last even longer when stored in an air-tight container in the freezer.

Dry goods e.g. flour, sugars, beans, rice, pasta: It does not happen often but occasionally there are little hitchhikers in a food package, who go on to colonize the offending package and, potentially, your entire pantry. Place new dry goods, in their original packaging, into airtight containers. These can be fancy canisters, Ziploc bags, or reused glass and plastic jars. For odd-shaped packages, wrap with plastic wrap. This will contain potential damage to just one package of food, so if you do bring home an unwanted guest or one gets in from the garden, it will discourage them from colonizing your kitchen.

Save Endangered Food!

There are occasions when time just slips away. You look at the fresh produce that you "just bought" – five days ago – and see it racing past its prime. Or you realize that you are not going to make those pork chops this week after all. If you act quickly, you may be able to save them from the landfill. The two primary last-ditch techniques to extend the viability of foods are Freeze It and Cook It. Let's look at these in action:

Fruit: Bananas, stone fruit, grapes, and berries can be frozen. Wash the fruit first. For the best result, fruit should be sliced no thicker than 1.5 inches, and then frozen quickly in an individual layer. Put frozen fruit in a Ziploc bag or container. Frozen fruit is great for cooking or making smoothies. Fresh citrus does not freeze well but the juice does. Many fruits can also be cooked down to form a compote, which will last for another week in the fridge.

Fresh meat: The easiest thing to do with meat is to simply toss it in the freezer. However, sometimes this is not practical. Perhaps it was already frozen and thawed once. If you are cooking meat to extend its useful life, the internal temperature needs to be high enough to kill most bacteria, about 160°F. In this case, your best bet is to cook the meat then freeze or refrigerate it. Ground meat (beef, turkey, pork or chicken) is particularly forgiving: you can brown it, freeze it and then use it in any saucy recipe later. Time permitting, the entire planned recipe can be prepared ahead of time since the cooked product will stay good longer than the raw ingredients.

If you simply don't have time to cook the meat according to your original plan, don't worry. You can save the meat without spending time preparing the whole dish. One relatively quick and low-impact method is poaching in water or broth. This works well for fish, shellfish, and chicken, which will then stay good in the refrigerator for a few more days.

Sausage and bacon: Partial packages of raw sausage and bacon are high risk for spoilage. Sometimes it is only the sloppy edges of the package that smell funny but …yuck, the whole package goes in the trash. If you cook the entire package when you open it, then your cooked meat will stay good quite a while in the fridge or freezer. It will save time for your next meal too! Sausage can be fried in a skillet, but roasting it in the oven requires less effort and attention.

Veggies: Many veggies may be frozen, although some should be blanched before freezing to keep them looking their best. To extend the life for a few days, the best bet is often to steam or parboil the vegetable to tender-crisp, and then rinse with cool water to avoid overcooking. The cooked veggies will stay good in the fridge for several days and can be quickly heated, used in a recipe, or included in a salad.

Dairy: Most dairy products can be frozen but may lose some texture and/or separate. Simply mix well upon thawing and use these in cooking, rather than serving on their own. Cheese can be frozen but will likely lose texture and/or taste, so plan to use frozen cheese in a cooked dish.

Eggs: Technically you can safely freeze certain types of beaten raw eggs. However, it may be easier to use them up by making French toast or breakfast egg cups that can be frozen. You could also whip up quick pudding.

Bread/baked goods: Bread that has become stale but not moldy can be made into croutons or breadcrumbs. Freeze them as they are, or dry further in the oven. Stale bread and sweet rolls work well in French toast or bread pudding. Crumbs made from oven-toasted stale cookies make a nice crust for pies or a crispy topping for desserts.

<u>Leftovers</u>: Before you put away leftovers after a meal, think about when they are going to be eaten and choose the appropriate storage method. If it is unlikely that they'll be eaten in the foreseeable future, put them in the freezer directly. Individual servings may offer the most flexibility.

The storage container you choose will affect if, when, and how leftovers may be eaten. If you expect the grazers in your family to find the leftover goodies, make it easy for them to do so. Firstly, clear or transparent containers will let anyone see what is hiding in the fridge. If you can't see what it is, consider putting a label on it. Secondly, tempered glass or ceramic containers allow leftovers to be warmed directly in the microwave or oven. If it is a single serving, it may even be eaten directly out of the same container. Both factors increase the likelihood that the leftovers will be consumed before they expire.

It is hard, if not impossible, to achieve zero food waste. However, if you are strategic about what you buy and how you store it, you can significantly reduce how much food goes into the garbage.

Strategies for Reducing Food Waste – Key Points

Better buying
  » **Reduce the number of unique items you buy, choose the least specific, most flexible option, focus on food longevity**

Enhanced storage
  » **Refrigerate or freeze items you use slowly**

The Save #1
  » **Freeze it *before* it expires**

The Save #2
  » **Cook it *before* it goes bad**

Utilize leftovers
  » **Make them *easy* to find and easy to eat with see-through containers and labels**

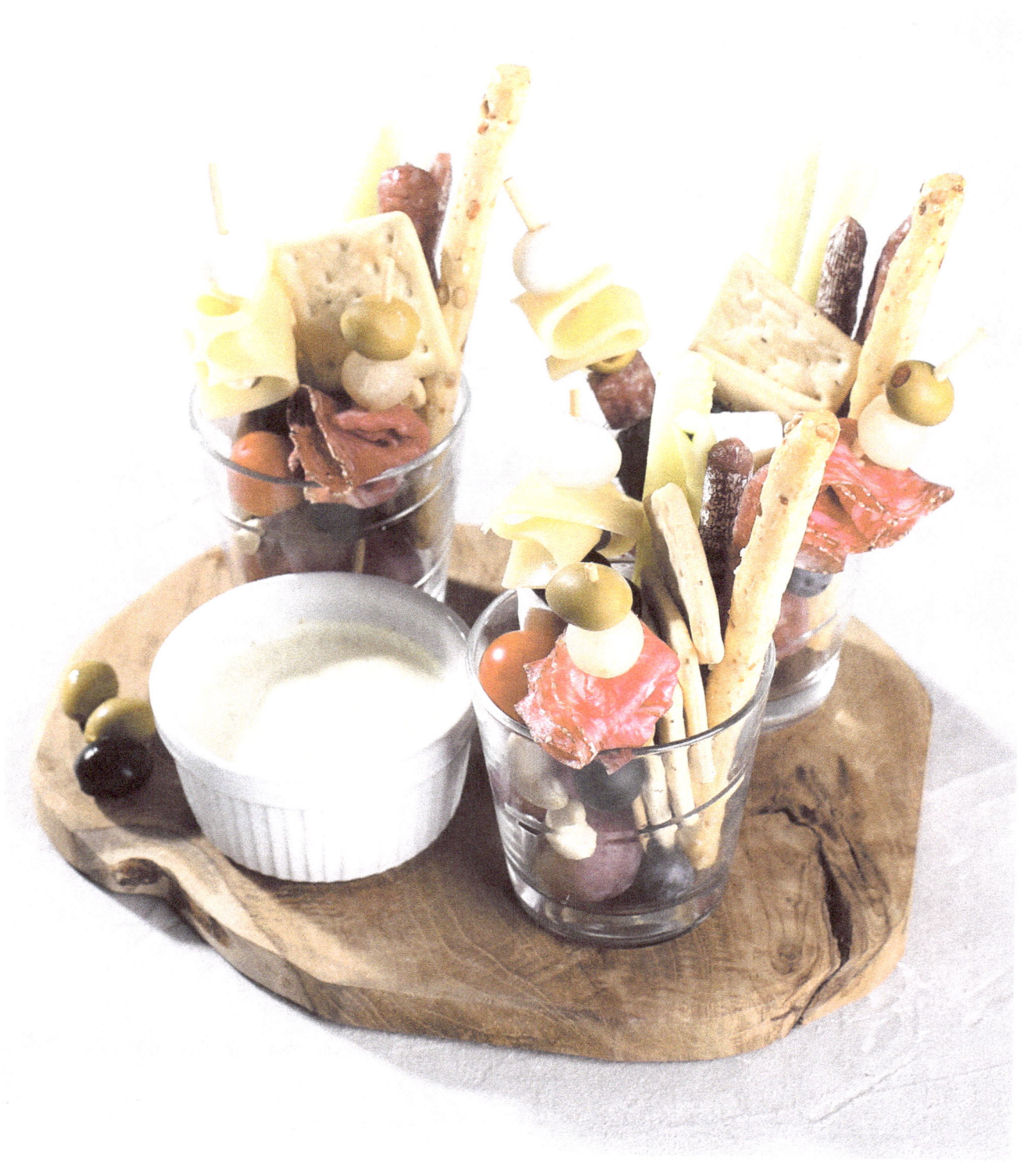

CHAPTER 23

FEEDING A CROWD: ENTERTAINING TIPS

Coming together over food is a cherished part of every culture. Almost everyone looks forward to the yummy food and socializing with friends and family. Almost everyone. Whether bringing a dish or creating a feast, the person preparing the food will probably experience some level of anxiety. What will people eat and enjoy? How much time and cost should I invest in this? Food is so personal and can be emotionally charged. Having your food rejected can feel like a personal snub.

Unfortunately, it often seems easiest and least risky to choose some combination of prepared snack foods. Everyone likes chips and dip, pizza, wings, brownies, or a bakery cake, right? Well, everyone does eat it, and probably more than they ever intended to. Even so, there are always too many leftovers that no one wants to take home with them. Guess who ends up either eating junk they don't want or throwing food away? Let's improve the process and discuss strategies to get the most from your entertainment efforts: less stress, better food, and less waste.

Communications vs Food Drama

I went to a dinner party at a friend's house, where she was cooking for six people. My friend is a wonderful cook, and the first course was a treat: shrimp bisque. One person simply did not eat it. He allowed the portion to be served to him, presumably knowing what it was, but then did not eat it. He never said a word. My friend was a little disappointed, to say the least. It turns out that this friend had a shellfish allergy. But why didn't anyone say anything?

We seem to feel a great inhibition about discussing our food needs and/or menu plans. Perhaps the host wants the food to be a wonderful surprise, and the guests don't want to seem ungrateful or demanding. I can't tell you how much wasted food and hurt feelings I've seen when there is a mismatch between what people will (can) eat and what has been served. (OK, to be honest, some of the misunderstandings were entirely intentional but that is a separate issue.)

It never hurts to ask for and to provide information beforehand. Food is an area where "don't ask, don't tell" is a poor policy. I remember one unforgettable potluck that had eight different macaroni and cheese casseroles, most of which were never eaten. However, you do want to walk that fine line between avoiding a major food mismatch and offering to take individual orders for each person. So, how can you manage the process, while keeping everyone happy?

You Are the Guest

You have been invited to take a dish. Contact your host (email, phone, text) and ask:

- » Are they aware of any food restrictions among the attendees?
- » If there is something in particular they'd like you to bring?
- » What are they serving and what are others bringing?

You Are the Host

Whether you are hosting a potluck, or a more formal meal, sharing more information is always better. In your invitation, ask your invitees:

- » To let you know of any food restrictions when they RSVP.
- » If it's a potluck, let everyone know what they are bringing. (There are several apps that make coordinating a potluck easy.)
- » Provide a menu of what you will be serving (with the invite or later).

Adding Labels

No matter whether you are hosting or just contributing a dish; if it is going on a buffet table put a label on it. Give it a good description, with the main ingredients listed: "Green Bean Salad with Goat Cheese, Pecans and Orange-Honey Vinaigrette" is better than "Bean Salad". People are more likely to eat something if they know what it is and how it's made. If there is anything special about your preparation, put it on your label. Is it gluten-free? Vegan? Did you use artificial sweeteners or low-fat mayo? Are those keto meatballs? Say so.

When you make the label, tape it to the side of the serving dish or make a little tent card to stand by it. Don't tape it to the lid, which will be out of sight once the dish is opened for serving. Another cute idea is to buy tiny, inexpensive stand-up picture frames for your labels.

Guests With Dietary Requirements

One last note about guests with serious food intolerances. It is essential to discuss food with them ahead of the event, but also don't take it personally regardless of how they choose to proceed. They may choose to simply bring their own food. They cannot come to inspect your kitchen or test every ingredient you might use. (Would you catch that "modified food starch" in the chili sauce which might contain a smidge of gluten?) On the other hand, they may be comfortable giving you very precise instructions on what and how their food must be prepared.

For my son's fourth birthday, we invited his preschool class over for a party. One of the children had a critical peanut allergy. I was eager to make our treats conform to his needs, but his mom was very honest with me. She said it was easier and less stressful for everyone if she packed his food to bring and if she could help through the party. She was just grateful for the child to be included since he was often not invited as people didn't want to deal with the complications. It broke my heart to think of a cute little 4-year-old being left out of anything. It also helped me better appreciate what people with critical food allergies must deal with.

Deconstruction is your Ally

A friend of mine went on a bit of a rant after an elaborate brunch, when her lovingly prepared meal was not a hit with her family. Her fancy egg casserole was too complicated for the kids and had unacceptable ingredients for some adults.

Of course, the first step is to ASK. You may have to accept that the wonderful mixed dish you wanted to serve is simply not going to work with this group. Save it until you have a bigger event to support a variety of dishes or your next dinner party with your favorite foodie couple.

With a better understanding of your audience, look for opportunities to serve things in as deconstructed a manner as necessary. Serve the salad with dressing on the side. Maybe the salad adders like tomatoes, cucumbers, and nuts on the side as well. Let people serve/assemble their own dessert. If the mushroom and sausage egg casserole doesn't work for everyone, then how about scrambled eggs with the mushrooms, sausage, and cheese on the side? Avoid putting gravy or sauce on everything. How about make-your-own individual pizzas? Think in terms of mix and match: grilled chicken goes with veggies or salad as well as it does with the rice and bread.

Sometimes the "bar" model is a good solution: pasta bar, soup bar, salad bar, ice cream sundae bar. One of the most popular dishes I've ever served for a group was a soup bar. The slow cooker had a butternut squash soup and then people could add goat cheese, spiced pumpkin seeds, croutons, or brown sugar as desired.

It is important to remember that you can't please all the people all the time. There may be some parts of the meal that some people will not eat. If you know that in advance, you can make sure that there is something that they will eat, and everyone can move on with less food drama.

Nutrition – Real Food

Why do we assume that people prefer to eat junk food at social events? Is that what you want? For every person with health issues and/or weight challenges, social events can feel like walking through a minefield. And who taught us that you are somehow failing your guests if you put out healthy food? Well, we know that the Better Broccoli Association is not sponsoring those football tailgate party commercials on TV!

My experience is that most social events are carb-fests, with a heavy complement of fats. What tends to be missing are vegetables, fruits, and quality protein; coincidentally, our Priority Foods. I encourage you to be brave and go with the Real Food.

When I go to events, I watch what people eat. I can assure you that things like a fresh fruit salad, Caprese skewers, blue cheese stuffed olives, carrot/raisin salad, and homemade meatballs are devoured with relish. People will rave about the small, lopsided homemade cupcakes with drippy frosting because they are fresh and taste like Real Food. You can make it fun and even make it rich – but make it real.

It is easy to assume that fresh produce and/or protein are going to be more expensive than your standard party fare. However, pre-made foods aren't cheap. For example, it costs about the same to serve a pound of homemade chicken salad to spread on baguette rounds or cucumber slices as it does a plastic tub of deli artichoke dip and a box of crackers. Keep an open mind and do the math.

Minimizing Waste

The first step to minimizing waste is to only serve foods that you will eat later. If you don't want or need double fudge brownies in your house, don't serve them. (Seriously.)

The next step is to have a plan for the leftovers before the event ever starts. If 30-40% of all food is wasted, you can bet that the percentage of food wasted from entertaining is even higher. Assume that up to half of the food served will be excess.

One strategy is to share the leftovers. If you are hosting a big get-together, sometimes you can get people to take leftovers with them. To do this, you need to have take-away containers and bags ready to go. You will also probably need to be a little pushy about it as people are reluctant to take food with them. They often try to leave whatever is left of their dish with you! My best efforts have resulted in a small fraction of the leftover food going home with guests. You may have family or neighbors who would enjoy the food. Of course, the break room at work is always a good home for those leftovers that travel easily.

The bottom line is that you are still going to be left with a pile of food after everyone has left. Hopefully, you have considered this earlier and have a plan. How long will it last and when are you going to eat it? What are you going to store it in and how?

» If it is food that you will not eat, be ruthless: throw it out now and save the calories, refrigerator space, and time.
» If you are going to keep your leftovers, get the food covered up and chilled asap. You might want to move it into clean, smaller containers, for ease of storage.
» If it is something you want but can't eat it all soon, consider freezing it. This works well for many things: cakes, brownies, bread, many casseroles, soups, and meatballs, to name a few. Freezing it in individual portions increases the likelihood of it being eaten later. I enjoyed my recent birthday cake for months, one small piece at a time.

A New Life for Leftovers

Having a plan for the leftovers includes determining how and when you are going to eat them. Perhaps it is as easy as pulling the leftover food out of the fridge for dinner the following day. However, sometimes you need to give the leftover food a new life. Here are some examples:

» Fruit from a platter – make a fruit salad.
» Berries and yogurt dip – mix together to make parfaits or smoothies.
» Cubed or sliced cheese – make a soup or casserole with cheese like Macaroni and Cheese.
» Vegetable crudités – roast to make a side dish, or stir-fry, or chop into salads.
» Cold shrimp – Unused shrimp that has been kept cold may be a candidate to incorporate into a stir-fry or make shrimp salad.
» Meatballs – make meatball subs or add some sauce and serve with pasta, veggies, or rice.
» Deli tray – incorporate into sandwiches, salads, or flatbreads.
» Less-fresh bread – use for grilled or toasted sandwiches, French toast, croutons, or bread pudding.

Donate your Leftovers

If you are organizing a major event, you may have the opportunity to donate leftover food to a local homeless shelter or another charitable facility. This must be planned well in advance as each facility will have its particular requirements and protocol. They may not be able to accept home-prepared foods but may welcome whole fruits and vegetables, unopened drinks, breads and other packaged foods. If you are using a caterer, they will likely be familiar with which organizations might benefit from your donation of food and how to accomplish this. Food sharing may be another possible way to avoid wasting leftovers. Started in the UK, the Olio app allows users to post items they wish to give away, including food.

Serving Strategies

How you serve food greatly influences how it is received and how much is wasted. We have all had the experience of passing on food from a buffet table based on appearance: messy, wilted, too warm, sloppy, congealed, or turning brown... No, gracias. The chilled shrimp looks great until half is left swimming in a warm pool of melted ice, shrimp tails, and soggy lettuce.

The first consideration is temperature. Keeping cold foods chilled will keep them looking fresh and help them to last longer. If the food will be served in a hot, sunny environment, you might choose more forgiving foods: a vinegar-based bean salad versus a bibb-lettuce salad, for instance. Take dishes out at the last possible moment and look at ways to keep them in peak condition (see below).

Another consideration is to minimize collateral damage. For many foods, the ingredients last longer separately than they do once mixed together: sandwiches and salads, for instance.

Here are some serving strategies to optimize freshness and minimize waste:

» Put out less food at a time. Stage refills or serve it in batches.
» Use individual servings where possible.
» Put sauces and condiments on the side.
» Let people assemble their own sandwiches, etc.
» Keep wet and dry foods separate, as much as possible.
» Keep food covered as much as possible.
» Keep fragile foods cold. You may have to be creative or sacrifice aesthetics to do this.
  • Freeze a marble/rock slab or another glass platter to set your cold food tray on.
  • Put crushed ice in a slightly larger container, then place your serving container on the ice within it.
  • Freeze a layer of water in a larger container. Use it as a tray for individual serving cups.
  • Place artificial ice ("blue ice") under the dish and on top of the cover, then leave in place as long as practical.

Single-use Serving Ware

We have talked about food waste, but minimizing materials is also important. Going with disposable cups and plates can be the right choice but give it some thought first. It is amazing how inexpensive glassware can be: a set of 12 wine glasses can cost less than buying plastic disposable cups four times. Keep an eye out for bargains on a few basics like sets of neutral cloth napkins or small glass serving bowls. These will serve you well for years to come and look much classier than paper or plastic. If you do decide to buy plastic for a special event, the higher-end plastic plates and utensils can be washed and reused several times.

Entertaining Tips – Key Points

Communications
   » Understand your audience to avoid major food drama

Deconstruction
   » Serve components separately to suit the widest audience

Nutrition
   » Serve Real Food and only serve food you'll eat

Serving tips
   » Individual servings
   » Staged refills
   » Keep it cold
   » Minimize collateral damage

Plan for leftovers

Keep up with the latest news and join the conversation on our website
www.ReEngineeringtheKitchen.com

Download Agile Recipes™

Download Templates

Submit Agile Recipe™ Ideas

Books in Progress

Read the Blog

Share Your Favorite Time-Saving Tip

Acknowledgments

This book represents the culmination of a five-year journey, only possible with the help and support of many people.

First and foremost, I need to thank my husband, Harv for his incredible patience and support – while writing this book and always. *Re-Engineering the Kitchen*® simply would not have come to fruition without him. From the very initial glimmers of a concept, he encouraged me to make the commitment and write it down. I appreciate the endless hours he spent listening to me talk about ideas and trying to find the words to communicate them clearly. His thoughtful questions and suggestions have been invaluable. I am eternally grateful.

Next, I need to acknowledge my illustrators. Guy Harvey brought Agile to life through his unique style of drawing. Simon Thompson created a cover design that conveys the focus of the book in a unique and visually interesting way.

I'd like to acknowledge my developmental and copy editor, Becky Alexander. Her insightful perspectives and suggestions made this a much better book than it would have been. Many thanks to my final copy and proofread editor, Emily Kearns. She did her best to catch my many writing shortcomings and errors. Any that remain are entirely my doing.

I'd like to thank my publisher, White Bear Publishing, for faithfully bringing my vision to print. They did an exceptional job with the graphic design and the layout. The visual aspects of this book are essential to communicating the concepts clearly and they did a fantastic job ensuring that the graphic elements hit the mark. The innovative book layout is integral to making the content navigable and approachable.

Lastly, I'd like to thank my family for their support and encouragement through this process. They have provided the essential service of being sounding boards and recipe taste-testers for years, although at times unwittingly. My two daughters-in-law, Marisa and Eldis, have generously shared ideas, kitchen tips, recipes, nutrition information, and are always available to talk with me about any food-related subject. My grandsons, Erik and Reid, have delighted me with their enthusiastic interest and encouragement through the many elements involved with writing and publishing this book. My amazing sons, Harvey and Brad, for always backing me in any endeavor, no matter how improbable. And of course, Smoky, my beloved English Cream Golden Retriever who spent countless hours in my office serving as my Chief Morale Officer.

Appendix A

ABOUT BUYING SUPPLEMENTS

If you do consider supplementing your diet, you might keep a few things in mind. First, be thoughtful about what supplement you are going to take. Do you have a reason to think you need it? Look at what foods naturally provide that nutrient and then consider whether you do (or could) eat enough of these foods. Be aware that supplements can interact with other supplements, over-the-counter (OTC) drugs and prescription medicines. Talking with your healthcare professional prior to starting a supplement regime is highly recommended, particularly if you are regularly taking prescription drugs, OTC drugs or other supplements. Similarly, it is important to let your doctor know what supplements you are taking.

If an advertisement about a supplement caught your eye, look at the company's website and critically evaluate their claims. They should tell you exactly what is in their supplement, the active and inactive ingredients. Look up the active ingredients on unbiased websites like the Dietary Supplement Fact Sheets (https://ods.od.nih.gov/factsheets/list-all/). If a manufacturer simply lists a "proprietary blend", you literally have no idea what is in there (snake oil?). If they indicate that their supplement is scientifically validated, do they give you links to the actual studies? Were the results published in reputable, peer-reviewed journals? Were the studies done by someone with financial ties to the company? When you look at some of these websites with a critical eye you will often realize that it is just a slick website with little substance.

You might be tempted to think that supplements are safe and effective because they fall under FDA regulations. However, the FDA does not have the authority to approve dietary supplements for safety and effectiveness before the supplements are sold to the public. (For more details see FDA 101: Dietary Supplements (www.fda.gov/consumers/consumer-updates/fda-101-dietary-supplements). Dietary supplements are classified as food and assumed to be GRAS (Generally Regarded as Safe). You will note that every supplement label includes a statement to the effect: "This product has not been evaluated by the FDA and is not intended to diagnose, treat, cure, or prevent any disease." Anything that is intended to treat a medical condition is classified as a drug and is subject to stringent approval requirements and exhaustive regulations.

It is the manufacturer's responsibility to ensure that the supplement meets the relevant safety standards and is not otherwise in violation of the law. All manufacturers are required to follow the GMP/CGMP (Good Manufacturing Practices/Current Good Manufacturing Practices) issued by the FDA which are intended to assure the quality, safety, purity, and validity of products.

Some supplement companies are extremely reputable and others... maybe not. It is up to you to determine which is trustworthy. This article from Consumer Reports "Shop Smarter for Supplements" (www.consumerreports.org/supplements/shop-smarter-for-supplements) is a useful, in-depth guide to buying supplements. One easy step to take is buying the named-brand product from a company that has a long-term reputation to protect. Another easy step is to buy supplements manufactured in GMP-certified facilities, which should give you more confidence in the product's production methods.

Once you've determined that the supplement has probably been manufactured properly, the next step is to verify that it contains what it says it does. Some supplements are verified by third-party labs.

The three certifying agencies are:

1. NSF International – NSF | The Public Health and Safety Organization

2. USP (US Pharmacopeia) – US Pharmacopeia (USP)

3. Consumer Lab – Independent Tests and Reviews of Vitamin, Mineral, and Herbal Supplements ConsumerLab.com

Third-party lab verification assures you that you are getting what you think you are: the exact ingredients, dosage, and no contaminants. The label should indicate which lab was used.

Appendix B

USEFUL CHARTS AND TEMPLATES

Estimated calorie needs per day for Sedentary Lifestyle, Moderate Lifestyle, and Active Lifestyle (data from DGA[7]).

Figure 65 – Estimated Calorie Needs per Day – Sedentary Lifestyle

Males		Females	
Age	Calories/Day	Age	Calories/Day
2-3	1,000	2-3	1,000
4-5	1,200	4-7	1,200
6-8	1,400	8-10	1,400
9-10	1,600	11-13	1,600
11-12	1,800	14-18	1,800
13-14	2,000	19-25	2,000
15	2,200	26-50	1,800
16-18	2,400	51+	1,600
19-20	2,600		
21-40	2,400		
41-60	2,200		
61+	2,000		

Sedentary lifestyle includes only physical activites associated with independent living.

Figure 9 – Estimated Calorie Needs per Day – Moderate Lifestyle

Males		Females	
Age	Calories/Day	Age	Calories/Day
2	1,000	2	1,000
3-5	1,400	3	1,200
6-8	1,600	4-6	1,400
9-10	1,800	7-9	1,600
11	2,000	10-11	1,800
12-13	2,200	12-18	2,000
14	2,400	19-25	2,200
15	2,600	26-50	2,000
16-25	2,800	51+	1,800
26-45	2,600		
46-65	2,400		
66+	2,200		

Moderate lifestyle also includes the equivalent of 1½ - 3 miles of brisk walking.

Figure 66 – Estimated Calorie Needs per Day – Active Lifestyle

Males		Females	
Age	Calories/Day	Age	Calories/Day
2	1,000	2	1,000
3	1,400	3-4	1,400
4-5	1,600	5-6	1,600
6-7	1,800	7-9	1,800
8-9	2,000	10-11	2,000
10-11	2,200	12-13	2,200
12	2,400	14-30	2,400
13	2,600	31-60	2,200
14	2,800	61+	2,000
15	3,000		
16-18	3,200		
19-35	3,000		
36-55	2,800		
56-75	2,600		
76+	2,400		

Active lifestyle includes equivalent of 3-4 miles of brisk walking.

Figure 67 – Calorie Requirements per Day Calculator

The Base Metabolic Rate (BMR) is the number of calories required to maintain a body at rest. We use the Mifflin-St. Jeor Equation[38] to estimate the BMR, which is the sum of the body weight, height, and age calculations plus or minus a correction factor as shown in the tables below. The BMR is then multiplied by the Activity Factor to estimate the individual's calorie requirements per day.

Example Daily Calorie Req't – Male

Weight, lb	230	x 4.54 =	1,044
Height, in	76	x 15.82 =	1,202
Age, yr	30	x (-5) =	-150
Correction Factor		5	
BMR = Sum of Above			2,102
Activity Factor		x	1.725
Calorie Req't = BMR x Activity			3,625

Daily Calorie Requirement – Male

Weight, lb		x 4.54 =	
Height, in		x 15.82 =	
Age, yr		x (-5) =	
Correction Factor		5	
BMR = Sum of Above			
Activity Factor		x	
Calorie Req't = BMR x Activity			

Example Daily Calorie Req't – Female

Weight, lb	115	x 4.54 =	522
Height, in	58	x 15.82 =	918
Age, yr	70	x (-5) =	-350
Correction Factor		-161	
BMR = Sum of Above			929
Activity Factor		x	1.2
Calorie Req't = BMR x Activity			1,114

Daily Calorie Requirement – Female

Weight, lb		x 4.54 =	
Height, in		x 15.82 =	
Age, yr		x (-5) =	
Correction Factor		-161	
BMR = Sum of Above			
Activity Factor		x	
Calorie Req't = BMR x Activity			

Activity Level Factor for Calorie Requirements Calculator	
Sedentary (little to no exercise)	1.2
Lightly Active (light exercise/sport 1-3 days/week)	1.375
Moderately Active (moderate exercise/sport 3-5 days/week)	1.55
Very Active (hard exercise/sport 6-7 days/week)	1.725
Super Active (very hard exercise/sport, physical job, training	1.9

Figure 55 – Household Priority Foods Requirements Worksheet

	Person =>	1	2	3	4	5	6	Total
1	Name							
2	Age/Gender							
3	Activity Level							
4	Cal/Day (Figure 7 and Appendix II)							
	Veggies, c-eq							
5	Weekly Requirement (Figure 16)							
6	Weekly Veggies Out (Figure 22 est.)							
7	Weekly Veggies Home (Req't – Out)							
	Fruit, c-eq							
8	Weekly Requirement (Figure 16)							
9	Weekly Fruit Out (Figure 20 est.)							
10	Weekly Fruit Home (Req't – Out)							
	Protein, gm							
11	Weekly Requirement (Figure 16)							
12	Weekly Protein Out (Figure 20 est.)							
13	Weekly Protein Home (Req't – Out)							

Figure 56 – Baseline Priority Foods Plan Worksheet

Row	Priority Foods	Total	Out	Total-Home	Longevity Distribution		
					Fast-Fade	Fresh-Med	Long
1	Ratio =>						
2	Veggies, c-eq						
3	Fruit, c-eq						
4	Protein, g						

Figure 57 – Baseline Priority Foods Shopping Guide Worksheet

Row		Total	Fast-Fade	Fresh-Med	Long
1	Veggie Target, c-eq =>				
2					
3					
4					
5					
6					
7					
8					
9					
10					
11					
12	Total				
13	Fruit Target, c-eq =>				
14					
15					
16					
17					
18					
19					
20	Total				
21	Protein Target, g =>				
22					
23					
24					
25					
26					
27					
28					
29					
30					
31					
32	Total				

Figure 58 – Daily Priority Foods Distribution Worksheet

Priority Foods Distribution				Requirement Check		
Day	Breakfast	Lunch	Dinner	Veggie	Fruit	Protein
Daily Targets =>						
1						
2						
3						
4						
5						
6						
7						

Appendix C

Resources for More Information

Websites

The Linus Pauling Institute at Oregon State University is focused on the role that vitamins and other essential micronutrients play in enhancing health and preventing disease.
lpi.oregonstate.edu

The USDA Dietary Guidelines for Americans website has an abundance of information and tables available to the public on the topics of food and health.
dietaryguidelines.gov/resources/2020-2025-dietary-guidelines-online-materials

If you are interested in knowing what is actually in the food you eat, this is a useful website.
codesearch.arsnet.usda.gov/(S(3xmvc3edodjhhaqf1voilkck))/CodeSearch.aspx

For more information on the NOVA Food Classification System visit
ecuphysicians.ecu.edu/wp-content/pv-uploads/sites/78/2021/07/NOVA-Classification-Reference-Sheet.pdf

To learn more about the Glycemic Index (GI) or to search for the GI of various foods, visit
glycemicindex.com

Books

Allport, Susan – *The Queen of Fats*

Cummins, Ivor and Gerber, Jeffrey – *Eat Rich, Live Long*

Eades, Michael R. and Mary Dan – *Protein Power*

Enig Ph.D., Mary G. – *Know Your Fats: The Complete Primer for Understanding the Nutrition of Fats, Oils and Cholesterol*

Hyman, Mark M. – *The Food Fix*

Lustig MD, Robert – *Fat Chance*

Lustig MD, Robert – *Metabolical*

Moss, Michael – *Hooked: Food, Free Will, and How the Food Giants Exploit our Addictions*

Moss, Michael – *Salt Sugar Fat: How the Food Giants Hooked Us*

Nestle, Marion – *What to Eat*

Pollan, Michael – *In Defense of Food – An Eaters Manifesto*

Wilson, Bee – *The Way We Eat Now*

GLOSSARY

AMINO ACID: A simple organic compound containing both a carboxyl and an amino group. Amino acids play an important role in performing several biological and chemical functions including building and repairing the tissues, the formation and function of enzymes, and food digestion.

ANTIOXIDANT: Molecules that fight free radicals in your body. Fruits and vegetables are high in antioxidants such as vitamins C and E, selenium, and beta-carotene.

BIOENGINEERED: Defined by U.S. Department of Agriculture as food that "contains detectable genetic material that has been modified through certain lab techniques that cannot be created through conventional breeding or found in nature." It is essentially how genetically modified organisms, or GMOs, are defined and the term used by the USDA since January 1, 2022.

CARBON EMISSIONS: In simple terms, carbon emissions are carbon dioxide that cars, planes, factories, etc., produce and are harmful to the environment.

DARK GREEN LEAFY VEGETABLES: Edible plant leaves that are identified by their green color and edible leaves. Some can be eaten raw, while others may require cooking. Examples are kale, spinach, collard greens, Swiss chard, arugula, cabbage, endive, romaine, bibb lettuce, dandelion greens, mustard greens, and turnip greens.

FLAVONOID: Phytonutrients found in plants, fruits, vegetables, grains, roots, flowers, tea, and wine. The beneficial properties of flavonoids include being antioxidants, reducing inflammation, preventing mutation, interfering with the development of cancer, and regulating cellular enzyme functions.

FORTIFIED FOODS: Per the World Health Organization (WHO), food fortification is the practice of increasing or adding essential vitamins and minerals to improve the nutritional quality of the food. While this may help improve nutrition, it can also make it easier to eat highly processed foods.

FREE RADICALS: Unstable molecules that can damage cell components, including the membrane, proteins, and DNA. They are linked to illnesses including diabetes, heart disease, and cancer.

GLYCEMIC INDEX: A system that ranks foods by the speeds at which their carbohydrates are converted into glucose in the body; a measure of the effects of foods on blood-sugar levels.

Genetically Modified Organism (GMO): Organism whose DNA has been changed through bioengineering techniques to exhibit specific traits in ways that do not occur naturally.

Greenhouse Gases: Gases that absorb infrared radiation emitted from the Earth's surface and reradiate it back, thereby contributing to the greenhouse effect. Includes carbon dioxide and methane.

MACRONUTRIENT: Any of the nutritional components of the diet that are required in relatively large amounts: protein, carbohydrates, fats, and the macrominerals.

MICRONUTRIENT: An essential nutrient, as a trace mineral or vitamin, that is required by an organism in minute amounts.

NOVA: A system developed to define the extent of processing for food. There are four categories: (1) unprocessed or minimally processed, (2) processed ingredients, (3) processed foods, and (4) ultra-processed foods.

PHYTOCHEMICALS: Phytochemicals are bioactive chemical compounds that occur naturally in plant-based foods. They are antioxidants, which means they can neutralize harmful free radicals. Eating a variety of fruits and vegetables is the best way to optimize getting these nutrients.

POLYUNSATURATED FAT: A type of fat that has at least two double bonds and includes omega-3 and omega-6 fatty acids. Polyunsaturated fats are liquid at room temperature and are referred to as oils. They can be found mostly in fatty fish, plant-based oils, seeds and nuts.

SATURATED FAT: A type of single-bond animal or vegetable fat, as found in butter, meat, egg yolks, and coconut or palm oil.

UNSATURATED FAT: A type of fat that has at least one double bond and contains a large amount of fatty acid molecules.

REFERENCES

Cited References

[1] P.R. Shukla, J. S.-D.-O. (2019). *Climate Change and Land: an IPCC special report on climate change, desertification, land degradation, sustainable land management, food security, and greenhouse gas fluxes in terrestrial ecosystems.* In Press: IPCC.

[2] Yu, Y. a. (2020). Estimating Food Waste as Household Production Inefficiency. *American Journal of Agricultural Economics, Vol. 102, Issue 2*, 525-547.

[3] EPA Landfill Methane Outreach Program. (2020, August). Basic Information about Landfill Gas. Retrieved from Environmental Protection Agency: https://www.epa.gov/lmop/basic-information-about-landfill-gas.

[4] *Monteiro CA, Cannon G, Moubarac JC, Levy RB, Louzada MLC, Jaime PC. The UN Decade of Nutrition, the NOVA food classification and the trouble with ultra-processing. Public Health Nutr. 2018 Jan;21(1):5-17. doi: 10.1017/S1368980017000234. Epub 2017 Mar 21. PMID: 28322183; PMCID: PMC10261019. pubmed.ncbi.nlm.nih.gov/28322183/.*

[5] Rico-Campà Anaïs, M.-G. M.-A.-A.-D. (May 2019). Association between consumption of ultra-processed foods and cause mortality: SUN prospective cohort study. *British Medical Journal*, 365:l1949.

[6] *British Medical Journal 2024*: 384; e077310. http://dx.doi.org/10.1136/bmj-2023-077310

[7] U.S. Dept. of Agriculture & U.S. Dept. of Health and Human Services. (December 2020). *Dietary Guidelines for Americans: 2020-2025.* 9th Edition. Washington DC: USDA.

[8] Institute of Medicine. (2006). *Dietary Reference Intakes: The Essential Guide to Nutrient Requirements.* Washington D.C.: National Academies Press.

[9] U.S. Department of Agriculture. (2024). Food Data Central. https://fdc.nal.usda.gov.

[10] WebMD. (2023, September 7). Food Sources for Vitamins and Minerals. www.webmd.com/food-recipes/vitamins-and-minerals-good-food-sources.

[11] Food & Drug Administration. (2017). *Frequently Asked Questions for Industry on Nutrition Facts Labeling Requirements.* www.fda.gov/media/99069/download.

[12] Healthline. (2023, July 13). *Micronutrients: Types, Functions, Benefits, and More.* www.healthline.com/nutrition/micronutrients.

[13] WebMB. (2022, November 2). *Vitamins and Minerals: How Much Should You Take?* www.webmd.com/vitamins-and-supplements/vitamins-minerals-how-much-should-you-take.

[14] Mayo Clinic. (2023, November 23). *Nutrition and Healthy Living: Chart of High-Fiber Foods.* www.mayoclinic.org/healthy-lifestyle/nutrition-and-healthy-eating/in-depth/high-fiber-foods/art-20050948.

[15] Linus Pauling Institute at Oregon State University. (2023). *Micronutrients for Health.* lpi.oregonstate.edu/sites/lpi.oregonstate.edu/files/pdf/mic/micronutrients_for_health.pdf.

[16] NIH National Library of Medicine. (July 2023). *Vitamin D Deficiency.* www.ncbi.nlm.nih.gov/books/NBK532266/.

[17] Nutrients. (2019, May 11). *Dietary Protein and Muscle Mass: Translating Science to Application and Health Benefit.* pubmed.ncbi.nlm.nih.gov/31121843/.

[18] U.S. Bureau of Labor Statistics. (2023, September 8). *Consumer Expenditures - 2022.* www.bls.gov/newsrelease/pdf/cesan.pdf.

[19] The Bean Institute. (2023) *Bean Nutrition Overview.* beaninstitute.com/nutrition-health/beans-nutrition-overview/.

[20] USA Pulses. (2024). *About Pulses.* usapulses.org/.

[21] University of California Television (2099, May 26). *Sugar: THE BITTER TRUTH.* YouTube. youtube.com/watch?v=dBnniua6-oM.

[22] American Heart Association. (2023). *How Much Sugar is Too Much?* www.heart.org/en/healthy-living/healthy-eating/eat-smart/sugar/how-much-sugar-is-too-much

[23] The University of Sydney Glycemic Index and GI News. (2023). *The International Glycemic Index (GI) Database.* glycemicindex.com.

24 Desmarchelier, Charles & Ludwig, Tobias & Scheundel, Ronny & Rink, Nadine & Bader, Bernhard & Klingenspor, Martin & Daniel, Hannelore. (2012). *Diet-induced obesity in ad libitum-fed mice: Food texture overrides the effect of macronutrient composition.* The British Journal of Nutrition. 109. 1-10. 10.1017/S0007114512003340.

25 USDA Agricultural Research Service. (2023). *Food Availability and Consumption.* ers.usda.gov/data-products/ag-and-food-statistics-charting-the-essentials/food-availability-and-consumption/.

26 Hypoglycemia Support Foundation. (2018). *Added Sugar Repository.* hypoglycemia.org/added-sugar-repository/

27 Teicholz N. *A short history of saturated fat: the making and unmaking of a scientific consensus.* Curr Opin Endocrinol Diabetes Obes. 2023 Feb 1;30(1):65-71. doi: 10.1097/MED.0000000000000791. Epub 2022 Dec 8. PMID: 36477384; PMCID: PMC9794145.

28 Index Mundi. (2024). *United States Sunflowerseed Oil Consumption by Year.* https://www.indexmundi.com/agriculture/?country=us&commodity=sunflowerseed-oil&graph=domestic-consumption

29 Technical Committee of The Institute of Shortening and Edible Oils. (2016). *Food Fats and Oils.* Washington DC: The Institute of Shortening and Edible Oils, Inc.

30 American Heart Association. (2021, November 21). *Saturated Fats.* www.heart.org/en/healthy-living/healthy-eating/eat-smart/fats/saturated-fats

31 Allport, Susan. (2006). *The Queen of Fats.* University of California Press.

32 National Institute of Health Office of Dietary Supplements. (2023, February 15). *Omega 3 Fatty Acids.* ods.od.nih.gov/factsheets/Omega3FattyAcids-HealthProfessional/

33 World Wildlife Fund. (2021, February 23). *Sustainable Agriculture – Palm Oil.* Retrieved from World Wildlife Fund: https://www.worldwildlife.org/industries/palm-oil/

34 Sowmya Kadandale, R. M. (2018, January 8). *The palm oil industry and noncommunicable diseases.* Retrieved from Bulletin of the World Health Organization: https://www.ncbi.nlm.nih.gov/pmc/articles/PMC6357563/

35 Science Direct. (2011). *Canola Oil.* https://www.sciencedirect.com/topics/agricultural-and-biological-sciences/canola-oil

36 PJ Kabobs. (2024). *Does olive oils smoke point matter when cooking?* https://www.oliveoil.com/is-olive-oil-smoke-point

[37] U.S. Food & Drug Administration. (2024, March 5). *GMO Crops, Animal Food, and Beyond.* https://www.fda.gov/food/agricultural-biotechnology/gmo-crops-animal-food-and-beyond

[38] Mifflin MD, St Jeor ST, Hill LA, Scott BJ, Daugherty SA, Koh YO. *A new predictive equation for resting energy expenditure in healthy individuals.* Am J Clin Nutr. 1990 Feb;51(2):241-7. doi:10.1093/ajcn/51.2.241. PMID: 2305711.

Additional Resources

[39] USDA Food and Nutrition Information Center. (2021, February 23). *DRI Calculator for Healthcare Professionals.* Retrieved from USDA National Agricultural Library: https://www.nal.usda.gov/fnic/dri-calculator/

[40] North Harvest Bean Growers Association. (2021, February 23). *Bean Nutrition Overview.* Retrieved from The Bean Institute https://beaninstitute.com/

[41] Technical Committee of the Institute of Shortening and Edible Oils. (2016). *Food Fats and Oils.* Washington DC: The Institute of Shortening and Edible Oils, Inc.

[42] NIH National Library of Medicine. (March 2016). *Dietary Protein Intake and Human Health.* pubmed.ncbi.nlm.nih.gov/26797090/.

[43] NIH National Library of Medicine. (March 2018). *Protein for Life: Review of Optimal Protein Intake, Sustainable Dietary Sources and the Effect on Appetite in Ageing Adults.* pubmed.ncbi.nlm.nih.gov/29547523/

[44] NIH National Library of Medicine. (May 2019). *Dietary Protein and Muscle Mass: Translating Science to Application and Health Benefit.* pubmed.ncbi.nlm.nih.gov/31121843/.

[45] NIH Office of Dietary Supplements. (2023). *Dietary Supplement Fact Sheets.* ods.od.nih.gov/factsheets/list-all/.

[46] Consumer Reports. (January 2020). *Shop Smarter For Supplements.* www.consumerreports.org/supplements/shop-smarter-for-supplements/.

INDEX

ABOUT THE AUTHOR

Alin (Alina) E. Steele

Alina writes nonfiction based on her life experiences and expertise including business, engineering, science, and food. She earned a BS in Chemical Engineering from Michigan State University and is a licensed Professional Engineer. She earned an MBA (Finance and Business Economics) from Wayne State University and a Certificate in Nutrition and Healthy Living from Cornell.

After a 30-year corporate career in the energy industry, Alina now focuses on food and the related processes that we employ in our everyday lives. She created the Re-Engineering the Kitchen™ program to provide practical methods to improve one's nutrition by translating vague goals into actionable plans. You can find more information at www.reengineeringthekitchen.com.

Alina lives in Minnesota with her husband, Harvey, and their amazing Golden Retriever, Smoky. She enjoys every adventure with her children and grandchildren, and loves to visit friends in Florida or wherever they may be.

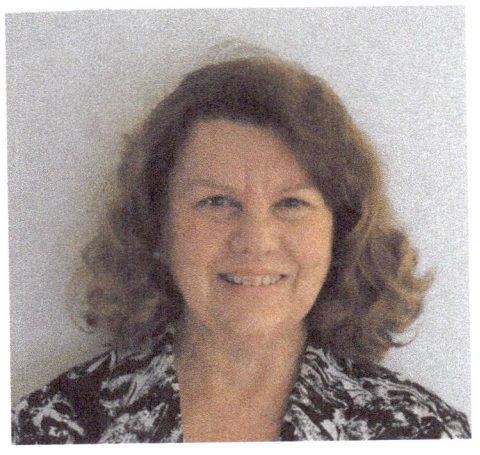

Notes

Notes

Notes

www.ingramcontent.com/pod-product-compliance
Lightning Source LLC
Chambersburg PA
CBHW080835120626

46553CB00009B/2440